CRC SERIES ON NUTRITION
IN EXERCISE AND SPORT

Editors, Ira Wolinsky and James F. Hickson, Jr.

Published Titles

Luke Bucci
Nutrients as Ergogenic Aids for Sports and Exercise

Ira Wolinsky & James F. Hickson, Jr.
Nutrition in Exercise and Sport, 2/E

Ronald R. Watson & Marianne Eisinger
Exercise and Disease

Luke Bucci
Nutrition Applied to Injury Rehabilitation and Sports Medicine

Catherine G. R. Jackson
Nutrition for the Recreational Athlete

Forthcoming Titles

James F. Hickson, Jr.
Sports Nutrition

Editor, Ira Wolinsky

Published Titles

Constance V. Kies and Judy A. Driskell
Sports Nutrition: Minerals and Electrolytes

Forthcoming Titles

Jaime S. Ruud
Nutrition and the Female Athlete

E. R. Buskirk & S. Puhl
Body Fluid Balance: Exercise and Sport

Jana Parizkova
Nutrition, Physical Activity and Health in Early Life

SPORTS NUTRITION
Minerals and Electrolytes

Edited by
Constance V. Kies
Judy A. Driskell

CRC Press
Boca Raton   Ann Arbor   London   Tokyo

Library of Congress Cataloging-in-Publication Data

Sports nutrition : minerals and electrolytes / editors, Constance
  V. Kies, Judy A. Driskell.
     p.   cm. — (Nutrition in exercise and sport)
  Includes bibliographical references and index.
  ISBN 0-8493-7916-4
  1. Athletes—Nutrition.   2. Sports.   I. Kies, Constance, 1934-
  II. Driskell, Judy A.   III. Series.
TX361. A8S674   1995
613.2′024796—dc20   94-18438
                                                                     CIP

This book contains information obtained from authentic and highly regarded sources. Reprinted material is quoted with permission, and sources are indicated. A wide variety of references are listed. Reasonable efforts have been made to publish reliable data and information, but the author and the publisher cannot assume responsibility for the validity of all materials or for the consequences of their use.

No claim to original U.S. Government works
International Standard Book Number 0-8493-7916-4
Library of Congress Card Number 95-18438
Printed in the United States of America 1 2 3 4 5 6 7 8 9 0
Printed on acid-free paper

SERIES PREFACE

The CRC Series on Nutrition in Exercise and Sport will provide a setting for detailed exploration of the diverse aspects of nutrition and exercise including sport. The topic of exercise and sports nutrition has been a focus of research among scientists since the 1960s and the healthful benefits of good nutrition and exercise have been appreciated. As our knowledge expands, it will be necessary to remember that there must be a range of diets, as well as a range of exercise regimes, that will support excellent physical condition and performance. There will not be a single diet/exercise treatment — a common denominator or a formula for health or a panacea for performance.

The CRC Series on Nutrition in Exercise and Sport is dedicated to providing a stage to explore these issues. Each volume will provide a detailed and scholarly examination of some aspect of the topic.

Contributors from any bona fide area of nutrition and physical activity, including sport, and including the controversial, are welcome.

Ira Wolinsky, Ph.D.
Series Editor

PREFACE

This volume addresses the relationships of mineral and electrolyte needs/interactions to sports and exercise. The book includes a collection of chapters written by individuals from several academic disciplines, some of whom have a long history of research in the area of mineral nutrition as it relates to sports and exercise. Some chapters describe specific research projects, while others are literature reviews. The book reviews convincing evidence that exercise and sport activities do affect the mineral status of individuals.

Editors
Constance V. Kies
Judy A. Driskell

THE EDITORS

Constance V. Kies, Ph.D. R.D., was Professor of Nutritional Science in the Department of Nutritional Science and Dietetics at the University of Nebraska–Lincoln. She received a B.S. degree in English from the then Wisconsin State College at Platteville (1955) and M.S. (1960) and Ph.D. (1963) degrees in human nutrition from the University of Wisconsin–Madison. Following receipt of her B.S. degree she taught in secondary schools in Wisconsin. After obtaining her Ph.D. degree, she joined the faculty of the University of Nebraska as an Assistant Professor and moved through the ranks to being appointed full Professor in 1968.

Dr. Kies was a member of many professional organizations including The American Institute of Nutrition, The American Society for Clinical Nutrition, The American Chemical Society, The American Dietetic Association and The American Association of Cereal Chemistry. She was editor-in-chief of the international journal *Plant Foods for Human Nutrition,* has published widely, and has received many research grants and contracts. Her research centered on human metabolic studies and most recently emphasized bioavailability of minerals. She taught many classes within the department including a mini-course on sports nutrition.

Judy Anne Driskell, Ph.D. R.D., is currently Professor of Nutritional Science and Dietetics at the University of Nebraska.

Dr. Driskell received her B.S. degree in Biology in 1965 from the University of Southern Mississippi; her M.S. and Ph.D. degrees were obtained from Purdue University in 1967 and 1970, respectively. She served as an Assistant Professor of Nutrition and Foods at Auburn University from 1970–1972, an Assistant Professor of Foods and Nutrition at Florida State University from 1972–1974, an Associate Professor and Professor of Human Nutrition and Foods at Virginia Polytechnic Institute and State University from 1974–1989, and Professor of Nutritional Science at the University of Nebraska from 1989 to present. She was the Nutrition Scientist for the U.S. Department of Agriculture/Cooperative State Research Service in 1981–1982, and part-time in 1985.

Dr. Driskell is a member of numerous professional organizations including the American Institute of Nutrition, the American Society for Clinical Nutrition, the Institute of Food Technologists, and the American Dietetic Association. In 1993 she received the Professional Scientist Award of the Food Science and Human Nutrition Section of the Southern Association of Agricultural Scientists. In addition, she was the 1987 recipient of the Borden Award for Research in Applied Fundamental Knowledge of Human Nutrition. She served as a member and chair of the Subcommittee for Human Nutrition of the Experiment Station Committee on Policy and Organization from 1981–1987. She is listed as an expert in B-Complex Vitamins by the Vitamin Nutrition Information Service. Her current research interests center around vitamin metabolism and requirements, including the interrelationships between exercise and water-soluble vitamin requirements.

CONTRIBUTORS

Okezie I. Aruoma, Ph.D., D.Sc.
Senior Scientist
Pharmacology Group
University of London King's College
Manresa Road
London, United Kingdom

John L. Beard, Ph.D.
Professor
Department of Nutrition
InterCollegiate Program in
  Physiology and Program in
  Biobehavioral Health
College of Human Development
Pennsylvania State University
University Park, Pennsylvania

Joan E. Benson, M.S., R.D.
Research Associate
School of Medicine
University of Utah
Salt Lake City, Utah

Lorraine R. Brilla, Ph.D.
Associate Professor
Department of Physical Education,
  Health and Recreation
Western Washington University
Bellingham, Washington

Steven S. Carroll, Ph.D.
Associate Professor
Department of Decision and
  Information Systems
Arizona State Unviersity
Tempe, Arizona

Walter Castellani, M.D.
Department of Clinical
  Physiopathology
University of Florence
Florence, Italy

Chaun-Show Chen, Ph.D.
Professor
Department of Physical Education
Chukyo University
Toyota City
Aichi, Japan

Douglas B. Clement, M.D.
Professor
School of Family Practice/Physical
  Education and Recreation
University of British Columbia
Vancouver, British Columbia, Canada

David Cummin, M.D.
Department of Human Nutrition and
  Food Management
Ohio State Unviersity
Columbus, Ohio

Steven C. Dennis, Ph.D.
Associate Professor
Bioenergetics of Exercise Research Unit
Department of Physiology
Medical Research Council and
  University of Cape Town Medical
  School
Observatory, Republic of South
  Africa

Judy A. Driskell, Ph.D., R.D.
Professor
Department of Nutritional Science
  and Dietetics
University of Nebraska
Lincoln, Nebraska

Patricia A. Eisenman, Ph.D.
Professor
Department of Exercise and Sports
  Science
University of Utah
Salt Lake City, Utah

Gülgün Ersoy
Associate Professor
College of Health Technology
Hacettepe University
Ankara, Turkey

Mikael Fogelholm, D.Sc.
Research Fellow
Division of Nutrition
Department of Applied Chemistry
  and Microbiology
University of Helsinki
Helsinki, Finland

Paola Galvan, D. Biol.
Laboratory of Pediatric Research
  and Prevention
Department of Pediatrics
University of Florence
Florence, Italy

Luca Gatteschi, M.D.
Consultant Nutritionist of Italian
  Federation of Tracks and Fields
Chair of Sports Medicine
University of Florence
Florence, Italy

Philip R. Good, M.S., R.D.
Department of Human Nutrition and
  Food Management
Ohio State University
Columbus, Ohio

Jennifer Grayzar, M.D.
Department of Human Nutrition and
  Food Management
Ohio State University
Columbus, Ohio

Barry Halliwell, D.Phil., D.Sc.
Professor
Pharmacology Group
University of London King's College
Manresa Road
London, United Kingdom

John A. Hawley, Ph.D., F.A.C.S.M.
Research Fellow
Bioenergetics of Exercise Research
  Unit
Department of Physiology
Medical Research Council and
  University of Cape Town Medical
  School
Observatory, Republic of South
  Africa

Katherine K. Heinrich, M.S., R.D.
Clinical Nutritionist
Division of Foods and Nutrition
University of Utah
Salt Lake City, Utah

Julie M. Helleksen, M.S., R.D.
Graduate Student
Department of Family Resources and
  Human Development
Arizona State University
Tempe, Arizona

Fumio Hirata, Ph.D.
Professor
Department of Sports Recreation
National Institute of Fitness and
  Sports
Kanoya City
Kagoshima, Japan

Naotake Inoue, M.S.
Associate Professor
Department of Sports Recreation
National Institute of Fitness and
  Sports
Kanoya City
Kagoshima, Japan

Herman L. Johnson, Ph.D.
Research Physiologist
United States Department of
  Agriculture, Agricultural Research
  Service
Western Human Nutrition Research
  Center
Presido of San Francisco, California

Ken-ichi Kaihatsu
Student
Department of Physiology and
  Biomechanics
National Institute of Fitness and
  Sports
Kanoya City
Kagoshima, Japan

Jayanthi Kandiah, Ph.D., R.D.
Assistant Professor
Department of Home Economics
College of Applied Sciences and
  Technology
Ball State University
Muncie, Indiana

Fumihiko Kariya, M.S.
Graduate Student
Department of Physiology and
  Biomechanics
National Institute of Fitness and
  Sports
Kanoya City
Kagoshima, Japan

Constance V. Kies, Ph.D., R.D.
Deceased
Professor
Department of Nutritional Science
  and Dietetics
University of Nebraska
Lincoln, Nebraska

Takako Kizaki, Ph.D.
Assistant Professor
Department of Hygiene
National Defense Medical College
Namiki, Tokorozawa, Japan

Kohji Koyanagi
Student
Department of Physiology and
  Biomechanics
National Institute of Fitness and
  Sports
Kanoya City
Kagoshima, Japan

Mihye Kym, Ph.D.
Department of Nutritional Science
  and Dietetics
University of Nebraska
Lincoln, Nebraska

V. Patteson Lombardi, Ph.D.
Research Assistant Professor
Department of Biology
University of Oregon
Eugene, Oregon

Henry C. Lukaski, Ph.D.
Research Leader for Mineral Nutrient
  Functions, Supervisory Research
  Physiologist
Department of Applied Physiology
United States Department of
  Agriculture, Agricultural Research
  Service
Grand Forks Human Nutrition
  Research Center
Grand Forks, North Dakota

Sante Mantovanelli, Ch.D.
Deceased
Head Chemist
Laboratory of Clinical Chemistry and
  Hematology
General Hospital
Verona, Italy

Jean Merkel, M.S., R.D.
Diabetes Educator
Cigna Health Plan of Arizona
Tempe, Arizona

Melinda M. Manore Ph.D., R.D.
Associate Professor
Food and Nutrition Laboratory
Department of Family Resources and
  Human Development
Arizona State University
Tempe, Arizona

Ian J. Newhouse, Ph.D.
Associate Professor
School of Physical Education and
  Athletics
Lakehead University
Thunder Bay, Ontario, Canada

Nweze Nnakwe, Ph.D., R.D.
Associate Professor
Department of Home Economics
College of Applied Science and
  Technology
Illinois State University
Normal, Illinois

**Timothy D. Noakes, M.B.Ch.B.,
M.D., F.A.C.S.M.**
Professor and Liberty Life Chair of
  Exercise and Sport Science
Bioenergetics of Exercise Research
  Unit
Department of Physiology
Medical Research Council and
  University of Cape Town Medical
  School
Observatory, Republic of South
  Africa

Yoshinobu Ohira, Ph.D.
Professor
Department of Physiology and
  Biomechanics
National Institute of Fitness and
  Sports
Kanoya City
Kagoshima, Japan

Hideki Ohno, M.D., Ph.D.
Professor
Department of Hygiene
National Defense Medical College
Namiki, Tokorozawa. Japan

Tomomi Ookawara, M.D., Ph.D.
Assistant Professor
Department of Hygiene
National Defense Medical College
Namiki, Tokorozawa, Japan

Giuseppe Parise, M.D.
Chair of Sports Medicine
University of Florence
Florence, Italy

Alberto Pattini, Ph.D.
Researcher
Institute of Human Physiology
University of Verona
Verona, Italy

Angelo Resina, M.D.
Deceased
Professor, Chair of Sports Medicine
University of Florence
Florence, Italy

Maria G. Rubenni
Chair of Sports Medicine
University of Florence
Florence, Italy

Yuzo Sato, M.D., Ph.D.
Professor
Research Center of Health, Physical
  Fitness, and Sports
Nagoya University
Nagoya, Japan

Federico Schena, M.D., Ph.D.
Senior Researcher
Institute of Human Physiology
University of Verona
Verona, Italy

James S. Skinner, Ph.D.
Professor
Department of Exercise Science and
  Physical Education
Arizona State University
Tempe, Arizona

Jean T. Snook
Professor
Department of Human Nutrition and
  Food Management
Ohio State University
Columbus, Ohio

Satoko Sugawara, B.S.
Student
Department of Physiology and
  Biomechanics
National Institute of Fitness and
  Sports
Kanoya City
Kagoshima, Japan

Brian W. Tobin, Ph.D.
Assistant Professor
Department of Pediatrics
Division of Basic Medical Sciences
Mercer University School of
  Medicine
Macon, Georgia

Hitoshi Yamashita, Ph.D.
Assistant Professor
Department of Hygiene
National Defense Medical College
Namiki, Tokorozawa, Japan

Wataru Yasui, B.S.
Graduate Student
Department of Physiology and
  Biomechanics
National Institute of Fitness and
  Sports
Kanoya City
Koagoshima, Japan

Yibo Zhu-Wood, Ph.D.
Nutritionist and Nutrition Education
  Training Coordinator
Child and Adult Nutrition Services
State Department of Education and
  Cultural Affairs
Pierre, South Dakaota

TABLE OF CONTENTS

DEDICATION

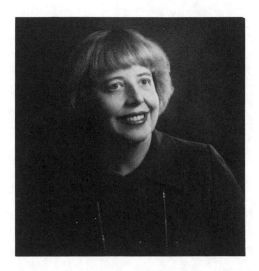

This book is dedicated to Constance V. Kies, Ph.D., one of the editors of the book. Connie died of cancer on November 30, 1993.

Constance Kies was an internationally renowned nutrition researcher and teacher. She was on the faculty at the University of Nebraska for over 30 years.

Connie's early research was centered around the protein requirements of humans with research in more recent years focused on protein-mineral interactions, including the relationships of the protein-mineral interactions and mineral metabolism to sports nutrition.

Connie was well known for producing graduate students with well rounded educations in the nutrition area. Approximately 36 Ph.D. and 177 M.S. (thesis) students have completed their programs under her direction. She has published well over 100 refereed journal articles, numerous book chapters, and edited a few of books. She also served as the editor of *Plant Foods in Human Nutrition.*

Connie organized several excellent symposias. The proceedings of many of these symposias have been published.

Connie dedicated her life to doing nutrition research, being active in the nutrition community, and working with her graduate students. She leaves behind three sisters (Cossette Kies, Camilla Chateen, and Carolyn Kies), numerous former students, and numerous colleagues who greatly appreciate what Connie did to help them.

Chapter 1

MINERAL AND ELECTROLYTE NEEDS IN EXERCISE, SPORT, AND AFTERWARDS: INTRODUCTION

Constance V. Kies

Over the last 20 years, a revolution has occurred in the U.S. relative to attitudes toward exercise and sport. While in the past these activities were of concern only to a small segment of the population, now all Americans are being strongly encouraged to participate in order to improve physical well-being.[1] The interests of the competitive athlete usually are directed toward performance; however, those of the recreational athlete may at least be motivated by achievement and maintenance of good health. In spite of advice and campaigns to increase exercise levels of all Americans, there still remains a sizeable portion of the population who may in theory accept the idea of health benefits of exercise, but still do not actually participate. Furthermore, with aging, individuals may move from one classification to another — usually toward a decline in physical activity.

With the evolution of exercise and sport as a concern of the general American population, there has been an increase in research interest in this general area and in interactions among exercise and sport with other scientific fields such as nutrition. Unfortunately, this has led to a fractionization of information.

In a recently revised book edited by Hickson and Wolinsky,[2] an excellent review of nutrition interactions with sports and exercise is given. The objective, scope, and approach of this current volume is different from that of the earlier Hickson and Wolinsky[2] book which gave in-depth review information by recognized experts in the field. This new volume presents research and papers on only a limited area of nutrition in sports and exercise: that of mineral and electrolyte needs/interactions. In addition, rather than being an in-depth review of this topic, an effort has been to bring together a collection of papers by individuals from a variety of academic disciplines, some of whom have had a long history of research in sport and exercise and whose work centers or touches on nutrition, as well as individuals whose work centers on mineral/electrolyte nutrition but whose research at least touches on sport and exercise. Papers included were largely presented in oral form in a symposium presented as part of the American Chemical Society (Agricultural and Food Chemistry Division) in Denver, Colorado, April, 1993, with some invited additional papers.

0-8493-7916-4/95/$0.00+$.50
© 1995 by CRC Press, Inc.

1

Much has been made in recent years of the health benefits of exercise and sports.[1] However, in relationship to mineral nutriture, although controversial, some negatives may exist. The high incidence of anemia among athletes, particularly female long distance runners, suggests at least secondary iron deficiency.[3-6] Although moderate amounts of exercise increase bone density, bone osteoporosis in amenorrheic female athletes suggests problems with calcium and/or other mineral utilization.[7-10] Blood plasma concentrations of zinc have been repeatedly demonstrated to be lower in athletes than in controls and to be reduced further following an event. This appears to be the result of compartmental location of zinc rather than a true zinc deficiency.[3,11-13]

Electrolyte needs of athletes and others involved in activities or climates generating high sweat losses is controversial.[14-20] It appears that replacement of sodium via, perhaps, sports drinks is desirable in events lasting more than 3 h, but that repletion following the event is more desirable in events of lesser length.[14-20]

Nutrients have been used by athletes as ergogenic aids to enhance performance. However, minerals have been used less often than other nutrients, such as vitamins. An excellent review of mineral supplement use by athletes and effects on exercise performance has been given in an article by Clarkson.[3]

In conclusion, many questions currently exist on the role of minerals and electrolytes on athletic performance and on the effects of sport and exercise on mineral status. Although receiving less research emphasis than many other nutrients, sufficient evidence does exist that exercise and sport activities do affect mineral status, and mineral status affects exercise and sports activities.

REFERENCES

1. U.S. Department of Health and Human Services, *Surgeon General's Report on Nutrition and Health,* 88-50210, U.S. Government Printing Office, Washington, D.C., 1988.
2. Hickson, J. F. and Wolinsky, I., *Nutrition in Exercise and Sport,* CRC Press, Boca Raton, FL, 1989.
3. Clarkson, P. M., Minerals: exercise performance and supplementation in athletes, *J. Sports Sci.,* 9, 91, 1991.
4. Sherman, A. R. and Kramer, B., Iron nutriture and exercise, in *Nutrition in Exercise and Sport,* Hickson, J. F. and Wolinsky, I., Eds., CRC Press, Boca Raton, FL, 1989, chap. 13.
5. Pattini, A. and Schema, F., Effects of training and iron supplementation on iron status of cross country skiers, *J. Sport Med. Phy. Fitness,* 30, 347, 1990.
6. Fogelholm, M., Jaakkola, L., and Lampisjavi, T., Effects of iron supplementation in female athletes with low serum ferritin concentrations, *Int. J. Sports Med.,* 13, 158, 1992.
7. Cree, C. D., Vermeulen, A., and Ostyn, M., Are high performance young women athletes doomed old wives?, *J. Sports Med. Phy. Fitness,* 31, 108, 1991.
8. Cann, C. E., Martin, M. C., and Genant, H. K., Decreased spinal mineral content in amenonheric women, *JAMA,* 251, 626, 1984.
9. Grandjean, A. C. and Rudd, J. S., Nutritional needs of the female athletes, in *Nutrition in Exercise and Sport,* Hickson, J. F. and Wolinsky, I., Eds., CRC Press, Boca Raton, FL, 1989, chap. 16.
10. Wolinsky, I. and Hickson, J. F., Calcium and bone in physical activity and sport, in *Nutrition in Exercise and Sport,* Wolinsky, I. and Hickson, J. F., Eds., CRC Press, Boca Raton, FL, 1989, chap. 12.

11. Lane, H. W., Some trace elements related to physical activity: zinc, copper, selenium, chromium, and iodine, in *Nutrition and Exercise and Sport,* Wolinsky, I. and Hickson, J. F., Eds., CRC Press, Boca Raton, FL, 1989, chap. 14.

12. Ohno, H., Sato, Y., Oshekawa, M., Yahata, T., Gasa, S., Doi, R., Yamamura, K., and Taniguchi, N., Training effects on blood zinc levels in humans, *J. Sports Med. Phy. Fitness,* 30, 247, 1990.

13. Singh, A., Moses, F. M., Smoak, B. L., and Deuster, P. A., Plasma zinc uptake from a supplement during submaximal running, *Med. Sci. Sports Exercise,* 24, 442, 1992.

14. Meyer, F., Bar-Or, O., MacDougall, D., and Heigenhaus, G. J. F., Sweat electrolyte losses during exercise in the heat: effects of gender and maturation, *Med. Sci. Sports Exercise,* 24, 776, 1992.

15. Millard-Stafford, M., Gender differences in fluid/electrolyte replacement during endurance exercise in heat, Paper, Am. Chemical Society national meeting, Denver, CO, March 28 to April 2, 1993, Denver, CO.

16. Millard-Stafford, M., Sparling, P. B., Rosskoff, L. B., and Dicarlo, L. J., Carbohydrate-electrolyte replacement improves distance running performance in the heat, *Med. Sci. Sports Exercise,* 24, 934, 1992.

17. Nagel, D., Seiler, D., and Franz, H., Biochemical, hematological, and endocrinological parameters during repeated intense short-term running in comparison to ultra-long distance running, *Int. J. Sports Med.,* 13, 337, 1992.

18. Noakes, T. D., Norma, R. J., Buck, R. H., Godlonton, J., Stevenson, K., and Pittaway, D., The incidence of hyponatremia during prolonged ultra-endurance exercise, *Med. Sci. Sports Exercise,* 22, 1655, 1990.

19. Rehrer, N. J., Beckers, E. J., Brouns, F., Saris, W. H. M., and Hoor, F. T., Effects of electrolytes in carbohydrate beverages on gastric emptying and secretion, *Med. Sci. Sports Exercise,* 25, 42, 1993.

20. Verde, T., Shephar, R. J., Corey, P., and Moore, R., Sweat composition in exercise and heat, *J. Appl. Physiol.,* 53, 1540, 1982.

Chapter 2

PHYSICAL EXERCISE AND IRON METABOLISM

Yoshinobu Ohira
Fumihiko Kariya
Wataru Yasui
Satoko Sugawara
Kohji Koyanagi
Ken-ichi Kaihatsu
Naotake Inoue
Fumio Hirata
Chuan-Show Chen
Hideki Ohno

CONTENTS

I. ABSTRACT

Effects of chronic exercise training and/or a single bout of strenuous exercise on hematological profiles were studied in elite sprinters and distance runners. Anemia accompanied by lower serum iron, ferritin, and haptoglobin was seen only in the distance runners. In distance runners, the total activities of serum creatine kinase (CK) and lactate dehydrogenase (LDH), with elevated percentages of Type I and decreased percentages of Type IV and V isozymes, were higher than normal levels, and haptoglobin concentration was subnormal. In response to an acute exhaustive treadmill run in distance runners, leakage of CK, LDH, and myoglobin from muscles was suggested. The serum iron level was elevated. The haptoglobin value in serum was lowered. These results suggest that distance runners are susceptible to iron deficiency in blood associated with hemolysis and iron loss during intensive training. However, tissue iron in distance runners may not be deficient, even though iron may be released from muscles in some degree in response to severe exercise.

II. INTRODUCTION

Sports anemia is induced by severe exercise or physical training. Yamaji[1,2] reported that anemia was induced approximately 10 d after the initiation of exercise training and was normalized when the physical fitness level was improved following the training. However, anemia is also noted even in Olympic athletes.[3] One of the causes of sports anemia may be hemodilution due to an increased plasma volume.[4-7] However, a reduction of serum iron with constant hemoglobin (Hb) level, for example, in response to physical training is also reported,[8,9] suggesting that hemodilution may not be the sole cause of sports anemia. Hemolysis may be another cause of sports anemia.[5,6,10] Further, it has been reported that sports anemia is generally associated with a lower iron status.[8,9,11,12] Such phenomena may be caused by an enhanced loss, or insufficient intake, of iron.[13,14] However, the mechanism responsible for the lower iron status in athletes is not well understood. Therefore, iron metabolism or cause of iron loss in response to physical exercise was investigated in the current study.

III. METHODS

Effects of different types of running exercise on hematological status were studied in elite distance runners and sprinters. The investigation was performed following the guiding principles for biomedical research in the institute. The purpose and possible risk in the study were explained, and agreements were obtained from the subjects. Following an overnight fast, approximately 10 ml of blood was withdrawn as pre-exercise samples from the brachial veins of 21 distance runners (15 males and 6 females) and 6 male sprinters. Urine samples were also collected after discarding the first urine in the morning.

A portion of blood was immediately transferred into a test tube containing ethylenediaminetetraacetic acid and mixed. The concentration of Hb, red blood cell (RBC) counts, hematocrit (Hct), mean corpuscular volume (MCV), mean corpuscular Hb (MCH), and mean corpuscular Hb concentration (MCHC) were measured immediately by using an autoanalyzer. The remaining blood was centrifuged and the supernatant was saved. In the serum, biochemical determinations were performed for iron (2,4,6-Tris(2-pyridyl)-s-triazine method), ferritin (radio-immunoassay, double antibody method), total protein (Biuret method), protein fractions (cellulose acetate electrophoresis), haptoglobin (nephelometry/polyacrylamide gel electrophoresis), myoglobin (radio-immunoassay, polyethylene glycol method), creatine kinase (CK) and lactate dehydrogenase (LDH) activities (ultra violet method), and isozymes of CK and LDH (cellulose acetate electrophoresis). In urine samples, protein and iron were analyzed.

The maximal capacities of oxygen consumption ($\dot{V}O_2$ max) in these athletes were also measured during treadmill run in a room where the temperature and humidity were regulated at approximately 20°C and 55%, respectively. The inclination of the treadmill was adjusted to 3 degrees. The speed was increased gradually every 2 min from 0 to 6 min and then every minute until the subject reached exhaustion. The expiratory gas was collected into Douglas bags and the percentages of oxygen, carbon dioxide (Perkin-Elmer, No. 1100) and gas volume were measured. An electrocardiogram was monitored throughout the study.

Since the results of whole blood analyses performed before exercise showed anemia only in the distance runners, effects of exercise were also studied in the distance runners. Second samplings of blood and urine were performed approximately 30 min after an exhaustive run on a treadmill to avoid the effects of hemoconcentration. The same parameters as in the pre-exercise samples were measured.

IV. RESULTS AND DISCUSSION

Physical characteristics of subjects are shown in Table 1. The mean ± SEM $\dot{V}O_2$ max values measured during exhaustive treadmill run were 71.2 ± 1.3, 63.0 ± 1.7, and 54.6 ± 1.5 ml·kg^{-1}·min^{-1} in male and female distance runners, and male sprinters, respectively. These results indicate that even sprinters had relatively high aerobic work capacities. However, anemia was seen only in the distance runners (Table 2). Especially Hct values were clearly less than the normal ranges. These parameters in the female runners were lower than other male athletes. These levels in the male distance runners were also significantly less than in sprinters who were normal hematologically. The MCV in the distance runners was less than the sprinters, although MCH levels were identical in all groups. Therefore, the MCHC in the distance runners were elevated. Small red cells, suggested by MCV, may explain why the reduction of Hct was more remarkable than Hb concentration or RBC counts.

The distance runners tended to be iron-deficient, although iron was not depleted (Table 3). Both serum iron and ferritin levels in the distance runners were less than in sprinters. These results suggest that anemia found in the distance runners is

TABLE 1   Physical Characteristics of Subjects

	n	Age (years)	Height (cm)	Weight (kg)	$\dot{V}O_2$ max (ml·kg^{-1}·min^{-1})
S–M	6	22.2 ± 0.3	171 ± 1	58.3 ± 1.1	54.6 ± 1.5
D–M	15	23.2 ± 1.0	168 ± 1	56.2 ± 1.1	71.2 ± 1.3***
D–F	6	20.1 ± 0.9	157 ± 1***,†††	47.0 ± 1.0***,†††	63.0 ± 1.7**,††

Note: Mean ± SEM. S: sprinters, D: distance runners, M: males, F: females, n: number
of subjects, and $\dot{V}O_2$ max maximal oxygen consumption. **: $p < 0.01$ and ***:
$p < 0.001$ vs. S–M. ††: $p < 0.01$ and †††: $p < 0.001$ vs. D-M by unpaired t-test.

associated with iron deficiency. But it is also indicated that iron deficiency is not
necessarily the sole cause of anemia. Our previous study showed that the Hb and
serum iron levels in distance runners were positively correlated if the serum iron is
less than a certain critical level (approximately 80 μg/100ml).[15] However, Hb concentration remained constant regardless of the serum iron levels, if serum levels were
above the critical level.

Oscai et al.[7] found an increased total Hb in response to training. It is also reported
that anemia, as well as erythropoietin, in sedentary women with lower erythropoietin
levels was improved when these subjects initiated physical training.[16] Plasma volume
is also increased following exercise training[4,7] and pseudoanemia is induced due to
hemodilution.[5,6] However, the levels of Hb, serum protein, iron, and/or ferritin were
not always correlated to each other in our study. If these parameters in the athletes
are influenced by the water content of plasma only, significant positive correlations
should be observed between them. Therefore, the current results suggest that the
cause of the sports anemia is not necessarily the hemodilution alone.

Serum levels of total protein in the distance runners were significantly lower
than in the sprinters (Table 3). However, the levels were not subnormal and the
protein fractions were normal, although enhanced loss of protein into urine was noted
after exhaustive exercise (data not shown). These results indicate that sports anemia
in elite athletes is not due to protein deficiency.

The haptoglobin concentration of male sprinters at rest in our study was normal,
although Haymes and Spillman[17] reported that its level and Hct were lower in women
sprinters. However, the haptoglobin levels in the distance runners were significantly
lower than in the sprinters (Table 3). Further, the total activity of LDH (Table 3) and
the distribution of Type I LDH isozyme, which was approximately 35% (not shown
in Table), exceeded the normal ranges. These data suggest that anemia in the distance
runners is also caused by a hemolysis within the circulation. Hemolysis is induced
by traumatic shock,[5,6,10] increased lysolecithin release from the spleen,[18] acidosis[19]
due to exercise, or lowered lipid content.[20] However, it is still unclear why such
phenomena were not seen in sprinters and soccer players, although the elevation of
serum LDH and CK levels and urinary protein loss were equally enhanced in
response to daily training or a soccer game suggesting that exercise intensities were
also high (unpublished observation).

The hemoconcentration estimated by the Hb level was not significant 30 min
after an exhaustive running. However, significant increases in serum iron ($p < 0.05$)

TABLE 2 Hematological Characteristics

	Hb (g/100ml)	RBC (10^4/mm^3)	Hct (%)	MCV (μ^3)	MCH ($\gamma\gamma$)	MCHC (%)
S–M	16.0 ± 0.1	529 ± 14	48.4 ± 0.4	91.7 ± 1.7	30.4 ± 0.7	33.1 ± 0.2
D–M	13.2 ± 0.2***	420 ± 10***	36.1 ± 1.1***	86.0 ± 1.1*	31.7 ± 0.4	37.1 ± 0.4***
D–F	11.0 ± 0.4***,†††	359 ± 15***,††	29.3 ± 1.1***,††	81.9 ± 1.5**	31.0 ± 0.9	37.5 ± 0.4***

Note: Mean ± SEM. S: sprinters, D: distance runners, M: males, F: females, Hb: hemoglobin, RBC: red blood cell, Hct: hematocrit, MCV: mean corpuscular volume, MCH: mean corpuscular hemoglobin, and MCHC: mean corpuscular hemoglobin concentration. *: $p < 0.05$, **: $p < 0.01$, and ***: $p < 0.001$ vs. S–M. and ††: $p < 0.01$ and †††: $p < 0.001$ vs. D–M by unpaired t-test.

TABLE 3 Parameters Determined in Serum

	TP (g/100ml)	Iron (μg/100ml)	Ferritin (ng/ml)	Mb (ng/ml)	Hapt (mg/100ml)	CK (IU/l)	LDH (IU/l)
S–M	7.4 ± 0.1	135.0 ± 9.5	86.9 ± 7.9	44.5 ± 7.6	126 ± 25	202 ± 27	307 ± 19
D–M	7.0 ± 0.1*	90.0 ± 7.3**	40.0 ± 2.5***	53.9 ± 6.6	55 ± 12**	428 ± 67	491 ± 39**
D–F	6.5 ± 0.1***,††	39.1 ± 8.0***,†††	27.8 ± 3.1***,†	14.6 ± 1.0**,††	43 ± 16*	512 ± 71**	559 ± 52**

Note: Mean ± SEM. S: sprinters, D: distance runners, M: males, F: females, TP: total protein, Mb: myoglobin, Hapt: haptoglobin, CK: creatine kinase, and LDH: lactate dehydrogenase. *: $p < 0.05$, **: $p < 0.01$, and ***: $p < 0.001$ vs. S–M, and †: $p < 0.05$, ††: $p < 0.01$. †††: $p < 0.001$ vs. D–M by unpaired t-test.

TABLE 4 **Responses of Serum Iron, Myoglobin, Total Protein, and Haptoglobin to an Exhaustive Treadmill Run in Distance Runners**

	Iron (μg/100ml)	Myoglobin (ng/ml)	Total protein (g/100ml)	Haptoglobin (mg/100ml)
Pre-ex	60.1 ± 9.8	36.2 ± 11.0	7.02 ± 0.07	45.9 ± 7.4
Post-ex	82.1 ± 6.5*	46.0 ± 13.5	7.18 ± 0.08**	40.4 ± 6.4*

Note: Mean ± SEM. n = 12. *: $p < 0.05$ and **: $p < 0.01$ by paired t-test.

and protein ($p < 0.01$) were noted (Table 4). The percentage of elevation of iron was greater than that of total protein or Hb, suggesting that these changes were not necessarily due to hemoconcentration. Serum haptoglobin was lower than the pre-exercise level ($p < 0.05$), therefore, one of the causes of the elevated iron and protein levels may be hemolysis.

Further, increased serum iron level after exercise may be related to an enhanced loss of tissue iron. For example, myoglobin concentration in serum tended to increase after exercise (Table 4, $p > 0.05$). Elevated serum ferritin was also seen after a marathon run.[21] It is also suggested that a 2 h exhaustive treadmill run increased loosely bound iron in rat gastrocnemius, although its magnitude was less in trained rats.[22] The responses of serum LDH and CK levels to exhaustive exercise are shown in Tables 5 and 6. The distributions of muscle-type isozymes were particularly increased. However, it was further suggested that these enzymes were also released from either heart or slow-twitch fibers of skeletal muscles with greater contents of iron-containing proteins. Similar results were observed after daily routine training in college distance runners (unpublished observation). An increased serum iron level may lead to iron loss, especially into urine. Although we could not detect any significant response of urinary iron to exercise, Kasugai et al.[14] reported that loss of iron into urine and sweat was increased during training.

Iron absorption into muscles may be increased in distance runners, although iron in muscle may be lost temporarily following an acute intensive exercise. Strause et al.[23] reported that absorption of iron into muscles was promoted by exercise training, although results from some studies do not always agree.[11,24] Such discrepancy may be caused, for example, by the level of physical fitness, type of training, or time after exercise. However, iron absorption into muscles may be stimulated when adaptation to training is induced in muscles generally, since synthesis of iron-dependent proteins in muscles is stimulated by endurance training.[25-27] Therefore, iron status in muscles may be increased in distance runners, even though the level of serum iron is lower.

Inadequate daily iron intake could cause iron deficiency.[13] However, it seems unlikely that the distance runners in the current study had lower iron intake than the RDI, because their diets were carefully checked by nutritionists. However, it is not clear whether iron intake was sufficient, because athletes may need more iron intake above the RDI.

In conclusion, effects of chronic exercise training, and/or a single bout of strenuous exercise, on hematological profiles were studied in elite sprinters and

TABLE 5   Responses of Serum Lactate Dehydrogenase Activity (IU/l) to
an Exhaustive Treadmill Run in Distance Runners

	Total	I	II	III	IV	V
Pre-ex	455 ± 26	195 ± 27	150 ± 12	102 ± 6	5.6 ± 1.0	2.1 ± 0.9
Post-ex	568 ± 39***	234 ± 31	154 ± 27	128 ± 13	26.8 ± 7.0*	25.6 ± 7.7*

Note: Mean ± SEM. n = 12. *: p <0.05 and ***: p <0.001 by paired *t*-test.

TABLE 6   Responses of Serum Creatine Kinase
Activity (IU/l) to an Exhaustive
Treadmill Run in Distance Runners

	Total	MB	MM
Pre-ex	477 ± 55	30.0 ± 4.8	448 ± 52
Post-ex	646 ± 71***	49.3 ± 9.6*	597 ± 65***

Note: Mean ± SEM. n = 12. *: p <0.05 and ***: p <0.001 by
paired *t*-test.

distance runners. Anemia accompanied by lower serum iron, ferritin, and haptoglobin was seen only in the distance runners. In distance runners, the total activities of
serum CK and LDH, with elevated percentages of Type I and decreased percentages
of Type IV and V isozymes, were higher than normal levels, and haptoglobin
concentration was subnormal. In response to acute exhaustive treadmill runs in
distance runners, leakage of CK, LDH, and myoglobin from muscles was suggested.
The serum level of iron was significantly increased. The serum haptoglobin value
was lowered. It is suggested that distance runners are susceptible to iron deficiency
in blood associated with hemolysis and iron loss during intensive training. However,
tissue iron of distance runners may not be deficient, even though some muscle irons
may be released in response to an exercise at a higher work load.

ACKNOWLEDGMENTS

This study was, in part, supported by the Teruo Namba Memorial Health Care
Foundation and the grant provided by the Ichiro Kanehara Foundation.

REFERENCES

1. Yamaji, R., Studies on protein metabolism during muscular exercise. I. Nitrogen metabolism in
   training for heavy muscular exercise, *J. Physiol. Soc. Jpn.*, 13, 476, 1951.
2. Yamaji, R., Studies on protein metabolism during muscular exercise. II. Changes of blood
   properties during training for heavy muscular exercise, *J. Physiol. Soc. Jpn.*, 13, 483, 1951.
3. Clement, D. B., Asmundson, R. C., and Medhurst, C. W., Hemoglobin values: comparative
   survey of the 1976 Canadian Olympic team, *Can. Med. Assoc. J.*, 117, 614, 1977.

4. Convertino, V. A., Greenleaf, V. E., and Bernauer, E. M., Role of thermal and exercise factors in the mechanism of hypervolemia, *J. Appl. Physiol.: Respirat. Environ. Exercise Physiol.*, 48, 657, 1980.

5. Eichner, E. R., Sports anemia, iron supplements, and blood doping, *Med. Sci. Sports Exercise*, 24 (*Suppl.*), S315, 1992.

6. Ohira, Y., Tabata, I., Shibayama, H., Maruyama, Y., Maruyama, I., Ebashi, H., Nishijima, Y., and Mitsudome, T., Investigation of the mechanism and preventive prescription for training-induced anemia, *Descente Sports Sci.*, 10, 258, 1989.

7. Oscai, L. B., Williams, B. T., and Hertig, B. A., Effect of exercise on blood volume, *J. Appl. Physiol.*, 24, 622, 1986.

8. Kilbom, A., Physical training with submaximal intensities in women. I. Reaction to exercise and orthostasis, *Scand. J. Clin. Lab. Invest.*, 28, 141, 1971.

9. Kilbom, A. and Astrand, I., Physical training with submaximal intensities in women. II. Effect on cardiac output, *Scand. J. Clin. Lab. Invest.*, 28, 163, 1971.

10. Streeton, J. A., Traumatic haemoglobinuria caused by karate exercises, *Lancet*, 2, 191, 1967.

11. Ehn, L., Carlmark, B., and Hoglund, S., Iron status in athletes involved in intense physical activity, *Med. Sci. Sports Exercise*, 12, 61, 1980.

12. Ohira, Y., Edgerton, V. R., Day, M. K., Gardner, G. W., Green, R., Hegenauer, J., and Ikawa, S., Responses of hematology and work capacity to iron in sedentary and trained women, in *Physical Fitness Research*, Ishiko, T., Ed., Baseball Magazine Sha, Tokyo, 1983, 65.

13. Clement, D. B. and Asmundson, R. C., Nutritional intake and hematological parameters in endurance runners, *Phys. Sportsmed.*, 10, 37, 1982.

14. Kasugai, A., Ogasawara, M., and Ito, A., Effects of exercise on the iron balance in human body examined by the excretion of iron into urine, sweat and feces, *Jpn. J. Phys. Fit. Sports Med.*, 41, 530, 1992.

15. Ebashi, H., Nishijima, Y., Maruyama, Y., Ohira, Y., Tabata, I., Takekura, H., Nishizono, H., Kurata, H., and Shibayama, H., Hematological characteristics and iron status in elite athletes, *Bull. Phys. Fit. Res. Inst.*, 73, 18, 1989.

16. Tanaka, N., Mayuzumi, M., Tanaka, N., and Hori, S., Effect of a moderate work for 7 successive days on concentrations of serum erythropoietin and hemoglobin of female university students, *Jpn. J. Phys. Fit. Sports Med.*, 42, 29, 1993.

17. Haymes, E. M. and Spillman, D. M., Iron status of women distance runners, sprinters, and control women, *Int. J. Sports Med.*, 10, 430, 1989.

18. Shiraki, K., The effect of splenectomy on sports anemia, *J. Physiol. Soc. Jpn.*, 30, 1, 1968.

19. Hiro, T., Studies on the osmotic fragility of erythrocytes influenced by a metabolic acidosis, *J. Phys. Fit. Jpn.*, 31, 279, 1982.

20. Sagawa, S. and Shiraki, K., Role of lipids in stabilizing red cell in rat, *J. Nutr. Sci. Vitaminol.*, 24, 57, 1978.

21. Lampe, J. W., Slavin, J. L., and Appl, F. S., Poor iron status of women runners training for a marathon, *Int. J. Sports Med.*, 7, 111, 1986.

22. Jenkins, R. R., Krause, K., and Schofield, L. S., Influence of exercise on clearance of oxidant stress products and loosely bound iron, *Med. Sci. Sports Exer.*, 25, 213, 1993.

23. Strause, L., Hegenauer, J., and Saltman, P., Effects of exercise on iron metabolism in rats, *Nutr. Res.*, 3, 79, 1983.

24. Ruckman, K. S. and Sherman, A. R., Effects of exercise on iron and copper metabolism in rats, *J. Nutr.*, 111, 1593, 1981.

25. Oscai, L. B., Mole, P. A., Brei, B., and Holloszy, J. O., Cardiac growth and respiratory enzyme levels in male rats subjected to a running program, *Am. J. Physiol.*, 220, 1238, 1971.

26. Pattengale, P. K. and Holloszy, J. O., Augmentation of skeletal muscle myoglobin by a program of treadmill running, *Am. J. Physiol.*, 213, 783, 1967.

27. Terjung, R. L., Winder, W. W., Baldwin, K. M., and Holloszy, J. O., Effect of exercise on the turnover of cytochrome c in skeletal muscle, *J. Biol. Chem.*, 248, 7404, 1973.

Chapter 3

IRON, EXERCISE AND GROWTH: IS EXERCISE CONTRAINDICATED IN IRON DEFICIENCY?

Brian W. Tobin
John L. Beard

CONTENTS

13

I. FUNCTIONAL CONSEQUENCES
OF IRON DEFICIENCY

A. HEME IRON

Iron deficiency is the most prevalent single nutrient deficiency in the world today.[1,2] At present it is estimated that worldwide, approximately 500 million individuals are iron-deficient. Historically, the clinical manifestations of iron deficiency are classically ascribed to a reduction in heme iron.[3,4] Approximately 70% of body iron resides in hemoglobin, and iron plays a central role in the transfer of oxygen from pulmonary to peripheral vascular beds. With adequate dietary iron and an absence of iron related pathophysiology, adequate heme iron concentrations are maintained and delivery of oxygen to metabolically active tissues remains uncompromised.

As iron supply becomes limited, however, a well characterized series of events occurs.[2] Initially, the erythron mass is protected against depletion of heme iron by mobilization of ferritin storage iron via transferrin. As body iron stores are depleted, however, an insufficient supply of iron to the developing erythron mass results in a progressive hypochromic, microcytic anemia (Table 1). With a decrease in hematocrit and hemoglobin, a decreased oxygen carrying capacity limits oxidative metabolism in peripheral tissues. Iron-deficient individuals, thus, have a dramatically reduced work performance which is related to decreased serum hemoglobin concentrations.[5,6] The influence of anemia vs. tissue iron deficiency has also been delineated in a series of elegant experiments by Finch et al.[7] and Davies et al.[8,9] These studies illustrate that hemoglobin concentration is an important determinant of maximal exercise performance, and non-heme tissue-associated iron is a primary determinant of endurance capacity at submaximal workloads.

B. NON-HEME IRON

While the effects of iron deficiency upon vascular iron have been classically described, a growing body of evidence has also suggested that there are functional consequences of iron deficiency beyond those attributable to oxyhemoglobin related deficits.[10] In addition to decreased oxidative capacity and impaired work performance, iron deficiency is associated with impairments in cognitive performance,[11] thermoregulatory capacity,[12] thyroid hormone kinetics,[13] sympathetic nervous system activation,[14] immune function,[15] glucose metabolism,[16] insulin sensitivity,[17] and growth.[18] A clear delineation between anemia and iron deficiency has been ascribed to only a limited number of these secondary consequences. Nonetheless, the diverse nature of these manifestations is testament to the variety of non-heme related physiologic and biochemical processes in which iron plays an important role. For example, iron is a necessary factor or co-factor in many enzymes including mitochondrial cytochromes, cytochrome p-450, ribonucleotide reductase, tyrosine and proline hydrolase, monoamine oxidase, catalase, glucose 6-phosphatase, and 6-phosphogluconate dehydrogenase.[10,20] It should not be surprising, therefore, that a deficit in non-heme body iron could lead to metabolic abnormalities which would ultimately affect

**TABLE 1   Hematologic Manifestations of the Progression into Overt
Iron Deficiency Anemia**

	Normal	Iron Depletion	Iron Deficiency Anemia
Transferrin iron binding capacity (µg/100 ml)	330	360	410
Plasma iron (µg/100 ml)	115	<115	<40
Plasma ferritin (ng/ml)	60	<12	<12
Transferrin saturation (%)	35	35	<16
Red blood cell protoporphyrin (µg/100 ml)	30	30	>100
Mean corpuscular volume (µ³)			<80
Hematocrit (%)	>30	<30	<30

From Beard, J.L., *Nutrition Today*, July/August 1986. With permission.

normal growth, development, and metabolic homeostasis. What is remarkable, however, is that the amount of iron associated with these enzymatic processes constitutes approximately only 1% of total body iron.

C. GROWTH

In infancy, iron deficiency is not normally associated with reduced growth rates. In fact, from a clinical perspective, it was once assumed that iron-deficient infants exhibited a moderate increase in body fat.[19] However, a closer examination of the literature illustrates that these children were often underweight at the time of diagnosis of iron deficiency. Schubert and Lahey[21] demonstrated that 56% of iron-deficient children they studied were below the tenth percentile for weight in their respective age group. This was similarly confirmed by Judisch et al.[22] who demonstrated that iron-deficient children less than 3 years of age were underweight for their height or age. Fifty percent of these children were below the twenty-fifth percentile for weight.

In young children there is good evidence that iron may play an important role in modulating normal growth rates. Aukutt et al.[18] and Chwang et al.[23] both reported an increase in the growth rate of iron-deficient children who were supplemented with iron, although two other studies showed no effect.[24,25] A recent study by Angeles et al.,[26] however, seems to strongly support a benefit of iron upon growth. In a double blind intervention trial, anemic Indonesian pre-school children received supplements of vitamin C or vitamin C plus iron. The latter group exhibited increased hematologic indices and increased height and weight compared to the vitamin C only group. Interestingly, the favorable effect of iron upon growth was not mediated through an increased food intake; however, there was a decreased morbidity. The rate of infectious diseases was lesser in the treatment group and may have additionally contributed to the favorable growth results.

Among adolescents, iron deficiency is the most prevalent nutritional deficiency in the world today.[10] Despite this fact, little is known regarding the impact of iron deficiency per se upon the growth rate of adolescents. It is well established, however, that during periods of rapid growth and development, increases in blood volume, lean body mass, and red blood cell mass increase the requirement for iron.[3,27] In older adolescent males, lean body mass accretion necessitates increased iron needs; in young women, the onset of menses is responsible for similar demands. As puberty ensues, the process of growth from infancy to adulthood requires a coordination of appropriate nutritional intake, commensurate to metabolic demands in light of a changing hormonal profile. Thus, if nutritional intake is insufficient to meet these needs, slowed growth may result by a variety of mechanisms. However, while it is well documented that chronic undernutrition will attenuate growth, a specific role of iron in growth stunting has not been established in adolescents.

Although studies in adolescent humans are somewhat incomplete, laboratory animal investigations illustrate growth stunting in iron-deficient animals.[28,29] Rats fed an AIN-76 diet with limited elemental iron (6 mg Fe/kg diet) show attenuated growth which is characterized by a lower body weight and a reduction in body protein content, when contrasted to control rats who received adequate iron (50 mg Fe/kg diet).[30] Absolute food intake is lesser in iron-deficient animals, which suggests possible neurobehavioral or cognitive defects. However, more recent data by Zahn[31] show that iron-deficient rats actually eat more per kg body weight than do controls when all are meal fed, and a pair fed group is included. The mechanism of this growth attenuation may be further related to altered energetic efficiency. That is, despite alterations in food intake, iron-deficient animals exhibit a reduced ability to retain ingested energy in their body mass during periods of growth.[30] This phenomenon may be explained by increased facultative thermogenesis, which may be altered in iron-deficient animals in a temperature-dependent fashion.[32] In addition, the hormones which regulate growth may very well be affected by iron deficiency, and this effect may be independent of tissue iron deficiency.[33]

1. Energy Metabolism

Aside from the oxygen transport role that heme iron plays in supplying oxygen to tissues, a number of laboratory animal studies now confirm that iron deficiency per se may be important to basic processes of energy metabolism. This was first observed by Henderson et al.[28] who demonstrated that iron-deficient animals are characterized by an increased basal metabolic rate and increased glucose oxidation. Later, Brooks et al.[34] confirmed that iron-deficient rats have an enhanced reliance upon glucose as a metabolic substrate as characterized by enhanced glucose turnover and oxidation. Further studies by Farrell et al.[17] illustrated that a part of the increased utilization of glucose in iron-deficient animals may be explained by enhanced insulin sensitivity. Borel et al.[35] expanded on this initial observation by demonstrating a significant left-shifting of the glucose-insulin sensitivity curve in iron-deficient rats through the use of hyperinsulinemic-euglycemic glucose clamp experiments. Overall, the iron-deficient animal is characterized by reduced growth, increased resting metabolic rate, reduced feed efficiency, and enhanced utilization of glucose as a metabolic substrate. The mechanisms of these adaptations have been partially elucidated and will be described in the following sections.

2. Thyroid Hormones

The thyroid hormones are responsible for maintaining basal metabolic rate and serve in a permissive role during periods of growth favoring lean body mass development.[36,37] It is clear that the thyroid hormones are critical for the action of growth hormone.[38] The thyroid hormones also act in concert with the sympathetic nervous system to regulate facultative thermogenesis.[39,40] Thus, body weight can be affected by hyperthyroid states which favor increased energy expenditure and a negative caloric balance. Conversely, hypothyroid states can also affect body weight since a reduced production of triiodothyronine (T_3) can limit lean body mass development during periods of rapid growth, such as in adolescence.

Martinez-Torres and Cubeddu,[41] Lukaski et al.,[42] and Beard et al.[43] illustrated that iron-deficient human subjects are functionally hypothyroid. Though only in the latter study were there sufficient numbers of subjects and control of body fat to demonstrate a significant decrease in circulating thyroid hormones. When cold stressed, iron-deficient subjects fail to adequately thermoregulate and core temperature drops. These data are consistent with earlier experiments in iron-deficient rats that illustrated a failure to thermoregulate at decreased environmental temperatures concurrent with a decreased plasma T_3 concentration.[44,45] Kinetic studies of T_3 metabolism illustrated that whole body T_3 production in iron-deficient animals was half that of control rats.[13] The mechanisms of a reduced T_3 production in iron deficiency may relate to altered T_4-5'-deiodinase activity;[13,46] this enzyme converts thyroid hormone (T_4) to T_3, the active form of the hormone. The central importance of iron in this lesion was established when iron repletion corrected this defect.[47] Additionally, a role of anemia was established when exchange transfusion failed to completely correct observed thermoregulatory defects. Although the T_4-5'-deiodinase enzyme has not been purified and the role of iron directly assessed, an early study by Stanbury et al.[48] showed that *in vitro* hepatic T_4 to T_3 conversion is markedly blunted when liver homogenates are devoid of iron. A more recent report by Fuchs et al.[49] illustrated a reduced glutathione peroxidase activity in HepG2 cells cultured in a media devoid of iron; such observations may additionally delineate a role of the transferrin receptor in hepatic enzyme regulation. Thus, iron deficiency of sufficient severity is associated with a biochemical and a functional hypothyroid state which may be related to an iron-linked enzymatic lesion. This state is characterized by reduced plasma T_3 production as well as a failure to thermoregulate at cold temperatures.

3. Sympathetic Nervous System

An enhancement in sympathetic nervous system activity can serve as a mechanism for heat dissipation and increased caloric expenditure. If increases in caloric expenditure are not met by an enhanced energy intake, however, a negative energy balance may result. Thus, an upregulation of sympathetic nervous system activity without increased caloric intake or enhanced energetic efficiency may be implicated in altered growth or body weight maintenance. The mechanisms which regulate autonomic nervous system function and energy balance, and hormonal factors which determine caloric expenditure have been extensively reviewed by others.[50–52]

A number of studies illustrate an enhancement of sympathetic activity in iron deficiency.[12,14,53] This hypernoradrenergic state is characterized by an increased plasma norepinephrine concentration and increased urinary norepinephrine excretion in iron-deficient human subjects and laboratory animals. Tissue-specific defects also exist. Beard et al.[30,32] demonstrated an increased norepinephrine turnover in heart and interscapular brown adipose tissue (IBAT) of iron-deficient animals. These studies suggest than an increase in sympathetic activity, characterized by an increased tissue norepinephrine turnover in the IBAT, might increase facultative thermogenesis. The upregulation of the sympathetic nervous system may be a means to control core temperature in light of deficits in thyroid hormone production.[54] Taken together, these adaptations could partially explain altered feed efficiency and attenuated growth in functionally hypothyroid, sedentary weanling iron-deficient animals.

II. FUNCTIONAL CONSEQUENCES OF EXERCISE

A. IRON AND EXERCISE

That modulations in heme and non-heme iron play significant roles in determining oxidative capacity and exercise performance should not be surprising. What is intriguing and somewhat paradoxical, however, is that exercise per se may detrimentally affect iron status. Studies performed in chronically exercising human subjects have illustrated a reduction in serum ferritin, hemoglobin, hematocrit, and serum iron binding capacity of athletes involved in intense physical activity (for recent reviews see References 55,56). A number of researchers have coined the phrase "sports anemia" to characterize the hematologic changes occurring during periods of intense physical activity.[57,58] The exact nature of a true sports anemia, however, has been debated in the scientific literature.[59]

1. Human Studies

A substantial body of research literature supports the notion of a detrimental effect of exercise on body iron status.[56] To review these investigations is not within the scope of the present manuscript, however, several studies are noteworthy. One study determined hemoglobin, packed cell volume, serum iron, and iron binding capacity of selected athletes during the 1968 Olympic games.[60] These data illustrated an iron-deficient anemia in 2% of male and 2.5% of female athletes and a mild anemia without signs of iron depletion in 3% of the general athletic population. A later study was performed specifically in middle and long distance runners, elite rowers, and professional racing cyclists.[61] These data illustrated that compromised iron status may be a sport-specific phenomenon, as only the runners had lower serum ferritin, serum iron, and haptoglobin. Sustained chronic exercise of moderate intensity may also affect hematologic variables. Soldiers who marched 35 km/d for 6 d at

35% of $\dot{V}O_2$ max were evaluated for changes in iron status.[62] Four days of marching produced a decrease in erythrocytes and hematocrit, which persisted 6 d into the post-march period. Although the previously stated reports suggest that exercise performance should be detrimentally affected by an altered hematologic status, this hypothesis has been questioned. Dresendorfer et al.[63] presented data on RBC count, hemoglobin and related hematological factors in 12 marathon runners during a 20 d, 312 mile road race. In these subjects, RBC number and hemoglobin were decreased during the race, however, running speeds were not affected. The possibility of a "pseudo anemia" secondary to alterations in blood volume during chronic physical training was suggested.

A number of investigators have proposed mechanisms by which iron balance could be affected by intense physical exercise. Explanations include increased gastrointestinal blood losses following running,[64] and hematuria as a result of erythrocyte rupture from footstrike.[65] Iron loss in sweat has been proposed, yet some investigations suggest such losses may be inconsequential.[66] Taken together, the data support an increased prevalence of iron deficiency in certain populations of chronically exercising individuals. The exact cause of these manifestations and the functional consequences, however, remain to be clearly elucidated.

2. Animal Studies

Animal studies are not totally in agreement with studies in humans since the former both support and refute a detrimental effect of exercise on iron status. Studies by Strause et al.[67] illustrate no effect of exercise on vascular iron; however, there was an increased redistribution of iron from liver to heart and skeletal muscle. Prasad and Pratt[68] also documented reduced liver iron in exercised rats. Some of these changes observed may be sex specific, as another study suggests gender differences in the hematologic response to exercise.[69] Several investigators corroborate a beneficial effect of exercise upon body iron physiology. Two studies document an increased hemoglobin concentration in treadmill exercised animals and suggest that the impact of dietarily induced anemia may be lessened by exercise training.[70,71] In addition, iron-deficient trained animals show some beneficial, functional adaptations to exercise. Willis et al.[29,72,73] determined that iron-deficient trained animals will increase TCA cycle activity, electron transport chain capacity, and pyruvate carboxylation compared to sedentary counterparts. These studies illustrate a 15% increase in cytochrome C, a 15% increase in TCA cycle enzymes, and a 33% increase in the manganese superoxide dismutase. These latter data suggest interactive adaptations in iron-deficient trained animals which enhance endurance performance and improve oxidative metabolism at rest.

B. GROWTH

When evaluating the influence of exercise upon body weight and/or growth, one must consider the biologic determinants of weight. The simplest partitioning of weight considers that the body can be described as two compartments:[74] one which is principally fat, and the other which is termed fat-free weight. This simplification is necessary because it is not clinically feasible to directly analyze the lipid, protein, carbohydrate, and mineral content of a human being, although such procedures can be performed in laboratory animals. In human subjects, however, a variety of techniques are utilized to determine body composition. The gold standard is currently densitometry. Based on Archimedes' principle and validations by Siri,[75] the density of the body is determined by weighing a subject in and out of water. Skinfold measurements are also used as estimates of body composition, assuming that external adiposity is related to total body fat.[76] These, and other methods have been extensively reviewed in the literature and the relative merits of each method have been ascribed.[77,78]

Despite the availability of techniques for assessing morphological changes in exercising subjects, there is currently a paucity of data regarding effects of exercise on prepubescent children.[79] One study illustrated little change in body density and skinfold measurements during a 12-week running program.[80] This may be due, in part, to the limits of detectability for indirect estimates of body composition. Parizkova studied the effect of 7 years of exercise training in children.[81] Although body fat was lower in the exercised group, there was no significant difference in body weight over the course of the study. Resistance training studies have provided somewhat contradictory results. In one study, prepubescent boys participated in a program which increased strength over a 14-week period.[82] Interestingly, mean body density increased in the control group and body density decreased in the trained group. These studies paradoxically suggest that strength training in children may lead to a decrease in fat-free mass. Other studies, however, have shown no change in muscle mass for children involved in strength training.[83,84] Taken together, these data indicate somewhat inconclusive results. The reliability of certain techniques for measurement of body composition in children may be problematic and has been discussed.[85]

In adults, prolonged intense exercise has generally been determined to decrease the percentage of total body fat. This effect is sometimes, but not consistently, combined with a decrease in total body weight. Parizkova and Poupa[86] determined that intense training in female Olympic athletes results in a weight-constant decrease in percent body fat and an increase in the percentage of fat-free mass. Studies involving less intense physical activity give somewhat conflicting results. Although most studies show body fat to be significantly reduced, total body weight is not always reduced.[87–89] One study reported no change in weight or body fat.[90] Another reported an increase in fat-free mass.[89] Taken together, however, most studies confirm that exercise will reduce body fat. If caloric intake is maintained commensurate to metabolic demands, body weight, and more importantly lean body mass, will not decrease.

1. Caloric Balance and Energy Metabolism

The concept of caloric balance asserts that if an individual is taking in sufficient calories to meet daily energetic demands, then body weight is maintained. Caloric demand can be divided into three constituents: basal metabolic rate, thermogenesis,

TABLE 2 Factors Which Affect Energy Metabolism and Caloric Balance

Basal Metabolic Rate	Thermogenesis	Voluntary Activity
Fat-free mass	Food intake	Duration of exercise
Age	Environmental temperature	Exercise intensity
Sex	Stress	
Thyroid hormones	Thermogenic substances	
Protein turnover		

and voluntary activity (Table 2). The determinants of basal metabolic rate are the fat-free mass, age, sex, thyroid hormones, and protein turnover. Thermogenesis is classified as facultative or obligatory and is influenced by food intake, environmental temperature, stress, and thermogenic substances. Voluntary activity is determined by the duration of exercise and its intensity. These concepts serve as a framework for describing metabolic influences which may control growth, development, and maintenance of body weight. These metabolic constructs have been extensively reviewed by others in the literature.[36,50,52]

2. Basal Metabolic Rate

Basal metabolic rate (BMR) constitutes approximately 70% of daily energy expenditure, thus, a number of laboratories have investigated the possibility that residual effects of exercise may influence BMR in athletes. Tremblay et al.[91] studied the effects of submaximal exercise on a similar construct, the resting metabolic rate (RMR). RMR was increased in highly trained subjects when studied 48 h post-exercise. Additionally, glucose-induced thermogenesis was reduced 47% in trained subjects. Bielinski et al.[92] evaluated energy metabolism during the post-exercise recovery period. Energy expenditure increased during the early recovery period and faded in the night following exercise. The following morning, however, energy expenditure was increased 4.7% in exercised subjects. Animal studies have provided additional insight into the effects of exercise upon metabolic rate. Hill et al.[93] differentiated an age effect illustrating that younger animals are more susceptible to exercise-induced increases in resting oxygen consumption than older counterparts.

The thyroid hormones are an important modulator of RMR. However, the effect of exercise training upon thyroid hormone physiology has not been clearly delineated. One study suggests that trained subjects have an increased reliance upon T_4.[94] Three days following exercise, the fractional clearance of T_4 was increased by 28% in trained individuals. These effects may be time dependent, however, since 10 d of rest seems to ameliorate the response. Other studies illustrate that T_4 turnover is blunted (11%) in trained subjects; factors such as exercise intensity and duration may influence the turnover of T_4.[95] Animal studies show that exercise enhances the rate of utilization of T_4 and suggest that trained individuals might be slightly hypermetabolic due to thyroid-linked energetic lesions. An increased metabolic clearance is proposed; however, this has not been consistently demonstrated.[96]

3. Thermogenesis

Thermogenesis accounts for approximately 15% of daily energy expenditure, thus, several laboratories have attempted to elucidate the influence of exercise and body composition on this determinant of caloric balance.[97] Balon et al.[98] determined that the thermogenic potential of insulin is enhanced in skeletal muscle following exercise. LeBlanc et al.[99] illustrated that dietarily induced thermogenesis (DIT) is reduced in trained subjects; this effect may be modulated by a decreased sympathetic nervous system activity. Gleeson et al.[100] and McDonald et al.,[101] however, showed that exercise-trained animals have an increased DIT, suggesting decreased energetic efficiency. Segal et al.[102] illustrated that body composition may confound estimates of DIT; subjects with a low percentage of body fat exhibited a greater effect of post-exercise DIT. Jequier[50,103] has elegantly illustrated that the proportion of lean body mass is positively correlated to energy expenditure. Klieber[104] suggests that metabolic body size (weight $^{-0.75}$) best estimates BMR, whereas Huesner[105] suggests that body weight$^{-0.67}$ is a better estimate. Taken together, these studies illustrate that exercise may alter resting thermogenesis or thermogenic capacity. However, estimates of resting metabolism are likely more influenced by metabolic body size and the relative proportion of lean body mass and body fat.

An increase in norepinephrine turnover can be an indicator of enhanced sympathetic nervous system activity and increased facultative thermogenesis, and thus, increased energy expenditure. In rodents, IBAT has been utilized as a site-specific model of facultative thermogenic capacity.[106,107] By uncoupling oxidative phosphorylation, IBAT dissipates heat and serves as an indirect mechanism for decreasing energetic efficiency. Hirata and Nagasaka[108] studied calorigenic response to cold in physically trained rats and illustrated an increased norepinephrine-stimulated peak thermogenic potential. Later experiments demonstrated an increased blood flow to IBAT, and fostered the hypothesis that physical training may increase calorigenic response through increased IBAT blood perfusion concurrent with enhanced Sympathetic nervous system activation.[109] Not all studies illustrate an increased thermogenic effect of norepinephrine in trained animals, however. LeBlanc[110] demonstrated that exercise training did not increase oxygen consumption following norepinephrine administration and Rickard et al.[111] illustrated that thermogenic capacity in IBAT is not altered by training. Taken together, these studies illustrate that facultative thermogenesis may be altered with training, but this adaptation may be a temperature-specific phenomenon. Some insightful studies were subsequently performed by LeBlanc[112] who investigated effects of hyperphagia and exercise upon calorigenic response. Although training had no effect upon thermogenic response, hyperphagia was associated with increased IBAT weight in sedentary animals. Physically trained rats, that were hyperphagic via feeding a cafeteria diet, had an increased norepinephrine stimulated-oxygen consumption yet a decrease in IBAT weight. Thus, these studies may imply that dietary factors are primary to the hypertrophy of IBAT and that training acts in a secondary, inhibitory manor to attenuate IBAT hypertrophy. The net effect of exercise in hyperphagia, thus, may be a reduction of Sympathetic nervous system derived IBAT facultative thermogenesis.

III. INTERACTIONS OF IRON DEFICIENCY AND EXERCISE TRAINING

A. DOES EXERCISE EXACERBATE FUNCTIONAL CONSEQUENCES OF IRON DEFICIENCY WHICH MAY ALTER GROWTH?

A chronic inadequate intake of dietary iron is associated with a gradual reduction in body iron stores, followed by a progressive hypochromic microcytic anemia. Among the functional consequences of iron deficiency are impaired work performance,[5,6] decreased thyroid hormone production,[13] increased sympathetic nervous system activation,[14] and decreased growth.[18] While diet certainly affects body iron stores, exercise may also be implicated in promoting a negative iron balance.[55] A number of laboratories have substantiated that the incidence of iron deficiency is increased in certain populations of chronically exercising individuals.[56] Exercise is generally associated with a decrease in body fat, and provided that caloric intake is not limited, lean body mass is preserved. Energetic mechanisms which alter caloric balance may be influenced by exercise.[51,52] Most noteworthy is the possible residual increase in resting metabolic rate, decreased reliance upon thyroid hormones, and enhanced sympathetic nervous system activation.

A question which must be asked therefore, is what is the potential interactive influence of a reduced iron intake and exercise training upon the functional consequences of both states? Are their combined effects simply additive, do they negate each other, or are they truly interactive, thus promoting a greater detrimental effect? While some animal studies have illustrated increases in oxidative metabolism[28,72,73] and enhanced endurance capacity[71] in exercise-trained iron-deficient animals, not all systems are beneficially affected. An inadequate intake of dietary iron and chronic exercise might concurrently interact to detrimentally alter growth. This in fact has been demonstrated in several laboratories. The effect of exercise upon reduction of growth rates in iron-deficient animals has been reported by ourselves[113] and by Willis et al.[72] Iron-deficient animals who were exercise trained for 6 or 12 weeks demonstrated a reduced body weight compared to sedentary counterparts (Figure 1).[113] Thus, there exists a somewhat paradoxical dichotomy here. The available data suggest a possible maladaptation in iron-deficient animals where exercise may enhance oxidative metabolism, yet this may occur at the expense of growth and development. How then is such an effect mediated? In order to answer these questions, we must return to our previously stated investigation in iron physiology, consequent to the premise of caloric balance assumptions as they relate to iron and exercise.

If exercise truly results in attenuated growth in iron deficiency several questions must be asked:

1. What is the effect of diet and exercise upon heme-iron status and the kinetic behavior of vascular iron?
2. Can altered growth be explained by neurohormonal factors which directly or indirectly alter caloric balance and/or anabolic states?

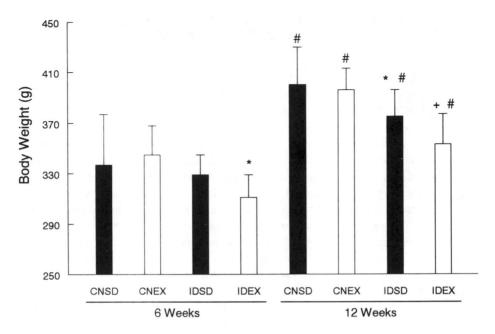

FIGURE 1.   Effects of 6 or 12 weeks treadmill exercise training (EX) or sedentary life (SD) upon the body weight of iron-deficient (ID) and control (CN) animals. Values are means ± SD for n = 7 to 10 animals per group. Significant differences between treatment groups are noted ($p \leq 0.05$) for effects of diet (*), exercise (+), and week of treatment (#).

3. If a growth deficit manifests, is this truly a growth deficit where protein mass is attenuated?
4. What are the energetic components of such a lesion?

To our knowledge, the laboratories of Drs. Brooks, Dallman, and Willis[28,70–73] and ourselves[113–115] are among the few groups to utilize an experimental paradigm designed to specifically isolate the independent and interactive influences of diet and exercise. This is accomplished in studies where four groups of animals are studied: iron-deficient sedentary, iron-deficient exercised, control sedentary, and control exercised. By introducing a dietary iron deficiency and superimposing exercise upon this paradigm, one can ask questions specific to diet or exercise, and/or interactions of diet and exercise. In addition, we have further refined this model by adjusting exercise workloads to correspond to 65 to 70% $\dot{V}O_2$ max respective to the treatment group. With this extended paradigm, one can isolate the independent and interactive effects of diet and exercise, yet do so in a model of calorically equivalent exercise intensity.

1.   Hematology and Ferrokinetics

In an initial series of experiments[113] we asked the question "what are the independent and interactive effects of diet and exercise upon hematology and kinetic behavior of vascular iron?" If exercise does detrimentally alter body iron status, then animals at risk (those already iron-deficient) should demonstrate the greatest detriment

**TABLE 3   Detrimental Effects of Dietary Iron
Deficiency and Exercise Training in Rats**

	Analysis of Variance Effects		
	Diet	Exercise	Interaction
Iron status:			
Hematocrit	⇓	≠	⇓
Hemoglobin	⇓	≠	≠
Fractional Iron Clearance	⇑	⇑	≠
Red Cell Associated Iron	⇑	≠	≠
Thyroid hormones:			
Liver $T_4 \rightarrow T_3$ Conversion	⇓	≠	≠
Nutritional factors:			
Digestible Energy Intake	⇓	≠	⇓
Caloric Retention	⇓	⇓	≠
Feed Efficiency	≠	⇓	≠
Carcass body composition:			
Caloric Content	⇓	⇓	≠
Protein Content	⇓	⇓	≠
Fat Content	⇓	⇓	≠
Mineral Content	⇓	≠	≠

Note: The symbols (⇑, ⇓) indicate a statistically significant increase
or decrease in the noted effect, $p \leq 0.05$; ≠ indicates a non-
significant effect, $p \geq 0.05$. Interaction effect direction (Diet ×
Exercise) is denoted for iron-deficient exercised animals relative
to other treatment groups.

in iron related measures. These studies illustrated that 12 weeks of submaximal
exercise training per se (treadmill running) at 65 to 70% $\dot{V}O_2$ max did not alter
hematocrit, hemoglobin, mean corpuscular hemoglobin, red blood cell mass, or
serum iron; however, an interactive effect of diet and exercise altered hematocrit
(Table 3). In addition, there were significant differences in the kinetic behavior of
plasma iron. That is, the rate of clearance of iron from the plasma pool (fractional iron
clearance) was increased 16% in iron-deficient exercised animals vs. sedentary iron-
deficient controls. A portion of this increase was attributable to an enhanced red
blood cell uptake of radiolabled iron (red cell associated iron). As previously discussed, we also observed that iron-deficient exercised animals exhibited attenuated
growth, which was interactively influenced by factors of diet and exercise. We were
unable to duplicate studies in humans, however, which suggested a more fragile
RBC;[65] in our paradigm, erythrocyte osmotic fragility was not altered by exercise.
Taken together, our studies illustrated that iron-deficient exercised animals behaved
in a ferrokinetic manner characteristic of a heightened state of iron deficiency. The
kinetic behavior suggests that exercise may alter certain aspects of the distribution of
iron, which is consistent with a previous hypothesis.[67]

2.   Metabolic Rate and Associated Factors

A second question is: What is the energetic state of these animals and can
alterations in resting metabolic rate, and influences of the thyroid hormones or

sympathetic nervous system activation serve as an explanation for slowed growth? To accomplish these ends we repeated the previous experiments with one addition: instead of carrying out studies to twelve weeks only, we additionally studied a subset of animals that received 6 weeks of exercise.[114] Again, animals were treadmill exercised at 65 to 70% $\dot{V}O_2$ max. Resting metabolic rate was determined by indirect calorimetry and illustrated that 6 weeks training did not induce a hypermetabolic state; yet 12 weeks of exercise training resulted in a significantly elevated resting oxygen consumption in iron-deficient animals. However, exercise exerted no independent or interactive effect upon RMR. Sympathetic nervous system activation was assessed by norepinephrine turnover techniques following inhibition of a rate-limiting enzyme, tyrosine hydroxylase. Norepinephrine turnover in heart and liver was less in iron-deficient animals, yet exercise had no effect. The IBAT responded differently, however. IBAT norepinephrine turnover of iron-deficient sedentary animals was 240% of iron sufficient sedentary controls, yet exercise normalized this indicator of Sympathetic nervous system activity in trained iron-deficient rats. The *in vitro* capacity for T_3 production via T_4-5'-deiodinase activity was assessed in liver and IBAT. Most noteworthy was a decreased *in vitro* hepatic T_4 to T_3 conversion in older animals, regardless of treatment, and a decreased conversion capacity in iron-deficient exercised rats during the initial 6 week period (Table 3). Since growth was also attenuated during the initial six weeks (Figure 1), yet tissue Sympathetic nervous system activity illustrated no net increase, the depressed T_3 production in liver was of particular interest.

3. Body Composition and Energetic Efficiency

The final questions which were asked related to feeding behavior, energetic efficiency, and body composition. To elucidate these queries, we utilized feed intake data which was collected prior to animal sacrifice, and then performed body composition analysis via proximate analysis procedures.[115] These studies illustrated an interactive effect of diet and exercise upon digestible energy content (DE: kcal consumed minus fecal energy; Table 3). That is, while control exercised animals tended to increase food consumption and thus DE content, iron-deficient exercised animals failed to respond to the caloric demands of exercise (Table 3). This lack of caloric availability was further complicated by a reduced feed efficiency. Feed efficiency was calculated as kcal retained in the carcass of the animal divided by kcal of DE during a 7-d growth period. These data illustrated that diet, and an interaction of diet and the treatment duration, resulted in a reduced feed efficiency due to iron deficiency, especially during periods of rapid growth.

Body composition data revealed that the reduction in body weight seen in iron-deficient exercised animals was due to a reduced fat and protein content (Table 3). Interestingly, exercise as an independent factor did not alter the protein content of control animals; however, it did result in a reduction of fat content. Thus, the additional weight loss seen in iron-deficient exercised animals was attributable to the additional decrement in body protein content (Figure 2). This may be related to previously discussed reductions in the capacity for hepatic T_3 production,[13,114] since

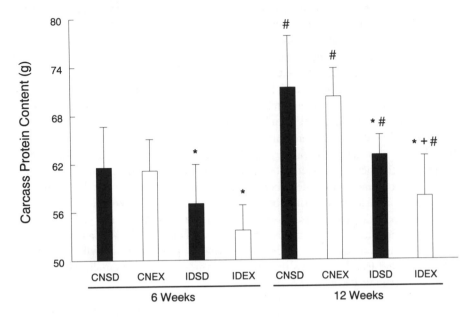

FIGURE 2. Effects of 6 or 12 weeks treadmill exercise training (EX) or sedentary life (SD) upon the carcass protein content of iron-deficient (ID) and control (CN) animals. Values are means ± SD for n = 7 to 10 animals per group. Significant differences between treatment groups are noted ($p \leq 0.05$) for effects of diet (*), exercise (+), and week of treatment (#).

the deficit in hepatic T_4-5'-deiodinase activity was observed during the initial 6 weeks of exercise training at a time when the animals were rapidly growing. With a lack of T_3 availability, lean body mass development may have been detrimentally attenuated. From a functional perspective, such an adaptation does not appear to make sense; however, a portion of the lean mass protein may have been utilized via increased hepatic gluconeogenesis,[72] which would be necessitated by the previously demonstrated enhanced glucose oxidation of iron deficiency.[28,34] In addition to fat and protein measures we also performed determinations of mineral content in these animals. Apparently, exercise has no statistically significant effect upon mineral content, however, iron-deficient animals had reduced mineral content. As would be expected, caloric content was reduced as a function of iron deficiency and exercise.

B. PROPOSED: EXERCISE IS CONTRAINDICATED IN IRON DEFICIENCY

Based on the discussion of our previous experiments and the reports of others, one is left with a somewhat paradoxical scenario. Exercise may negatively influence selected hematologic indices of iron status, may exacerbate selected functional consequences of iron deficiency such as growth and development, yet may improve selected oxidative consequences such as mitochondrial oxidative capacity. Thus, one must conclude a benefit or detriment which is specific to the system in question. The query, thus, becomes somewhat philosophical.

Certainly, it is well documented by a number of laboratories that chronic exercise will raise $\dot{V}O_2$ max and endurance capacity,[70,71] and increase oxidative enzyme activity in iron-deficient exercised animals,[72,73] suggesting a benefit of exercise. However, we and others have conversely demonstrated an attenuation of growth in iron-deficient exercised rats, illustrating a detrimental effect of exercise on iron-related consequences.[113–115] Studies to elucidate this phenomenon demonstrated that iron-deficient exercised animals had a reduced capacity for hepatic T_3 production.[114] The implications of a decreased T_3 availability, as well as a decreased energetic efficiency, are evidenced by a deficit in the caloric content of the carcass, decreased body fat, and less-lean body mass in iron-deficient exercised animals.[115] Thus, while a historic, important body of literature supports a beneficial effect of exercise upon oxidative and exercise-related function in iron deficiency,[70–73] studies of growth and nutritional energetics argue against a benefit.[113–115] When considering the functional consequences of peripheral tissue T_3 production, growth, energetic efficiency, and lean body mass development in iron-deficient animals, exercise is clearly contraindicated in iron deficiency.

REFERENCES

1. Beard, J. L., Finch, C. L., Iron deficiency, in *Iron Fortification of Foods*, Clyde, F. M., Ed., Academic Press, New York, 1985, pp. 3–16.
2. Finch, C. A., Huebers, M. D., Perspectives in iron metabolism, *New Engl. J. Med.*, 25, 1520, 1982.
3. Bowering, J., Sanchez, A. M., A conspectus of research on iron requirements of man, *J. Nutr.*, 7, 987, 1976.
4. Cook, J. D., Lynch, S. R., The liabilities of iron deficiency, *Blood*, 68, 803, 1986.
5. Gardner, G. W., Edgerton, V. R., Barnard, R. J., Bernauer, E. H., Cardiorespiratory, hematological and physical performance responses of anemic subjects to iron treatment, *Am. J. Clin. Nutr.*, 28, 982, 1975.
6. Gardner, G. W., Edgerton, V., Senenwiratne, B., Barnard, R., Ohira, Y., Physical work capacity and metabolic stress in subjects with iron deficiency anemia, *Am. J. Clin. Nutr.*, 30, 910, 1977.
7. Finch, C. A., Miller, L., Inamdar, A. R., Person, R., Seiler, K., Mackler, B., Iron deficiency in the rat: physiological and biochemical studies of muscle dysfunction, *J. Clin. Invest.*, 58, 447, 1976.
8. Davies, K. J. A., Maquire, J. J., Brooks, G. A., Dallman, P. R., Muscle mitochondrial bioenergetics, oxygen supply, and work capacity during dietary iron deficiency and repletion, *Am. J. Physiol.*, 242, E418, 1982.
9. Davies, K. J. A, Donovan, C. M., Refino, C. J., Brooks, G. A., Packer, L., Dallman, P. R., Distinguishing effects of anemia and muscle iron deficiency on muscle bioenergetics in the rat, *Am. J. Physiol.*, 246, E535, 1984.
10. Dallman, P. R., Manifestations of iron deficiency, *Semin. Hematol.*, 19, 19, 1982.
11. Soemantri, A. G., Pollitt, E., Insum, K., Iron deficiency anemia and educational achievement, *Am. J. Clin. Nutr.*, 42, 1221, 1985.
12. Dillman, E., Johnson, D. G., Martin, J., Mackler, B., Finch, C. A., Catecholamine elevation in iron deficiency, *Am. J. Physiol.*, 237, R297, 1979.

13. Beard, J. L., Tobin, B. W., Green, W., Evidence for thyroid hormone deficiency in iron-deficient anemic rats, *J. Nutr.*, 119, 772, 1988.
14. Vorhees, M. L., Stuart, M. J., Stockman, J. A., Oski, F. A., Iron deficiency anemia and increased urinary NE excretion, *J. Ped.*, 86, 542, 1975.
15. Dallman, P. R., Iron deficiency and the immune response, *Am. J. Clin. Nutr.*, 46, 324, 1987.
16. Brooks, G. A., Henderson, S. A., Dallman, P. R., Increased glucose dependence in resting, iron-deficient rats, *Am. J. Physiol.*, 250, E414, 1987.
17. Farrell, P. A., Beard, J. L., Druckenmiller, M., Increased insulin sensitivity in iron-deficient rats, *J. Nutr.*, 118, 1104, 1988.
18. Aukett, M. A., Parks, Y. A., Scott, P. H., Wharton, B. A., Treatment with iron increases weight gain and psychomotor development, *Arch. Dis. Child.*, 61, 849, 1986.
19. Oski, F. A., The nonhematologic manifestations of iron deficiency, *Am. J. Dis. Child.*, 133, 315, 1979.
20. Arthur, C. K., Isbuster, J. P., Iron deficiency: misunderstood, misdiagnosed, and mistreated, *Curr. Ther.*, 23, 1986.
21. Schubert, W. K., Lahey, M. E., Copper and protein depletion complicating hypoferremic anemia of infancy, *J. Pediatr.*, 24, 710, 1959.
22. Judisch, J. M., Naiman, J. L., Oski, F. A., The fallacy of the fat iron-deficient child, *Pediatrics*, 37, 987, 1966.
23. Chwang L., Soemantri, A, Pollitt, E., Iron supplementation and physical growth of rural Indonesian children, *Am. J. Clin. Nutr.*, 47, 496, 1988.
24. Gershoff, S. N., McGandy, R. B., Nondasuta, A., Tantiwongse, P., Nutrition studies in Thailand: effects of calories, nutrient supplements, and health interventions on growth of preschool Thai village children, *Am. J. Clin. Nutr.*, 48, 1214, 1988.
25. Migasena, P., Thurnham, D. I., Jintakanon, K, Pongpaew, P., Anemia in Thai children: the effect of iron supplement on haemoglobin and growth, *Southeast Asian J. Trop. Med. Public Health*, 3, 255, 1972.
26. Angeles, I. T., Schultink, W. J., Matulessi, P., Gross, R., Sastroamidjojo, S., Decreased rate of stunting among anemic Indonesian preschool children through iron supplementation, *Am. J. Clin. Nutr.*, 58, 339, 1993.
27. Dwyer, J. T., Nutrition and the adolescent, in *Textbook of Pediatric Nutrition*, Suskind, R. M. and Lewinter-Suskind, L., Eds., Raven Press, New York, 1993, 257.
28. Henderson, S. A., Dallman, P. R., Brooks, G. A., Glucose turnover and oxidation are increased in the iron-deficient rat, *Am. J. Physiol.*, 250, E414, 1986.
29. Willis, W. T., Brooks, G. A., Henderson, S. A., Dallman, P. R., Effects of iron deficiency and training on mitochondrial enzymes in skeletal muscle, *J. Appl. Physiol.*, 62, 2442, 1987.
30. Beard, J. L., Tobin, B.W., Norepinephrine turnover and energetic efficiency in iron deficiency anemia, *Proc. Soc. Exp. Biol. Med.*, 184, 337, 1987.
31. Zahn, C., Effect of iron deficiency anemia on the regulation of metabolic rate, hormonal responses to cold, and growth rates in rat, Masters thesis, The Pennsylvania State University, 1993.
32. Beard, J. L., Tobin, B. W., Smith, S. M., Altered sympathetic nervous system activity in iron-deficient rats: effects of environmental temperature, *Am. J. Physiol.*, 255, R90, 1988.
33. Hostettler-Allen, R., Tappy, L., Blum, J. W., Enhanced insulin-dependent glucose utilization in iron-deficient veal calves, *J. Nutr.* 123:1656, 1993.
34. Brooks, G. A., Henderson, S. A., Dallman, P. R., Increased glucose dependence in resting, iron-deficient rats, *Am. J. Physiol.*, 250, E414, 1987.
35. Borel, M. J., Beard, J. L., Farrell, P. A., Hepatic glucose production and insulin sensitivity and responsiveness in iron-deficient anemic rats, *Am. J. Physiol.*, 264, E380, 1993.
36. Danforth, E., Burger, A., The role of thyroid hormones in the control of energy expenditure in man, *Clin. Endo. Metab.*, 13, 581, 1984.
37. Chopra, L. J., Soloman, D. H., Chopra, U., Wu, S. Y., Nakamura, Y., Pathways of metabolism of thyroid hormones, *Rec. Prog. Horm. Res.*, 34, 521, 1977.

38. Sterling, K., Thyroid hormone action at the cellular level, in *The Thyroid.* Ingbar, S. H. and Braverman, L. E., Eds., J.B. Lippincott Company, Philadelphia, 1986, 221.
39. Galton, V. A., Thyroid hormone catecholamine interrelationships, *Endocrinology*, 77, 278, 1965.
40. Spaulding, S. W., Noth, R. H., Thyroid-catecholamine interactions, *Med. Clin. N. Am.*, 59, 1123, 1975.
41. Martinez-Torrez, C., Cubeddu, L., Effect of exposure to cold on normal and iron-deficient subjects, *Am. J. Physiol.*, 246, R380, 1984.
42. Lukaski, H. C., Hall, C. B., Nielsen, F. H., Thermogenesis and thermoregulatory function of iron-deficient women without anemia, *Aviat. Space Environ. Med.*, 61, 913, 1990.
43. Beard, J. L., Borel, M. J., Derr, J., Impaired thermoregulation and thyroid function in iron-deficiency anemia, *Am. J. Clin. Nutr.*, 52, 813, 1990.
44. Dillman, E., Gale, C., Green, W., Johnson, D. G., Mackler, B., Finch, C., Hypothermia in iron deficiency due to altered triiodothyronine metabolism, *Am. J. Physiol.*, 239, R377, 1980.
45. Beard, J., Finch, C. A., Green, W. L., Interactions of iron deficiency, anemia, and thyroid hormone levels in the response of rats to cold exposure, *Life Sci.*, 30, 691, 1982.
46. Smith, S. M., Lukaski, H. C., Estrous cycle and cold stress in iron-deficient rats, *J. Nutr. Biochem.*, 3, 23, 1992.
47. Beard, J. L., Tobin, B. W., Smith, S. M., Effects of iron repletion and correction of anemia on norepinephrine turnover and thyroid metabolism in iron deficiency, *Proc. Soc. Exp. Biol. Med.*, 193, 306, 1990.
48. Stanbury, J., Morris, M. L., Corrigan, H. J., Lassiter, W. E., Thyroxine deiodination by a microsomal preparation requiring Fe^{++}, oxygen, and cysteine or glutathione, *Endocrinology*, 67, 353, 1960.
49. Fuchs, O., Borova, J., Neuwirt, J., The regulation of the transferrin receptor in glutathione peroxidase mRNA's synthesis by changes in intracellular iron levels, *Biomed. Biochim. Acta*, 49, S47, 1990.
50. Jequier, E., Energy expenditure in obesity, *Clin. Endocrinol. Metab.*, 13, 563, 1985.
51. Pacey, P. J., Webster, J., Garrow, J. S., Exercise and obesity, *Sports Med.*, 3, 89, 1986.
52. Sims, E. A. H., Danforth, E., Expenditure and storage of energy in man, *J. Clin. Invest.*, 79, 1019, 1987.
53. Groeneveld, D., Smeets, H. G. W., Kabra, P. M., Dallman, P. R., Urinary catecholamines in iron-deficient rats at rest and following surgical stress, *Am. J. Clin. Nutr.*, 42, 263, 1985.
54. Sata, T., Imura, A., Murata, A., Igarashi, N., Thyroid hormone-catecholamine interrelationship during cold acclimation in rats: compensatory role of catecholamines for altered thyroid states, *Acta Endocrinol.*, 113, 536, 1986.
55. Weaver, C. M., Rajaram, S., Exercise and iron status, *J. Nutr.*, 122, 782, 1992.
56. Newhouse, I. J., Clement, D. B., Iron status in athletes. An update, *Sports Med.*, 5, 337, 1988.
57. Clement, D. B., Sawchuck, L. L., Iron status and sports performance, *Sports Med.*, 1, 65, 1984.
58. Pate, R. R., Sports anemia and its impact on athletic performance, in *Nutrition and Athletic Performance*, Haskell, W., Ed., Bull Publishing Company, Palo Alto, 1982, 202.
59. Sweringen, J. V., Iron deficiency in athletes: consequence or adaptation in strenuous activity, *J. Orth. Sp. Phys. Ther.*, 7, 192, 1986.
60. Wijn, J. F., De Jongste, J. L., Mosterd, W., Willebrand, D., Hemoglobin, packed cell volume, and iron binding capacity of selected athletes during training, *Nutr. Metab.*, 13, 129, 1971.
61. Dufaux, B., Hoederath, A., Streitberger, I., Hollman, W., Assman, G., Serum ferritin, transferrin, haptoglobin and iron in middle and long distance runners, elite rowers, and professional racing cyclists, *Int. J. Sports Med.*, 2, 43, 1981.
62. Radomski, M. W., Sabiston, B. H., Isoard, P., Development of sports anemia in physically fit men after daily sustained submaximal exercise, *Aviat. Space Environ. Med.*, 51, 41, 1980.
63. Dressendorfer, R. H., Wade, C. E., Amsterdam, E. A., Development of a pseudoanemia in marathon runners during a 20-day road race, *J. Am. Med. Assoc.*, 246, 1215, 1981.
64. Stewart, J. G., Ahlquist, D. A., McGill, D. B., Ilstrup, D. M., Schwartz, S., Owen, R. A., Gastrointestinal blood loss and anemia in runners, *Ann. Int. Med.*, 100, 843, 1984.

65. Siegel, A. J., Hennekens, C. H., Solomon, H. S., Van Boeckel, B. V., Exercise-related hematuria, findings in a group of marathon runners, *J. Am. Med. Assoc.*, 241, 391, 1979.
66. Brune, M., Magnusson, B., Persson, H., Hallberg, L., Iron losses in sweat, *Am. J. Clin. Nutr.*, 4, 438, 1986.
67. Strause, L., Hegenauer, J., Saltman, P., Effects of exercise on iron metabolism in rats, *Nutr. Res.*, 3, 79, 1983.
68. Prasad, M. K., Pratt, C. A., The effects of exercise and two levels of dietary iron on iron status, *Nutr. Res.*, 10, 1273, 1990.
69. Ruckman, K. S., Sherman, A. R., Effects of exercise on iron and copper metabolism in rats, *Nutr. Res.*, 3, 79, 1983.
70. Perkkio, M.V., Jansson, L. T., Brooks, G. A., Refino, C. J., Dallman, P. R., Work performance in iron deficiency of increasing severity, *J. Appl. Physiol.*, 58, 1477, 1985.
71. Perkkio, M. V., Jansson, L. T., Henderson, S., Refino, C., Brooks, G. A., Dallman, P. R., Work performance in the iron-deficient rat: improved endurance with exercise training, *Am. J. Physiol.*, 249, E306, 1985.
72. Willis, W.T., Dallman, P.R., Brooks, G. A., Physiological and biochemical correlates of increased work performance in trained iron-deficient rats, *J. Appl. Physiol.*, 65, 256, 1988.
73. Willis, W. T., Chengson, J. R., Dallman, P. R., Hepatic adaptations to iron deficiency and exercise training, *Am. J. Physiol.*, 73, 510, 1992.
74. Brozek, J., Body composition. Parts I and II., *N. Y. Acad. Sci.*, 110, 1, 1963.
75. Siri, W. E., The gross composition of the body, in *Advances in Biological and Medical Physics*, Vol. 4, Tobias, C. A., Lawrence, J. H., Eds., Academic Press, New York, 1956, 239.
76. Allen, T. H., Peng, M. T., Chen, K. P., Huang, T. F., Chang, H. C., Fang, H. S., Prediction of total adiposity from skinfolds and the curvilinear relationship between external and internal adiposity, *Metabolism*, 5, 346, 1956.
77. Garrow, J. S., New approaches to body composition, *Am. J. Clin. Nutr.*, 35, 1152, 1982.
78. Lukaski, H. C., Methods for the assessment of human body composition: traditional and new, *Am. J. Clin. Nutr.*, 46, 537, 1987.
79. Lohman, T. G., Exercise training and body composition in childhood, *Can. J. Sport Sci.*, 17, 284, 1992.
80. Lussier, L., Buskirk, E. R., Effects of an endurance training regimen on assessment of work capacity in prepubescent children, *Ann. NY Acad. Sci.*, 30, 734, 1977.
81. Parizkova, J., Interrelationships between body size, body composition and function, *Adv. Exp. Med. Biol.*, 49, 119, 1974.
82. Weltman, A., Janney, C., Clark, B. R., Strand, K., Berg, B., Tippilt, S., Wise, J., Cahill, B. R., Fatch, F. I., The effects of hydraulic resistance strength training in prepubescent males, *Med. Sci. Sports Exercise*, 18, 629, 1986.
83. Vrijens, J., Muscle strength development in the pre- and post-pubescent age, in *Medicine and Sport, Pediatric Work Physiology*, Vol. 11, Borms, J., Hebbelinck, M., Eds., Kerger, New York, 1978, 152.
84. Ramsey, J. A., Blimkie, C. J. R., Smith, K., Garner, S., MacDougall, J. D., Sale, D. G., Strength training effects in pre-pubescent boys, *Med. Sci. Sports Exercise*, 22, 605, 1990.
85. Figueroa-Colon, R., Clinical and laboratory assessment of the malnourished child, in *Texbook of Pediatric Nutrition*, Suskind, R. M. and Lewinter-Suskind, L., Eds., Raven Press, New York, 1993, 191.
86. Parizkova, J., Poupa, O., Some metabolic consequences of adaptation to physical work, *Br. J. Nutr.*, 17, 342, 1963.
87. Bjornthorp, P., Holm, G., Jacobson, B., Schiller-de Jounge, K., Lundberg, P. A., Physical training in human hyperplastic obesity. IV. Effects on the hormonal status, *Metabolism*, 26, 319, 1977.
88. Sidney, K. H., Shepard, R. J., Harrison, J. E., Endurance training and body composition in the elderly, *Am. J. Clin. Nutr.*, 30, 326, 1977.
89. Franklin, B. A., Buskirk, E., Hodgson, J., Gahagan H., Kollias, J., Effects of physical conditioning on cardiorespiratory function, body composition and serum lipids in relatively normal-weight and obese middle aged women, *Int. J. Obes.*, 3, 97, 1979.

90. Girandola, R. N., Body composition changes in women: effects of high and low exercise intensity, *Arch. Phys. Med.*, 57, 297, 1976.
91. Tremblay, A., Fontaine, E., Nadeau, A., Contribution of postexercise increment in glucose storage to variations in glucose induced thermogenesis in endurance athletes. *Can. J. Physiol. Pharmacol.*, 63, 1165, 1985.
92. Bielinski, R., Shutz, Y., Jequier, E., Energy recovery during the postexercise recovery in man, *Am. J. Clin Nutr.*, 42, 69, 1985.
93. Hill, J. O., Davis, J. R., Tagliaferro, A. R., Dietary obesity and exercise in young rats, *Physiol. Behav.*, 33, 321, 1984.
94. Irvine, C. H. G., Effect of exercise on thyroxine degradation in athletes and non-athletes, *J. Clin. Endocrinol. Metab.*, 28, 942, 1968.
95. Balsam, A., Leppo, L. E., Effect of physical training on the metabolism of thyroid hormones in man, *J. Appl. Physiol.*, 38, 212, 1975.
96. Terjung, R. L., Winder, W. W., Exercise and thyroid function, *Med. Sci. Sport Exercise*, 7, 20, 1975.
97. Segal, K. R., Pi-Sunyer, F. X., Exercise, resting metabolic rate, and thermogenesis, *Diab. Metab. Rev.*, 2, 19, 1986.
98. Balon, T. W., Zorzano, A., Goodman, M. N., Ruderman, N. B., Insulin-enhanced thermogenesis in skeletal muscle after exercise: regulatory factors, *Am. J. Physiol.* 251, E294, 1986.
99. LeBlanc, J., Diamond, P., Cote, J., Labrie, A., Hormonal factors in reduced postprandial heat production of exercise-trained subjects, *J. Appl. Physiol.*, 56, 772, 1984.
100. Gleeson, M., Brown, J. F., Waring, J. J., The effects of physical exercise on metabolic rate and dietary induced thermogenesis, *Br. J. Nutr.*, 47, 173, 1982.
101. McDonald, R. B., Wickler, S., Horwitz, B., Stern, J. S., Meal-induced thermogenesis following exercise in the rat, *Med. Sci. Sports Exercise*, 20, 44, 1988.
102. Segal, K. R., Gutin, B., Nyman, A. M., Pi-sunyer, F. X., Thermic effect of food at rest, during exercise, and after exercise in lean and obese men of similar body weight, *J. Clin. Invest.*, 76, 1107, 1985.
103. Jequier, E., Carbohydrates: energetics and performance, *Nutr. Rev.*, 44, 44, 1986.
104. Klieber, M., *The Fire of Life; An Introduction to Animal Energetics*, Robert Krieger, New York, 1975, 128.
105. Huesner, A. A., Biological simultude: statistical and functional relations in comparative physiology, *Am. J. Physiol.*, 15, R839, 1985.
106. Canon, B., Nedergaard, J., The biochemistry of an inefficient tissue: brown adipose tissue, *Essays in Biochem*, 20, 111, 1985.
107. Himms-Hagen, J., Thermogenesis in brown adipose tissue, an energy buffer, *New Engl. J. Med.*, 311, 1549, 1985.
108. Hirato, K., Nagasaka, T., Enhancement of calorigenic response to cold and to norepinephrine in physically trained rats, *Jpn. J. Physiol.*, 31, 657, 1981.
109. Hirata, K., Blood flow to brown adipose tissue and norepinephrine induced calorigenesis in physically trained rats, *Jpn. J. Physiol.*, 32, 279, 1982.
110. LeBlanc, J., Dussalt, J., Lupien, D., Richard, D., Effect of diet and exercise on norepinephrine induced thermogenesis in male and female rats, *J. Appl. Physiol.*, 52, 556, 1982.
111. Richard, D., Arnold, J. D., LeBlanc, J., Energy balance in exercise trained rats acclimated at two environmental temperatures, *J. Appl. Physiol.*, 60, R1054, 1986.
112. LeBlanc, J., Thermogenesis in relation to feeding and exercise training, *Int. J. Obes.*, 9, 75, 1985.
113. Tobin, B. W., Beard, J. L., Interactions of iron deficiency and exercise training in male Sprague-Dawley rats: ferrokinetics and hematology., *J. Nutr.*, 119, 1340, 1989.
114. Tobin, B. W., Beard, J. L., Interactions of iron deficiency and exercise training relative to tissue norepinephrine turnover, triiodothyronine production, and metabolic rate in rats, *J. Nutr.*, 120, 900, 1990.
115. Tobin, B. W., Beard, J. L., Kenney, W. L., Exercise training alters feed efficiency and body composition in iron-deficient rats, *Med. Sci. Sports Exercise*, 25, 52, 1993.

Chapter **4**

IRON DEFICIENCY AFFECTS EXERCISE AND EXERCISE AFFECTS IRON METABOLISM: IS THIS A CHICKEN AND EGG ARGUMENT?

John L. Beard
Brian W. Tobin

CONTENTS

0-8493-7916-4/95/$0.00+$.50

I. INTRODUCTION

There is abundant literature documenting the effect of iron deficiency on human populations. These effects of iron deficiency have been recently reviewed by ourselves[1-3] and others.[4] The functional consequences of iron deficiency are most significantly related to the severity of anemia, though numerous animal studies and some human studies demonstrate dramatic effects of tissue iron depletion and individual organ function. Relevant to this paper is the literature relating iron deficiency to decreased oxygen transport and poor muscle function,[5-7] poor temperature regulation,[3] heart hypertrophy,[7] increased catecholamine metabolism,[8-10] and decreased thyroid metabolism.[11-13] A additional issue concerns the importance of anemia vs. tissue iron deficiency causing alterations in glucose metabolism and insulin sensitivity.[5,14-16]

The prevalence of iron deficiency is reported to be higher in segments of the population that chronically exercise compared to segments that do not exercise (see references 17 and 18 for recent reviews). While the prevalence of iron deficiency can be as high as 80% in some studies,[19] others report 5% of women and 2% of athletic men are iron-deficient.[20] None of the published studies, however, are sufficiently powerful and have a sufficient design to allow an accurate estimate of the prevalence of iron-deficiency anemia in exercising populations. Nonetheless, there is evidence that the anemia being detected is in fact iron-deficiency anemia.[17,21] The strongest evidence is frequently generated from clinical trials in which an iron intervention is performed and a response is noted. This approach has been utilized to test the effectiveness of large doses of iron, greater than 300 mg/d,[22] as well as minimal effective dose of 39 mg/d.[23] To understand the documented negative effects of iron deficiency on exercise, it is best to first describe the biologic model of iron deficiency, how iron deficiency is detected, and then to consider how exercise might alter normal metabolism of iron.

II. BIOLOGIC MODEL

Iron deficiency can be defined as that moment in time when body stores of iron become depleted and a restricted supply of iron to various tissues becomes apparent (Figure 1).[2,5] This depletion of iron stores can occur rapidly or very slowly, and is dependent on the balance between iron intake and iron requirements. The former part of the balance equation is dependent on food composition and the quantity of iron in the diet. A number of inhibitors, and a smaller number of enhancers, of iron absorption are now known to exist.[4] While we used to consider these components of the diet as central to overall iron balance, it is now apparent that long-term administration of as much as 1000 mg of ascorbic acid per day for several years has no impact on iron status.[24] This forces us to consider that it is iron status itself that is the key determinant of the amount of iron absorbed in a meal. This strong inverse correlation between percentage absorption and iron status is the key regulatory step that prevents excess accumulation of iron with subsequent toxic effects.[4]

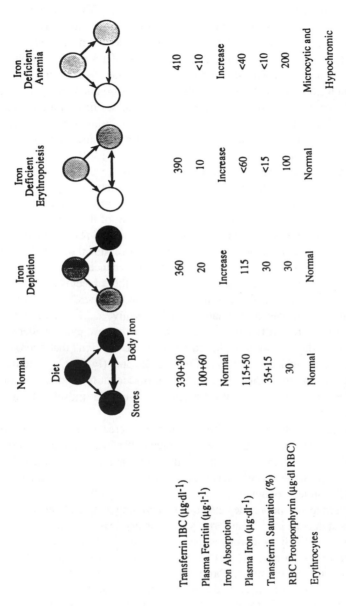

	Normal	Iron Depletion	Iron Deficient Erythropoiesis	Iron Deficient Anemia
Transferrin IBC (μg·dl^{-1})	330+30	360	390	410
Plasma Ferritin (μg·l^{-1})	100+60	20	10	<10
Iron Absorption	Normal	Increase	Increase	Increase
Plasma Iron (μg·dl^{-1})	115+50	115	<60	<40
Transferrin Saturation (%)	35+15	30	<15	<10
RBC Protoporphyrin (μg·dl RBC)	30	30	100	200
Erythrocytes	Normal	Normal	Normal	Microcytic and Hypochromic

FIGURE 1. Schematic diagram of the relationship of iron status measurements to changes in dietary iron intake and stores. The darkness of the circles and the thickness of the lines refer to the amount of iron.

The latter part of the iron balance equation is dependent on body requirements for growth, tissue requirements for maintenance of the essential body iron pool, and replacement of any iron losses from the body. Iron requirements for the adult male vary between 0.7 to 1.2 mg/d or about 14 μg/kg of body mass.[5] The requirements for the menstruating female are about double this, 20 to 40 μg/kg of body mass, with the larger requirement due to monthly blood losses. Iron losses from the body are not highly regulated and are in stark contrast to the regulation of absorption of iron. Iron losses in sweat are now known to be very small,[25] while losses in feces and urine are variable depending on gastrointestinal bleeding or intravascular hemolysis of red cells.[26] There is some literature that suggests that fecal losses of iron are increased after exercise and that urine iron losses are large, especially after a very stressful event, but carefully controlled studies in individuals at moderate levels of exercise fail to observe any effect.[27]

A long-term negative iron balance eventually leads to the depletion of the storage iron pool and plasma ferritin concentrations drop dramatically. The storage iron is bound to either ferritin or hemosiderin and can comprise a storage pool of 0 to greater than 1500 to 2000 mg in older adults. Depletion of the storage iron pool is generally without influence on functional outcomes, with a few exceptions. To date, the most realistic tool in a non-clinical setting for assessment of the size of the storage pool is the measurement of serum or plasma ferritin concentrations. Each μg/l of ferritin is thought to represent 1 mg of storage iron, if the subject is not also in an inflammatory state.[28] The plasma ferritin concentration can increase dramatically with both acute and chronic inflammations and thus give sizable false positive indications of iron stores sufficiency.[3,4] In addition, it is now evident there is a considerable day-to-day variation in plasma ferritin concentrations that approaches 25 to 40%, and is independent of the size of the storage pool (Figure 2).[30] Studies of iron status in exercising individuals frequently fail to account for concurrent infections or the effects of acute inflammatory states associated with muscle damage on this index of storage iron.

The measurement of serum transferrin receptor holds great promise for detection of the depletion of iron stores, as this receptor "fragment" concentration increases in the plasma with iron deficiency and is insensitive to inflammation.[31] No studies to date have utilized this indicator, which is very sensitive to erythropoiesis and may be of great benefit in athletic populations.

Once the storage iron pool is depleted due to a prolonged or acute negative iron balance, there is a decline in the transferrin saturation and less than adequate iron is available for essential body iron proteins. Individuals in this stage of iron depletion have a transferrin saturation below 15 to 16% and an inadequate supply of iron to bone marrow to support normal erythropoiesis. The amount of erythropoiesis is clearly an important aspect in this iron delivery scheme, as decreased erythropoiesis can lower iron transport requirements by 50 to 80%. Increased erythropoiesis can also lead to an increased iron requirement and would be an expected consequence of exercise training.[32]

The last "stage" of iron deficiency is when stores are depleted and there is no longer sufficient iron to meet daily requirements. This stage of iron-deficient

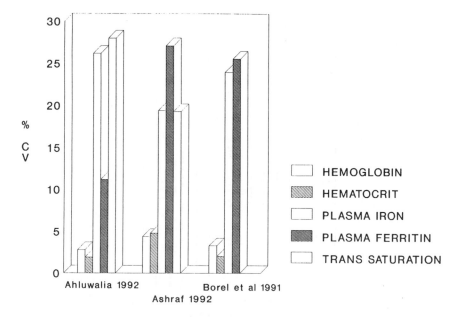

FIGURE 2.   Variation in iron status indicators expressed as coefficient of variation (%CV) in three studies. The study of Borel et al.[30] examined young men and women, that of Ahluwalia et al.[44] examined healthy elderly women, and Ashraf[48] examined elderly women with chronic diseases.

erythropoiesis leads to a significant compromise of cellular function in many organs.[5] The rate at which individual tissues and cellular organelles within those tissues develop a true "deficit" in iron is dependent on the rate of turnover of iron-containing proteins, the rate of cell growth, as well as the intracellular mechanisms for recycling iron. The manifestations of depletion of essential body iron have profound effects in skeletal muscle, with a significant decrease in mitochondrial iron-sulfur content, mitochondrial cytochrome content, and in total mitochondrial oxidative capacity.[5] The activity of tricarboxylic acid cycle enzymes and oxidative capacity of mitochondria in other organs is less strongly affected. Our ability to measure severity of iron deficiency in this stage has relied on the measurement of various hematologic variables such as hemoglobin concentration, red cell number, hematocrit, red cell protoporphyrin content, and others.[30] Since the red cell has a lifetime of approximately 120 d in man, and lesser times in other species, it is apparent that certain tissues and organelles may actually experience some functional lack of iron prior to measurable changes in hematologic parameters.

III. IRON DEFICIENCY AND EXERCISE

The early studies of effects of iron deficiency centered on whether the relationship of anemia to decreased work performance was linear or curvilinear with a "plateau".[33] This is exemplified by the data presented in Figure 3. The one data set

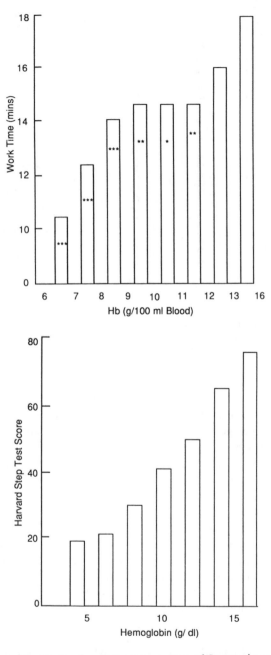

FIGURE 3. Harvard Step Test performance among a group of Guatemalan agricultural laborers. Impaired performance occurred even with mild anemia (left panel). Maximum treadmill work time in different Hb groups. Means (± SEM) were compared using an unpaired t test between the highest Hb group and each of the lower Hb groups ($p < 0.05^*$, $p < 0.01^{**}$, $p < 0.001^{***}$).

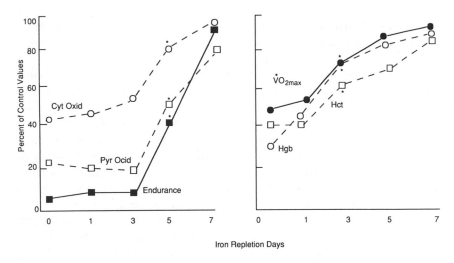

FIGURE 4.   Rates of recovery of work performance parameters in iron-deficient rats after initiation of an iron-sufficient diet. Cytochrome oxidase and pyruvate oxidase activity and endurance in a prolonged, sub-maximal exercise did not increase significantly until 5 d after the start of iron administration (left panel). In contrast, significant recovery of $\dot{V}O_2$ max and anemia occurred more rapidly, after 3 d of iron administration (right panel). The stars indicate the day on which values were significantly higher ($p < 0.01$) than before treatment.

is that of Viteri and Torun in Latin America[33] who used a Harvard Step Test to demonstrate, in a laboratory setting, that performance was linearly and positively correlated with Hb over the entire Hb range normally seen in man. In contrast, the data of Gardener et al.[34] clearly demonstrates that the duration, or time to exhaustion, of submaximal exercise has a curvilinear relationship to Hb. The apparent conflict between these two sets of data is most easily resolved when the animal experiments of Davies et al. are considered (Figure 4).[35] Extensive studies showed that repair of iron deficiency in rats correlated with an improvement in exercise performance in two different fashions. Peak aerobic performance ($\dot{V}O_2$ max) was strongly correlated with Hb or Hct, while the improvement in endurance performance was related to the improvement of myoglobin content in the muscle. The basis of this observation is the known decrease in muscle content of all heme and nonheme iron containing proteins during iron deficiency. Finch et al. argued that α-glycerol phosphate dehydrogenase was the single key-rate limited step in iron-deficient muscle, which when exercising at a substantial rate, led to an increase in lactic acid.[36] Additional studies demonstrate that lactate dehydrogenase is increased in activity in iron-deficient skeletal muscle, and that isozyme adaptations occur to maximize this capacity for anaerobic metabolism.[5] In contrast, other, more recent experiments suggest that a number of nonheme iron-sulfur proteins, especially aconitase, may be very susceptible to cellular variations of cellular iron content.[37] Dallman's laboratory demonstrated that this key enzyme in gluconeogenesis can be restored to full activity within 15 h of an iron injection in the rat model with a rapid return of lactate and glucose concentrations toward normal. It is perhaps ironic that the cytoplasmic version of aconitase plays a role in the genetic regulation of iron storage proteins, as does ferritin.[1,38] Aconitase is the reputed "iron-response-element-binding protein" that regulates the synthesis of several proteins through a highly specific binding to a stem motif in the 5' untranslated region (UTR) of the mRNA. The effects of exercise on aconitase concentrations are not directly known, nor are the interactive effects of iron status and exercise on the genomic regulation of this protein understood.

A number of human studies note that there is an elevation in lactate concentrations in iron-deficient subjects relative to controls.[39] A difficulty that is frequently overlooked, however, is the difference in absolute work load that an iron-deficient subject is performing at vs. the load that a control subject is using. This difference often amounts to more than a 30% differential. For example, Celsing et al.[39] noted that iron-deficient subjects had higher blood lactate concentrations than matched controls at a certain work load. As we noted in our report several years ago,[40] when iron-deficient subjects are allowed to work at an identical relative effort (percentage of $\dot{V}O_2$ max) as matched controls, they often have the identical lactate concentrations as the controls. These comments are not meant to diminish in any way the animal studies of several research groups, including our own, on changes in carbohydrate homeostasis with iron deficiency.[5,6,14,15,35] In fact, it is clear from these very elegant studies that glucose production and utilization rates are dramatically increased by iron deficiency. Several investigations from the laboratories of Peter Dallman and George Brooks have demonstrated that a systematic increase in hepatic gluconeogenesis occurs with iron deficiency.[16,41] We have also demonstrated that this increased glucose uptake is, in part, explained by an increased insulin concentration and an increased sensitivity[14,15] Similar studies have not yet been conducted in humans.

IV. INTERVENTION STUDIES

The possible causes of iron deficiency during athletic training are attributed to decreased absorption, increased excretion, increased hemolysis of red cells, and poor dietary quality.[17,18,25,26] Few of these studies, in and of themselves, seem convincing, based on methodologic problems of timing of blood samples, no control groups, no dietary assessment or control, poor methods for the determination of dependent variables, and other reasons.

A decreased haptoglobin has been suggested to indicate an increased intravascular hemolysis and an increased loss of iron.[26] This plasma protein is produced by the liver at a fairly constant rate and momentary declines in concentration due to a temporary increase in intravascular breakdown of red cells. This does not necessarily translate into increased whole body losses of iron. Increased hemolysis of red cells has also been reported in swimmers, suggesting that muscular contraction, apart from "foot-strike" hemolysis, is a component of iron metabolism in exercise.[42]

Others have suggested an increased loss of iron in sweat and feces with exercise training (see reference 17). The sweat losses, even in the extreme of heavy exercise during high heat, are insignificant if careful analyses of iron content are conducted.[25] It is likely that other, higher concentrations of iron in sweat are due to laboratory contamination of samples. Fecal blood loss may occur with the regional ischemia that can occur with very heavy exertion. These losses may be significant in individuals who are exercising heavily. One would expect, however, that if a continued fecal blood loss occurred and iron status dropped that compensatory iron absorption would occur. The failure of this compensatory system to maintain iron status over a long term has not been adequately explored in exercising individuals.

Convincing data now demonstrate that the moderate exercise-induced decline in iron status can be prevented by appropriate dietary or supplementary iron intakes.[17,21] A number of intervention trials have used large doses of oral iron to demonstrate that increased iron intake could alleviate the drop in serum-ferritin frequently associated with exercise (i.e., reference 43). Recently published studies show that even small amounts of exercise (aerobic dance for 5 d/week) caused a significant fall in serum-ferritin, and in some subjects a fall in hemoglobin.[17,21] This could be alleviated by the consumption of a small amount of meat or 50 mg of iron/d. A longer follow-up study, currently near completion, is investigating the possible causes of this drop in iron.[45]

We used a different approach to examine effects of exercise on iron metabolism, using careful weekly examinations of the iron status of competitive female college-age swimmers and blinded iron-supplement intervention.[23] We determined that 39 mg of iron, in the form of ferrous sulfate, was sufficient to prevent the decline in iron status associated with the competitive swimmer over the duration of a season. In Figure 4, it is apparent that in this cross-over design, in which each subject acts as her own control, the non-iron supplemented period was associated with a significant decline in plasma ferritin. There was in fact an increased prevalence of anemia in the unsupplemented group, suggesting that marginal iron status was the norm in these young women and persisted if vigorous intervention was not used.

Our laboratory has conducted several in-depth animal studies in an attempt to clarify these issues.[13,32] Initial studies demonstrated that exercise interacted with iron status to affect the kinetics of iron movement in the plasma and its disappearance from the plasma pool. Iron deficiency led to a dramatic increase in the fractional rate of removal of iron from the plasma pool with an additional effect of exercise (Figure 5). There was no effect of exercise in the control animals who were also training at 70% of maximal aerobic capacity for 5 d/week for 12 weeks. There is also a clear effect of iron status on red cell utilization (RCU) of iron (Figure 5). These observations have now been confirmed using an identical exercise protocol with additional data on red cell lifetime, estimated from noncompartmental modeling of the red cell mass over 14 d, fecal and urinary iron losses, and heme and nonheme iron absorption. These experiments show that the mean red cell lifetime, in control sedentary animals, is approximately 102 d, and is decreased to 95 d with exercise training. Iron deficiency leads to a further decrease in red cell lifetime to approximately 60 d with

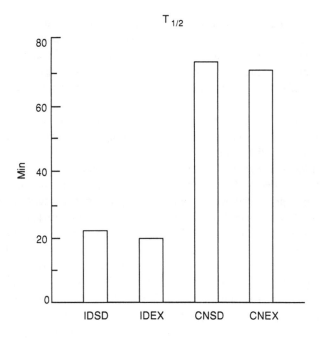

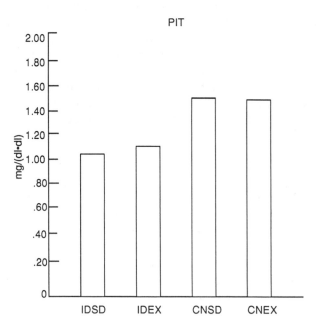

FIGURE 5. Plasma iron kinetic parameters of rats determined by ^{59}Fe bolus injection 48 h postexercise following 12 weeks of training.

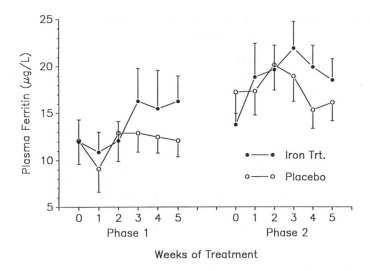

FIGURE 6.   Changes in plasma ferritin in female college swimmers over the course of the fall (Phase 1) and winter (Phase 2) components of their competitive season. Intervention consisted of 39 mg $FeSO_4$ per day. (From Brigham, D. E., Beard, J. L., Krimmel, R., and Kenney, W. L., *Nutrition,* 9, 418, 1993. With permission.)

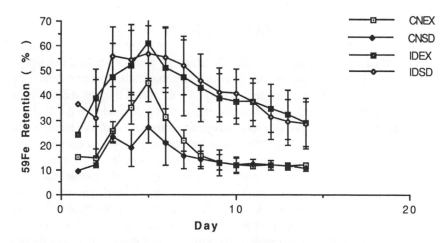

FIGURE 7.   Percent retention of radioactive iron over 14 d after oral doses between days 1 to 4. There was a significant effect of iron status on retention, but not exercise. CN refers to control diet, ID refers to iron-deficient diet, EX refers to exercise, SD refers to sedentary. There were 12 rats per group.

exercise training, leading to an additional shortening of life span to 45 d. The dietary treatment effect is highly significant, as is the effect of exercise in the iron-deficient animals (Figure 6). While iron deficiency has the profound effect of increasing iron absorption, there is little, separate impact of exercise on heme iron or nonheme iron

**TABLE 1. Effect of Exercise Training
on Iron Absorption**

	Heme Iron Absorption (% dose)	Non-Heme Iron (% dose)
ID EX	26.8 ± 3.4*	21.1 ± 2.9*
ID SD	26.7 ± 3.8	21.7 ± 3.1
CN EX	10.8 ± 1.2	3.0 ± 0.3
CN SD	10.7 ± 1.8	2.9 ± 0.2

Note: *Significant effect of diet, but not exercise, on percentage absorption. n = 12 to 15 rats/group. Training consisted of 12 weeks of treadmill running at 70% $\dot{V}O_2$ max for 90'/d, 5 d/week. Absorption was measured by isotope retention by rats over a 14-d period after dietary administration.

absorption, loss of iron in feces or urine, incorporation of iron into red cells, liver, or spleen, or concentration of haptoglobin in blood (Table 1). The argument of increased losses of iron associated with increased rates of turnover of red cell iron were not upheld when the fecal excretion data were examined. No effect of exercise was observed.

V. CONCLUSION

The initial question put forth in this manuscript revolved around the interaction of iron and exercise. We have reviewed the literature that shows that iron deficiency clearly decreases exercise performance. This probably occurs through a complexity of influences of anemia and tissue iron depletion on muscle oxidative metabolism, fuel availability, oxygen delivery, blood flow, and hormonal control of metabolism. Secondly, we have examined the information that seeks to show that exercise leads to a negative iron balance, and eventually to iron deficiency. While careful animal studies fail to replicate the human studies, they do suggest that exercise leads to a increased rate of red cell destruction in individuals already under iron-nutritional stress. These conclusions are similar to the careful studies from Purdue.[17,21] We conclude that it is likely that exercise affects iron status in a deleterious fashion, and that this poor iron status leads to profound metabolic and cognitive changes if dietary patterns are not adjusted to increase iron intake. Since these alterations are not observed in iron-adequate individuals, it behooves the athlete to avoid poor iron status since strenuous exercise likely decreases iron status over a prolonged period.

REFERENCES

1. Beard, J., Dawson, H., Iron, in Handbook on Minerals, Sunde, R. and O'Dell, B., Eds., in press, 1994.
2. Beard, J. L., Connor, J. R., and Jones, B. C., Iron in the brain, *Nutr. Rev.*, 51, 157, 1993.
3. Beard, J. L., Neuroendocrine alterations in iron deficiency anemia, in *Progress in Food and Nutrition Science*, 4, 45, 1990.
4. Baynes, R. D. and Bothwell, T. H., Iron deficiency, *Annu. Rev. Nutr.*, 10, 133, 1990.
5. Dallman, P. R., Biochemistry of iron deficiency, *Annu. Rev. Nutr.*, 6:13, 1986.
6. Davies, K. J. A., Maguire, J. J., Brooks, G. A., Dallman, P. R., and Packer, L., Muscle mitochondrial bioenergetics, oxygen supply, and work capacity during dietary iron deficiency and repletion, *Am. J. Physiol.*, 242, E418, 1982.
7. Smith, S. M., Smith, S. H., and Beard, J. L., Heart norepinephrine content in iron deficiency anemia, *J. Nutr. Biochem.*, 3, 167, 1992.
8. Beard, J. L., Tobin, B., and Smith, S. M., Norepinephrine turnover in iron deficiency at three environmental temperatures, *Am. J. Physiol.*, 255, R90, 1988. (Regulatory Integrative Comp. Physiol.)
9. Smith, S. and Beard, J., Norepinephrine turnover in iron deficiency: effect of two semi-purified diets, *Life Sci.*, 45, 341, 1989.
10. Beard, J. L., Tobin, B. W., and Smith, S. M., Effects of iron repletion and correction of anemia on norepinephrine turnover and thyroid metabolism in iron deficiency, *Proc. Soc. Exp. Biol. Med.*, 193, 306, 1990.
11. Beard, J., Tobin, B., and Green, W., Evidence for thyroid hormone deficiency in iron-deficient anemic rats, *J. Nutr.*, 119, 772, 1989.
12. Beard, J. L., Borel, M. J., and Derr, J., Impaired thermoregulation and thyroid function in iron deficiency anemia, *Am. J. Clin. Nutr.*, 52, 813, 1990.
13. Tobin, B. W. and Beard, J. L., Interactions of iron deficiency and exercise training on tissue norepinephrine turnover, triiodothyronine production and metabolic rate, *J. Nutr.*, 120, 900, 1990.
14. Farrell, P. A., Beard, J. L., and Druckenmiller, M., Increased insulin sensitivity in iron-deficient rats, *J. Nutr.*, 118, 1104, 1988.
15. Borel, M. J., Beard, J. L., and Farrell, P. A., Hepatic glucose production and insulin sensitivity and responsiveness in iron-deficient anemic rats, *Am. J. Physiol.*, 264, E380, 1993.
16. Linderman, J. K., Dallman, P. R., Rodriguez, R. E., and Brooks, G. A., Lactate is essential for maintenance of euglycemia in iron-deficient rats at rest and during exercise, *Am. J. Physiol.*, 264, E662, 1993.
17. Weaver, C. M. and Rajaram, S., Exercise and iron status, *J. Nutr.*, 122, 782, 1992.
18. Telford, R. D., Cunningham, R. B., Deakin, V., and Kerr, D. A., Iron status and diet in athletes, *Med. Sci. Sports Exerc*ise, 25, 796, 1993.
19. Clement, D. B. and Asmundson, R. C., Nutritional intake and hematological parameters in endurance runners, *Phys. Sportsmed.*, 10, 35, 1982.
20. DeWijn, J. F., DeJongste, J. L., Mosterd, W., and Willebrand, D., Hemoglobin, packed cell volume, serum iron and iron binding capacity of selected athletes during training, *J. Sports Med.*, 11, 42, 1971.
21. Lyle, R. M., Weaver, C. M., Sedlock, D. A., Rajaram, S., Martin, B., and Melby, C. L., Effect of oral iron therapy vs. increased consumption of muscle food on iron status in exercising women, *Am. J. Clin. Nutr.*, 56, 1049, 1992.
22. Newhouse, I. J. and Clement, D. B., Iron status in athletes. An update, *Sports Med.*, 5, 337, 1988.
23. Brigham, D. E., Beard, J. L., Krimmel, R., and Kenney, W.L., Changes in iron status during a competitive season in college female swimmers, *Nutrition*, 9, 418, 1993.
24. Cook, J. D., Dassenko, S. A., and Lynch, S. R., Assessment of the role of nonheme-iron availability in iron balance, *Am. J. Clin. Nutr.*, 54, 717, 1991.

25. Brune, M., Magnusson, B., Persson, H., and Hallberg, L., Iron losses in sweat, *Am. J. Clin. Nutr.*, 43, 438, 1986.
26. Eichner, E. R., Sports anemia, iron supplements and blood doping, *Med. Sci. Sports Exercise*, 24, 315, 1992.
27. Rajaram, S., Weaver, C. M., Lyle, R. M., Sedlock, D. A., Martin, B., Templin, T. J., Beard, J. L., and Percival, S. S., Changes in iron status of young women induced by moderate exercise, *Am. J. Clin. Nutr.*, in press, 1994.
28. International Nutritional Anemia Consultative Group, *Measurements of Iron Status*, Nutrition Foundation, Washington, D.C., 1985.
29. Lipschitz, D. A., Cook, J. D., and Finch, C. A. A clinical evaluation of serum ferritin as an index of iron stores, *Nutrition*, 8, 443, 1992.
30. Borel, M. J., Smith, S. M., Beard, J. L., and Derr, J., Day-to-day variation in iron status parameters in healthy men and women, *Am. J. Clin. Nutr.*, 54, 729, 1991.
31. Cook, J. D., Skikne, B. S., and Baynes, R. D., Serum transferrin receptor, *Annu. Rev. Med.*, 44, 63, 1993.
32. Tobin, B. and Beard, J. L., Interactions of iron deficiency and exercise training in male Sprague-Dawley rats: ferrokinetics and hematology, *J. Nutr.*, 119, 1340, 1989.
33. Viteri, F. L. and Torun, B., Anemia and physical work capacity, *Clin. Haemat.*, 3, 626, 1974.
34. Gardner, G. W., Edgerton, V. R., Senewiratne, B., Barnard, R. J., and Ohira, Y., Physical work capacity and metabolic stress in subjects with iron deficiency anemia, *Am. J. Clin. Nutr.*, 30, 910, 1977.
35. Davies, K. J. A., Donovan, C. M., Refino, C. J., Brooks, G. A., Packer, L., and Dallman, P. R., Distinguishing effects of anemia and muscle iron deficiency on exercise bioenergetics in the rat, *Am. J. Physiol.*, 246, E535, 1984.
36. Finch, C. A., Miller, L. R., Inamdar, A. R., Person, R., Seiler, K., and Mackler, B. Iron deficiency in the rat: physiologic and biochemical studies of muscle function, *J. Clin. Invest.*, 58, 447, 1976.
37. Willis, W. T., Gohil, K., Brooks, G. A., and Dallman, P. R., Iron deficiency: improved exercise performance within 15 hours of iron treatment in rats, *J. Nutr.*, 120, 909, 1990.
38. Aziz, N. and Munro, H. N., Iron regulates ferritin mRNA translation through a segment of its 5′ untranslated region, *Proc. Natl. Acad. Sci.*, 84, 8478, 1987.
39. Celsing, F., Blomstrand, E., Werner, B., Pihlstedt, P., and Ekblom, B., Effects of iron deficiency on endurance and muscle activity in man, *Med. Sci. Sports Exercise*, 18, 156, 1986.
40. Beard, J. L., Haas, J. D., Tufts, D., Spielvogel, H., Vargas, E., and Rodriguez, C., Iron deficiency anemia and steady-state work performance at high altitude, *J. Appl. Physiol.*, 64, 1878, 1988.
41. Johnson, J. A., Willis, W. T., Dallman, P. R., and Brooks, G. A., Muscle mitochondrial ultrastructure in exercise-trained iron-deficiency rats, *J. Appl. Physiol.*, 68, 113, 1990.
42. Selby, G. B. and Eichner, E. R., Endurance swimming, intravascular hemolysis, anemia, and iron depletion, *Am. J. Med.*, 81, 791, 1986.
43. Rowland, T. W. and Kelleher, J. F., Iron deficiency in athletes. Insights from high school swimmers, *Am. J. Dis. Child.*, 143, 197, 1989.
44. Ahluwalia, N., Lammi-Keefe, C. J., Haley, N. R., Beard, J. L., Day-to-day variation in iron status indexes in elderly women, *Am. J. Clin. Nutr.*, 57, 414, 1993.
45. Weaver, C., Personal communication, 1993.
46. Ashraf, M., Assessment of iron nutrition in elderly females with chronic health disorders, Doctoral Dissertation, Penn State University, 1992.

Chapter 5

THE EFFICACY OF IRON SUPPLEMENTATION IN IRON DEPLETED WOMEN

Ian J. Newhouse
Douglas B. Clement

CONTENTS

0-8493-7916-4/95/$0.00+$.50
© 1995 by CRC Press, Inc.

I. ABSTRACT

Two research projects in our laboratories have examined different aspects of the efficacy of iron supplementation in iron-depleted women. The questions addressed have been:

1. Will iron supplementation improve physical work capacity?
2. Will iron supplementation negatively affect other blood mineral levels?
3. What are the effects of discontinuing iron supplementation?

Results indicate that in iron-deplete, but not iron-deficient, women (serum-ferritin <20 µg/l, hemoglobin >120 g/l) iron supplementation (320 mg ferrous sulfate/d for 8 weeks) will improve serum ferritin values (12.4 ± 4.5 to 37.7 ± 19.7 µg/l) but will not significantly enhance work capacity. The second study investigated the response of hemoglobin and the serum levels of ferritin, iron, copper, zinc, calcium, and magnesium to 12 weeks of iron supplementation followed by 12 weeks of discontinuation. While the supplementation period raised mean serum-ferritin levels from 15.9 ± 22.5 to 36.5 ± 32.9 µg/l, there were no significant effects on any of the other minerals. There was, however, a slight decrease in serum zinc and magnesium levels, with these 2 indices dropping further during the discontinuation period to a point of significance. Serum-ferritin values remained significantly elevated (32.7 ± 23.5 and 32.4 ± 26.7 µg/l at 18 and 24 weeks, respectively) throughout the 12-week discontinuation period.

II. INTRODUCTION

Justification for the use of iron supplementation comes from the fact that iron deficiency is the most common form of nutritional deficiency in many populations. It is estimated that, worldwide, over 500 million individuals are suffering from iron-deficiency anemia. While the problem is most severe in developing countries, it is not uncommon in affluent countries, and even more so among female athletes.[1,2]

Serum ferritin measurements accurately reflect the size of the body iron stores,[3,4] with levels below 64 µg/l possibly indicating an iron-deficient state.[1] The median serum ferritin level in normal adult females is about 35 µg/l, equivalent to only 280 mg storage iron.[4,5] There is great individual variability in serum ferritin measurements, with values between 10 and 160 µg/l considered normal. Female endurance athletes tend to be more susceptible to the development of iron deficiency.[6] In a large sampling of U.S. adult females, controls had a mean ferritin level of 69.6 µg/l, while runners had a mean ferritin of 17.8 µg/l.[7] Duester et al.[8] confirmed these values as 35% of their sample of elite female marathoners had serum ferritins below 12.0 µg/l. Clement and Asmundson[9] found 82% of elite Canadian female distance runners had serum ferritin levels below 25 µg/l, while a more recent study of recreational Canadian female runners noted a 60% incidence of serum ferritin levels below 30µg/l.[10]

The causes of jeopardized iron balance in endurance athletes may be an inadequate dietary intake, malabsorption from the gut, or increased iron losses in the sweat, urine, or feces. Women are at increased risk due to menstrual blood loss. A thorough review of the iron status of athletes and the proposed etiologies can be found in the work of Newhouse and Clement.[1]

It has been estimated that 37% of the general adult population uses nutrient supplements, and of these, 58% use a multivitamin containing iron and/or other minerals.[11] Iron supplements are easily obtained without prescription in amounts equal to 5 to 6 times the recommended dietary allowance for most adults. Read et al.[12] observed that over 50% of individuals who use iron supplements consume 5 to 10 times the recommended dietary allowance (RDA). Highly competitive female distance runners may be especially prone to using iron supplementation as a study by Durstine et al.[13] noted half of these women regularly ingested a dietary iron supplement. Whether prescribed or not, iron supplementation is very common and is usually undertaken without a full investigation into the efficacy of this treatment. Research in our laboratories has examined three aspects of iron supplementation efficacy:

1. Does iron supplementation improve work capacity in iron deficient, but not anemic, female runners?
2. Will iron supplementation negatively affect other blood mineral levels?
3. What are the effects of discontinuing iron supplementation?

III. STUDY ONE:
THE EFFECTS OF IRON SUPPLEMENTATION ON PHYSICAL WORK CAPACITY IN WOMEN

The most apparent physiological consequences of iron deficiency are those that can be attributed to anemia. Approximately 70% of the body's iron exists in hemoglobin, and as such, is responsible for the transport of O_2 from the lungs to the tissues and CO_2 from the tissues to the lungs. An inability to transport O_2 would limit the oxidative capacity of the muscles; whereas an inability to clear CO_2 from the working muscle would reduce muscle pH and thereby limit metabolic processes. The negative health effects of iron deficiency can also be ascribed to a drop in other iron-containing compounds, such as enzymes in various sites.[14] Heme iron compounds in muscles include myoglobin, the cytochromes, catalase, and peroxidase. Cytochromes a, b, and c are located within the mitochondria and are responsible for the oxidative production of energy. Other cytochromes are present in the membranous structures of the endoplasmic reticulum, and these assist functions such as oxidative degradation of drugs and endogenous substances (cytochrome p-450 in the liver), or protein synthesis (cytochrome b5). Non-heme iron compounds include the iron-sulfer proteins of the electron transport system in the mitochondria.

Iron deficiency decreases work capacity through the combined effects it has on O_2/CO_2 transport and iron-dependent enzymatic reactions. Decrements in endurance performance are proportional to the degree of anemia,[15-17] with higher than normal hemoglobin further increasing performance.[18,19] Apart from the vulnerable position, in terms of impaired erythropoiesis, that a low serum-ferritin places an endurance athlete in, evidence to suggest that the prelatent/latent stage of iron deficiency affects performance has been equivocal.[10,20-23] Our first study on iron supplementation examined this topic.

The purpose of the first investigation into the efficacy of iron supplementation was to assess the physical work capacities of physically active females who were iron deplete, but not iron-deficient, anemic before and after 8 weeks of oral iron supplementation.

A. METHODOLOGY[a]

Forty volunteers between the ages of 18 and 40 were selected after screening 155 females for being iron deplete but not iron-deficient (i.e., serum ferritin below 20 µg/l and a hemoglobin level of 120 g/l or greater). The subjects were primarily recreational runners with a mean estimate of five workouts per week and 40 min per workout.

The hematological data collected on the subjects included: hemoglobin, serum ferritin, serum iron, and unsaturated iron binding capacity. The physiological tests consisted of the Wingate cycle ergometer test (30 sec of all-out cycling with mean power and peak power recorded),[24] the anaerobic speed test (a time-to-exhaustion run with the treadmill set at a 20% incline and 7 mi/h)[24] and a progressive workload treadmill test where $\dot{V}O_2$ max and ventilatory threshold were estimated from gas exchange variables.

Seventeen subjects consented to pre- and post-treatment muscle biopsies. The enzymes assayed were citrate synthase and cytoplasmic å-glycerophosphate dehydrogenase.[26]

The experimental treatment consisted of oral iron supplementation (320 mg ferrous sulfate = 100 mg elemental iron), taken as Slow-Fe® one tablet twice a day, as tolerated. The control group took a placebo in the same manner. A double-blind method of administration and random assignment to treatment groups was used. Treatment continued for 8 weeks, with retesting upon completion of treatment. Appropriate controls and exclusion criteria were in place.

The experimental design was a 2 × 2 (treatment × time) factorial design experiment, with repeated measures on the second factor. Two multivariate analyses of variance were used. An alpha level of 0.05 was chosen.

B. RESULTS AND DISCUSSION

The only significant difference between the iron-treated and the placebo-treated groups was the change in serum ferritin levels. Both groups started with mean serum ferritin levels around 12.3 µg/l. The control group's mean level rose to 17.2 µg/l, while the iron group's rose to 37.7 µg/l.

---

[a] For a thorough description of the methodologies, the reader is referred to the original studies.[10,25] Just brief summaries are presented here.

Although there was a trend that favored the iron-treated group on the work capacity tests, this was not statistically significant. The conclusion to be reached was that "eight weeks of iron supplementation (a daily dose of 100 mg elemental iron (320 mg $FeSO_4$ taken as Slow-Fe® twice a day as tolerated) to prelatent/latent iron-deficient, physically active females did not significantly enhance work capacity."

What implications does this study have regarding the efficacy of iron supplementation? Iron supplementation intervention programs are predicated on the assumption that nutritional iron deficiency does indeed lead to significant disability. What this study helps do is to draw the line on the continuum of iron deficiency where work capacity may start to be impaired. It would appear from this data that until hemoglobin levels start to drop, low iron stores do not significantly affect work capacity. Further research could institute a lower criterion for serum-ferritin (e.g., 10 or 12 µg/l) to draw this line with more precision.

IV. STUDY TWO:
THE EFFECTS OF IRON SUPPLEMENTATION AND DISCONTINUATION ON IRON STATUS AND THE BLOOD LEVELS OF OTHER MINERALS IN WOMEN

Based on the results of the previously described study, individuals may conclude that it would be prudent to take iron supplements "just to be on the safe side". While a low serum ferritin may not necessarily impair performance, iron supplementation may raise iron stores, and thus remove the individual's vulnerability to impaired erythropoiesis. This conclusion could be premature, for efficacy should address any negative side effects of the treatment. One potential side effect is the interference iron may have on other minerals. The interaction of minerals is a well-known characteristic.[27,28] An excess of almost any mineral can inhibit the absorption of another mineral. The biologic interactions of elements could be due to the physiochemical properties of their ions. Therefore cations with similar valences would be antagonist to each other biologically as they compete for protein-metal binding sites during absorption from the gastrointestinal tract.[27,28] Iron supplementation could thus, theoretically, further jeopardize low copper and zinc levels in female athletes. The ferroxidase activity of the major plasma copper protein, ceruloplasmin, adds another question regarding the efficacy of iron supplementation. An integral step in the absorption of iron is the oxidation of ferrous iron (Fe^{2+}) to the ferric state (Fe^{3+}) prior to its binding by plasma transferrin for transport. Ceruloplasmin is responsible for oxidizing ferrous iron, and a depletion of copper could thus impair iron absorption and lead to iron supplementation non-response. Iron supplementation non-response has been documented in previous studies on humans[10,23] although its mechanism remains unknown.

Few studies have addressed the possibility that iron stores may diminish shortly after the discontinuation of the supplementation program. A study by Hercberg et al.[29] examined the iron status of 54 women after 30 d of iron supplementation (105 mg/d of elemental iron) and 30 d of subsequent discontinuation. Mean ferritin levels significantly increased with supplementation, while subsequent discontinuation significantly decreased ferritin levels from 46.4 ± 30.3 to $40.6 \pm 23.4\,\mu g/l$ ($p < .05$). There are obvious implications in the efficacy of iron supplementation, if the pattern of fall in iron status can be predicted more accurately. A rapid return to baseline serum ferritin values would imply that the supplementation effort was somewhat futile.

The purpose of this study was thus:

1. To establish the prevalence of depleted iron stores, iron deficiency, and low serum copper, zinc, calcium, and magnesium levels in a healthy female population.
2. To examine the effects of iron supplementation and discontinuation on the hemoglobin levels and the serum levels of ferritin, copper, zinc, calcium, and magnesium.
3. To gain some insight into the reason behind iron supplementation nonresponse.

A. METHODOLOGY

One hundred and eleven healthy women between the ages of 18 to 40 were recruited to take part in this study. No fitness or regular training criteria was imposed, but the majority of the subjects trained regularly (three times per week at 75% of maximal effort for at least 120 min). The subjects reported for fasted morning blood sampling for hemoglobin and the serum values of ferritin, copper, zinc, calcium, and magnesium. Four subjects were iron-deficient as defined by a hemoglobin level below 120 g/l[30] while 43 subjects were iron-deplete as defined by a serum ferritin value below 20 µg/l.[10,31] Two subjects fit both criteria. Thus, 45 of the original 111 subjects were either iron-deplete or iron-deficient, and were prescribed a normal therapeutic iron dose (320 mg ferrous sulfate or 100 mg elemental iron per day, taken as two Slow-Fe® tablets/d for a period of 12 weeks). Serving as their own controls, the subjects then discontinued the iron supplementation for a further 12 weeks. The response of hemoglobin, and the serum levels of ferritin, iron, copper, zinc, calcium, and magnesium was monitored at 6-week intervals. Twenty-five subjects completed the full 24-week treatment and these formed the pool for statistical analysis.

Several variables that may have influenced the efficacy of iron supplementation were controlled. One control factor of note was oral contraceptive use. Estrogenic oral contraceptives can affect trace mineral status.[32] They produce elevated serum-copper levels due to increased plasma ceruloplasmin synthesis in the liver. Serum-iron levels have been noted to be higher in women ingesting oral contraceptives, and this has been speculated to be due to either decreased menstrual blood loss and/or increased iron absorption from the gut. Additionally, the use of oral contraceptives may decrease plasma zinc,[33] with an increase in erythrocyte zinc. For this reason, the taking of oral contraceptives (type and dosage) was monitored with a pooling of subjects for statistical comparisons. Forty-eight of the 111 screened subjects took oral contraceptives while 6 of the 25 completed subjects were oral contraceptive users.

A repeated measures analysis of variance design was employed with seven dependant variables (hemoglobin, and the serum values for ferritin, iron, copper, zinc, calcium, and magnesium) and five time periods. Follow-up multiple comparisons used the Duncan method. For comparing values between oral contraceptive users vs. non-users, an unpaired t-test was used while a paired t-test was used to compare pre- to post-nutritional intakes. Correlations were computed between the iron status measurements. Descriptive statistics are expressed as the mean ± the standard deviation. An alpha level of 0.05 was used for all statistical comparisons.

B. RESULTS AND DISCUSSION

The main conclusions to be made from this study were that:

1. For this sample population of women, iron depletion was quite common (39%), although low hemoglobin values (<120 g/l) were only seen in 3.6%. No subjects fell below the criteria for low serum copper levels (<13.3 µmol/l) nor low serum magnesium levels (<0.6 mmol/l). Seven subjects (6.5%) fell below the criteria for low serum zinc levels (<11.5 µmol/l) while 2 subjects (1.8%) were below the criteria for low serum calcium levels (<2.20 mmol/l).

2. Therapeutic oral iron supplementation (320 mg = 100 mg elemental iron, taken as Slow Fe® twice a day for 12 weeks) was successful in raising mean serum ferritin values from 15.9 µg/l to 36.5 µg/l, but was not associated with decrements in serum copper or calcium levels.

3. The treatment did not significantly affect serum zinc and magnesium levels during the supplementation period, but a downward trend continued through the discontinuation phase so that at 18 and 24 weeks serum zinc and magnesium levels were significantly lower than baseline.

4. Serum ferritin levels remained significantly elevated (32.4 µg/l) after 12 weeks of discontinued iron therapy.

5. Iron supplementation non-response was observed in three subjects and the mechanism cannot be attributed to a copper deficiency.

6. Oral contraceptive use was associated with elevated serum copper and ferritin values and lowered serum magnesium levels.

1. Mineral Response to Iron Supplementation

The main objective of this study, in terms of iron supplementation efficacy, was to determine if a therapeutic iron dose affected blood mineral levels. As serum ferritin is the most sensitive indicator of iron status,[3] it was not surprising to see a significant improvement in this index when iron-deficient or iron-deplete subjects were given a therapeutic iron dose for 12 weeks. It was also expected that non-anemic subjects would show little change in their hemoglobin values. Although it is known that correction of anemia will take precedence over repletion of iron stores, it appears that in some individuals the raising of hemoglobin levels to an individual set point still receives priority over raising serum ferritin values. Four non-anemic individuals who failed to raise their serum ferritin levels more than 10 µg/l responded to the treatment by bringing their hemoglobin levels up by more than 5 g/l. The literature has no definition for iron supplementation non-response. For the purposes of this study, non-response can be defined as a failure to raise serum ferritin levels by 10 µg/l or hemoglobin values by 5 g/l. Non-response of serum ferritin levels is a mystery. The large standard deviation of post-supplementation serum ferritin levels has been observed in other studies,[10,23] and was once again evidenced here. Not all subjects respond to iron treatment in a predictable fashion. It was speculated that some of the non-responders would be simultaneously low in serum copper. Without the ferroxidase activity of the copper-containing plasma protein, ceruloplasmin, iron cannot be absorbed into the body. Seven of the 25 subjects who completed the study failed to raise their serum ferritin levels by 10 µg/l, and 3 of these subjects were also unsuccessful in raising their hemoglobin values by 5 g/l. With no subjects being low in copper it would appear that reasons other than low serum copper levels account for iron supplementation non-response. Differences in absorption are likely the largest contributing factor to this variability.

In the present study, serum ferritin responded to iron supplementation with the mean values rising from 15.9 ± 5.3 µg/l at baseline to 36.5 ± 14.9 after 12 weeks. Values remained significantly higher than baseline throughout the discontinuation period (32.7 and 32.4 µg/l at 18 and 24 weeks, respectively). This would imply that 12 weeks of discontinued oral iron supplementation does not pose a threat to iron status in iron-repleted women.

Serum copper levels did not change significantly over the 24 weeks of this study. Animal studies have shown that in certain situations, copper absorption and retention can be significantly depressed in the face of iron supplementation.[34] Johnson and Murphy[34] fed copper-deficient rats or copper-adequate rats a moderate or high level of iron and a low or high level of ascorbic acid for 20 d. High iron intake decreased copper absorption only in copper-deficient rats. High ascorbic acid significantly decreased tissue copper levels in copper-adequate rats. The combination of high iron plus ascorbic acid caused severe anemia in the copper-deficient rats and decreased plasma ceruloplasmin by 44% in copper-adequate rats. If comparisons to animal studies can be made, the fact that the individuals in the present study were not copper-deficient, nor taking ascorbic acid supplements at the same time as the iron supplements, could account for the lack of change in serum copper levels. It can be concluded that iron supplementation of the dosage and duration administered in this study does not have a negative impact on serum copper levels.

While zinc levels dropped over the latter half of the supplementation period, the change was not significant. During the discontinuation period though, zinc levels continued to fall, with 5 of the 25 subjects having below normal values (<11.5 µmol/l) by week 24. It was hypothesized that due to competitive interactions between iron and zinc, zinc levels would fall during the supplementation period and then rebound during the discontinuation period. Adverse effects of high iron intakes on zinc absorption have been shown in experimental animals and in most studies on humans.[27,35,36] The present results are thus a puzzle. Two possible explanations can be suggested; (1) a drop in dietary zinc over the study duration, and (2) a drop in zinc absorption due to improved iron status. Dietary intake of zinc, according to 3 d analyses at baseline, and at 18 weeks, did not show any decline. The improved iron status, which was maintained throughout the study, may have had a continuing negative impact on zinc absorption. Yadrick et al.[37] have shown in adult women that higher pretreatment values for iron status (hemoglobin and hematocrit) resulted in less zinc absorption with zinc supplementation. It seems plausible that since serum ferritin remained significantly elevated in this study, a similar effect may be occurring. Absorption of iron and zinc may be through a common carrier ligand.[35] Increased iron nutriture will increase the saturation of this ligand and thus inhibit both iron and zinc absorption.

The downward trend during discontinuation that was seen with serum zinc was also apparent with serum magnesium. Magnesium levels remained at about .80 mmol/l over the first 12 weeks but dropped to .73 and .70 mmol/l at 18 and 24 weeks, respectively. Changes in dietary intake do not appear to account for this, as the change in dietary intake from baseline to 18 weeks (341 ± 85 mg/d to 314 ± 93 mg/d) was not significant ($.1 < p \le .375$). While mean dietary intakes did not change significantly, examination of individual scores suggests that diet may still have played a role in the observed drop. At 24 weeks, three subjects could be classified as borderline low (serum magnesium of .6 mmol/l or lower). For all three of these subjects, magnesium intake dropped from above RDA (280 mg/d) at baseline to below RDA at 18 weeks. Another possible mechanism for the drop in magnesium status follows the speculative reasoning noted above for decreased zinc absorption. The maintenance of iron status could also impair magnesium absorption, but it has not been reported previously that iron and magnesium are major mineral antagonists.[28]

V. CONCLUSIONS

As iron deficiency and iron supplementation regimens (whether prescribed or not) are extremely common, it is prudent to address all potential issues of their efficacy. One question of efficacy is whether work capacity can be improved by improving iron status. Previous studies have proven that even slight drops in hemoglobin levels will affect work capacity. Both studies have shown that iron-deplete (serum ferritin below 20 µg/l), but not iron-deficient anemic (hemoglobin above120 g/l) females can significantly raise their serum ferritin levels with an 8 to 12 week therapeutic iron dose. Study two revealed that these ferritin levels remain at an elevated state for at least 12 weeks. Study one indicated that the low iron stores alone of these females will not significantly impair work capacity. The justification of iron supplementing individuals in this state of iron-deficiency would thus be to alleviate the potential risk of any further drops in iron stores and the resultant iron-deficient erythropoiesis.

Another concern of iron supplementation regards the competitive inhibition of ingested minerals. Large doses of iron could theoretically impair other mineral levels. The main conclusion to be reached in study two is that supplementation, of the dosage and duration of this study, does not pose a threat to serum copper and calcium levels but the continued drop in serum zinc and magnesium values over 12 weeks of discontinuation deserves further investigation.

REFERENCES

1. Newhouse, I. J. and D. B. Clement, Iron status in athletes: an update, *Sports Med.*, 5, 337–352, 1988.
2. Van Swearingen, J., Iron deficiency in athletes: consequence or adaptation in strenuous activity, *J. Orthopaed. Sports Phys. Ther.*, 7:4, 192–195, 1986.
3. Jacobs, A., Serum ferritin and iron stores, *Fed. Proc.* 36:7, 2024–2027, 1977.
4. Jacobs, A., E. Miller, M. Warwood, M. R. Beamish and C. A. Wardrop, Ferritin in the serum of normal subjects and patients with iron deficiency and iron overload, *Brit. Med. J.*, 4: 206–208, 1972.
5. Cook, J. D., D. A. Lipschitz, E. M. Laughton and C. A. Finch, Serum ferritin as a measure of iron stores in normal subjects, *Am. J. Clin. Nutr.*, 27: 681–687, 1974.
6. Magazanik, A., Y. Weinstein, R. A. Dlin, M. Derin, S. Schwartzman and D. Allalouf, Iron deficiency caused by 7 weeks of intensive physical exercise, *Eur. J. Appl. Physiol.*, 57, 198–202, 1988.
7. Colt, E. and B. Heyman, Low ferritin levels in runners, *J. Sports Med.*, 24, 13–17, 1984.
8. Duester, P. A., S. B. Kyle, P. B. Moser, R. A. Vigersky, A. Singh and E. B. Schoomaker, "Nutritional survey of highly trained women runners, *Am. J. Clin. Nutr.*, 45, 954–962, 1986.
9. Clement, D. B. and R. C. Asmundson, Nutritional intake and hematological parameters in endurance runners, *Phys. Sports Med.*, 10:3, 37–43, 1982.
10. Newhouse, I. J., D. B. Clement, J. E. Taunton and D. C. McKenzie, The effects of prelatent and latent iron deficiency on physical work capacity, *Med. Sci. Sport Exercise*, 21:3, 236–268, 1989.
11. The Gallup Organization, *The Gallup Study of Vitamin Use in the United States,* Survey VI, Vol. 1, Princeton, N.J., The Gallup Organization, 1982.
12. Read M. H., D. Medeiros and M. A. Bock., Mineral supplementation practices of adults in seven western states, *Nutr. Res.*, 6, 375–383, 1986.
13. Durstine, J. L., R. R. Pate, P. B. Sparling, G. E. Wilson, M. D. Senn and W. P. Bartoli, Lipid, lipoprotein, and iron status of elite women distance runners, *Int. J. Sports Med.,* Suppl. 8, 119–123, 1987.
14. Dallman, P. R., E. Beutler and B. A. Finch, Effects of iron deficiency exclusive of anemia, *Bri. J. Haematol.*, 40, 179–184, 1978.
15. Anderson, H. T. and H. Barkve, Iron deficiency and muscular work performance, *Scand. J. Clin. Lab. Invest.*, 25, Suppl. 114, 1–62, 1970.
16. Gardner, G. W., V. R. Edgerton, B. Senewiratne, R. J. Barnard, and Y. Ohira, Physical work capacity and metabolic stress in subjects with iron deficiency anemia, *Am. J. Clin. Nutr.*, 30: 910–917, 1977.
17. Ohira, Y., V. R. Edgerton, G. W. Gardner, K. A. Gunawardena, and B. Sinewirante, Characteristics of blood gas in response to iron treatment and exercise in iron deficienct and anemic subjects, *J. Nutr. Sci. Vitaminol.*, 27, 87–96, 1981.
18. Edgerton, V. R., S. L. Bryant, C. A. Gillespie, and G. W. Gardner, Iron deficiency anemia and physical performance and activity of rats, *J. Nutr.*, 102, 382–400, 1972.
19. Ekblom, B., A. Goldburg and B. Gullbring, Response to exercise after blood loss and reinfusion, *J. Appl. Physiol.*, 33, 175–180, 1972.

20. Celsing, F., E. Blomsted, B. Werner, P. Pihlstedt and B. Ekblom, Effects of iron deficiency on endurance and muscle enzyme activity in man, *Med. Sci. Sport and Exercise*, 18: 2, 156–161, 1986.
21. Pate, R. B., M. Maguire and J. V. Wyk, Dietary iron supplementation in women athletes, *Phys. Sports Med.*, 7: 9, 81–88, 1979.
22. Rowland, T. W., M. B. Deisroth, G. M. Green and J. F. Kelleher, The effect of iron therapy on the exercise capacity of nonanemic iron deficient adolescent runners, *Am. J. Dis. Child.*, 142, 165–169, 1988.
23. Schoene, R. B., P. Escourrov, H. T. Robertson, K. L. Nilson, J. R. Parsons, and N. J. Smith, Iron repletion decreases maximal exercise lactate concentrations in female athletes with minimal iron deficiency, *J. Lab. Clin. Med.*, 102:2, 306–312, 1983.
24. Bouchard, C., A. W. Taylor, S. Dulac, Testing maximal anaerobic power and capacity, in *Physiological Testing of the Elite Athlete*, J. D. MacDougall, H. A. Wenger, H. J. Green, Eds., Canadian Assoc. Sport Sciences, Mutual Press, Canada, 1982, 61–74.
25. Newhouse, I. J., D. B. Clement and C. Lai, The effects of iron supplementation and discontinuation on serum copper, zinc, calcium and magnesium levels in women, *Med. Sci. Sport and Exercise*, 25:5, 562–571, 1993.
26. Newsholme, E. A. and C. Start, *Regulation in Metabolism*, John Wiley and Sons, London, 1973, 132–141.
27. Aggett, P. J., R. W. Crofton, C. Khin, S. Gvozdanovic and D. Gvozdanovic, The mutual inhibitory effects on their bioavailability of inorganic zinc and iron, in *Zinc Deficiency in Human Subjects*, Alan R. Liss, New York, 1983, 117–124.
28. Spallholz, J. E., Minerals in *Nutrition: Chemistry and Biology*, Prentice Hall, Englewood Cliffs, N. J. 1989, 91–132.
29. Hercberg, S., P. Galan, Y. Soustre, M. C. Dop, M. Devanlay and H. Dupin, Effects of iron supplementation on serum ferritin and other hematological indices of iron status in menstruating women, *Ann. Nutr. Metab.*, 29, 232–238, 1985.
30. Young, D. S., Implementation of SI units for clinical laboratory data, *Ann. Med.*, 106, 114–129, 1987.
31. Pakarinen, A., Ferritin in sports medicine, *NordiLab Newsl.*, 4, 20–28, 1980.
32. Tyrer, L. B., Nutrition and the pill, *J. Reprod. Med.*, 29:7, 547–550, 1984.
33. Haralambie G., Serum zinc in athletes in training, *Int. J. Sports Med.*, 2, 135–138, 1981.
34. Johnson, M. A. and C. L. Murphy, Adverse effects of high dietary iron and ascorbic acid on copper status in copper-deficient and copper-adequate rats, *Am. J. Clin. Nutr.*, 47, 96–101, 1988.
35. Solomons, N. W., O. Pineda, F. Viteri and H. H. Samdstead, Studies on the bioavailability of zinc in humans: mechanism of the intestinal interaction of nonheme iron and zinc, *J. Nutr.*, 113, 337–349, 1983.
36. Valberg, L. S., P. R. Flanagan and M. J. Chamberlain, Effects of iron, tin and copper on zinc absorption in humans, *Am. J. Clin. Nutr.*, 40, 536–541, 1984.
37. Yadrick, M. K., M. A. Kenney and E. A. Winterfeldt, Iron, copper and zinc status: response to supplementation with zinc or iron and iron in adult females, *Am. J. Clin. Nutr.*, 9, 145–150, 1989.

Chapter 6

NUTRIENT INTAKES AND IRON STATUS OF TURKISH FEMALE HANDBALL PLAYERS

Gülgün Ersoy

CONTENTS

0-8493-7916-4/95/$0.00+$.50

I. INTRODUCTION

Iron deficiency is probably the most common nutritional problem in Turkey.[1,2] The prevalence of clinical iron deficiency in athletes is not as high as in the general population, however, subclinical deficiencies have often been reported in athletes.[3,6]

It is known that physical training, inadequate nutrition, increased iron loss by sweating, menstruation, or urination affects the iron status. Iron status seems to be related mainly to the intensity of exercise, although the type of the exercise (especially running training) may also be of importance. [3,7-10]

Subclinical iron deficiency seems to be an important problem in female athletes. As in many other countries, handball is a popular sport in Turkey and running plays an essential role in handball training. However, little is known about changes in iron status of female athletes, especially in Turkey.

The purpose of this study is to examine the nutrient intakes and iron status of female handball players and to give some information on these subjects.

II. SUBJECTS AND METHODS

This study was conducted in Ankara, Turkey during the training season (between January–March 1992) on 10 elite female handball players, aged 19 to 25 years. The players were trained regularly for about 1.5 h per day, 6 times per week during the season.

The subjects were taught how to keep accurate records and then asked to record the kinds and amounts of food and beverages they would consume in three successive days (including one weekend day) on a standard form. The amounts of food and beverages were recorded by the subjects in terms of portions, plates, or numbers which were then converted into grams by the researcher. The energy and other nutrients provided by the daily dietary intake were calculated by using the food composition table.[11] The values were compared with the Recommended Dietary Allowances (RDA) for Turkey.[12]

Body mass index (BMI) was calculated as the quetelet index from the formula: weight (kg)/height (cm)^2 × 1000.

Hemoglobin (hb) and hematocrit (hct) levels were measured directly from whole blood in the Coulter Counter, model S-Plus VI, serum iron and serum total iron-binding capacity (TIBC) were measured using colorimetric method (Bathophen-anthroline, $FeCl_3 + MgCO_3$). Transferrin saturation was calculated by dividing serum iron concentration by serum TIBC. Serum ferritin was measured by radioimmunoassay method.

III. RESULTS

The characteristics of the players are summarized in Table 1.

TABLE 1   Characteristics of Female Handball Players

	Age (y)	Weight (kg)	Height (cm)	B.M.I Weight/Height^2 ×1000
Handball players (*n* = 10)				
Mean	22.1	62.3	170	21.6
Standard error	1.5	2.9	2.9	1.1
Range	19–25	52–79	160–185	19.6–23.0

TABLE 2   Serum Iron Parameters in Handball Players

Parameters	Handball Players (*n* = 10)		
	Normal Range	Mean*	Range
Hb (g/dl)	12–16	13.1 ± 1.0	11.5–14.3
Hct (%)	37–47	39.3 ± 1.6	35.7–42.7
Serum iron (µmol/ml)	6.6–25.9	20 ± 4.1	3–59
TIBC (µmol/ml)	44.7–71.6	63 ± 3.5	36–72
Transferrin saturation (%)	23–38	33 ± 5.3	4–93
Serum ferritin (ng/ml)	14–150	23 ± 4.5	9.9–79.8

* Mean ± standard error.

The iron status of the players is summarized in Table 2. Two players had iron-deficiency anemia with hemoglobin values of 11.5 and 11.6 g/dl, serum ferritin levels below 14 ng/ml (9.9 and 13.3 ng/ml) and serum iron level below 6.6 µmol/ml (3 and 3 µmol/ml). Two of the eight females had lower levels of serum ferritin (10.1 to 13.0 ng/ml) and transferrin saturation (4 and 14%). As it is seen in Table 2, most of these trained players had baseline iron values.

Table 3 shows the subjects' daily dietary intakes of energy and other nutrients, and the comparison with the RDA for Turkey proposed for this age and sex group. This table shows that the subjects generally consumed less than 100% of the RDA for most nutrients, with the exception of thiamin, vitamin A, and vitamin C.

IV. DISCUSSION

Iron deficiency seems to impair work capacity. [3,8,9,13] It is known to occur more frequently in women than in men performing physical activity. Endurance running is clearly a prognostic factor in iron deficiency.

Clinical iron deficiency is diagnosed by low blood hemoglobin concentration (<12 g/dl). In this study, two of the ten players, hemoglobin (11.5 and 11.6 g/dl), hematocrit (35.7 and 36.7%), serum iron (3 and 3 µmol/ml), and serum ferritin (9.9 and 13.3 ng/ml) levels were below normal range. According to these results, clinical evidence of anemia was found in two players. Hematological values of the other players were near the baseline.

TABLE 3   The Handball Players' Mean Daily Intakes
of Energy and Other Nutrients (*n* = 10)

Energy and Other Nutrients	Mean Daily Intakes*	% of RDA for Turkey
Energy (k.cal)**	1746	75.91
Protein (g)	51.1	85.16
% of energy from protein	11.7	—
Fat (g)	68.1	—
% of energy from fat	35.1	—
Carbohydrate (g)	229	—
% of energy from carbohydrate	52.5	—
Calcium (mg)	603	75.37
Iron (mg)	11.4	51.81
Vitamin A (IU)	6290	125.80
Thiamin (mg)	0.99	110.00
Riboflavin (mg)	0.88	73.33
Niacin (mg)	6.9	49.28
Ascorbic acid (mg)	105	140.00
Fiber (g)	4.1	—

*   The data shown do not include vitamin or mineral supplements.
** Based on 2300 kcal.

Subclinical iron deficiencies were preciously diagnosed by serum iron concentrations, TIBC, or transferrin saturation. The level of serum ferritin reflects the earliest stages of true iron deficiency or a decrease in body iron stores.[3,14,15] In this study, two of the eight players showed low serum ferritin level (10.1 to 13.0 ng/ml) and transferrin saturation (4 to 14%). Hemoglobin values of these subjects were 12.7 and 12.8 g/dl. According to these results, subclinical iron deficiencies were found in these two players. These results were similar to those reported by other authors.[16-18]

Season seems to affect iron balance, and thus needs testing and probably also supplements. The effects of training on iron balance has recently been studied in two Finnish studies.[3] These studies revealed that serum ferritin levels of athletes were below normal range, therefore supplements may be useful during extremely intense training periods. Diet may be a protective factor which counteracts proposed negative effects of exercise volume on iron balance.[19,20]

Adequate nutrition is a protective factor for subclinical iron deficiency,[3,21] therefore it is advisable for all female athletes to pay attention to dietary iron intake qualitatively or quantitatively. Different training at different stages of the training season seems to affect the iron balance.

Table 3 summarizes the mean energy intake of subjects, which was 1746 kcal/d. This level was lower than the mean value reported for women of the same age group in the Turkish population.[12] The subjects' mean intakes of two nutrients, iron and niacin, were less than 50% of the RDAs. Three nutrients, protein, calcium, and riboflavin were less than 75% of the RDAs. The overall mean intakes of vitamins A, C, and thiamin exceeded the RDAs. The average intakes of total fat were higher than the levels recommended.[22]

Daily dietary iron intakes were below all recommendations. The mean iron intake was 11.4 mg/d. However, vitamin C intake was significantly higher (105 mg/d). It is important to point to the positive effects of vitamin C in enhancing the dietary non-heme iron absorption.

In this study, specific nutritional inadequacies in relation to the RDAs are observed in athletes. The findings were consistent with studies of similar population samples.[23-25]

A strong effort should be made by all those involved in female handball sport, including coaches, parents, and health professionals, to emphasize the importance of consuming a nutrient-dense diet.

In conclusion, the findings in this report suggest that inadequate nutrition and regular training are associated with an increased risk of iron deficiency. Therefore all female athletes should monitor their diet and iron status regularly.

REFERENCES

1. Köksal O., Türkiye'de beslenme (Nutrition in Turkey), *Türk. 1974 Beslenme Sağlık ve Gıda Tüketimi Araştırması Raporu,* Aydın Matbaası, Ankara, 1977.
2. Tönük, B., Gültürk, H., Güneyli, U., Arikan, R., Kayim, H., Bozkurt, Ö., *1984 Gıda Tüketimi ve Beslenme Araştırması,* Tarım Orman ve Köy İşleri Bakanlığı/UNICEF, Ankara, 1987.
3. Fogelholm, M., The effect of training volume on serum ferritin in long-distance runners, *Nutr. Metab. Phys. Exercise, Proc. Int. Symp.,* Parizková, J., Ed., Charles University, Prague, p. 57, 1988.
4. Ersoy, G., Paker, S., Bayan koşucuların beslenme ve bazı hematolojik bulgularının değerlendirilmesi, *Spor Bilimleri Dergisi,* 2, 6, 1991.
5. Ersoy, G., Kız cimnastikçilerimizin beslenme ve bazı hematolojik bulgularının değerlendirilmesi, *Spor Hekimliği Dergisi,* 27, 101, 1992.
6. Turnagöl, H., Mercanlıgil, S.M., Kirazlı, Ş., Güreşçilerin hematolojik durumları, *Spor Hekimliği Dergisi,* 24, 49, 1989.
7. Selby, G.B., Eichner, E.R., Endurance swimming, intravascular hemolysis, anemia, and iron depletion, *Am. J. Med.,* 81, 791, 1986.
8. Eichner, E.R., The anemias of athletes, *Phys. Sports Med.,* 14, 122, 1986.
9. Colt, E., Heyman, B., Low ferritin levels in runners, *J. Sport Med. Phys. Fit.,* 24, 13, 1984.
10. International Olympic Committee, *Sport medicine manual,* Lausanne, Switzerland 73, 1990.
11. Baysal, A., Keçecioglu, S., Arslan, P., Yuçecan, S., Pekcan, G., Güneyli, U., Birer, S., Saglam, F., Yurttagül, M., Gehreli, R., Besinlerin bileşimleri, *Türkiye Diyetisyenler Derneği Yayını: l,* Ankara, 1991.
12. Baysal, A., Beslenme, *Hacettepe Üniversitesi Yayınları, A-13,* İleri Matbaası, Ankara, 1990.
13. Nutritional anaemia with special reference to iron deficiency, *WHO Tech. Rep. Ser.,* p. 580, Geneva, 1975.
14. Beutler, E., Sık Karşılaşılan Anemiler, *Gelişim JAMA,* 1, 542, 1988.
15. Walters, G.O., Miller, F.M., Worwood, M., Serum ferritin concentration and iron stores in normal subjects, *J. Clin. Pathol.,* 26, 770, 1973.
16. Manore, M.M., Besenfelder, P. D., Wells, C. L., Carroll, S. S., Hooker, S. P., Nutrient intakes and iron status in female long-distance runners during training, *J. Am. Diet. Assoc.,* 89, 257, 1989.
17. Mahlamaki, E., Mahlamaki, S., Iron deficiency in adolescent female dancers, *Br. J. Sports Med.,* 22, 55, 1988.
18. Matter, M., et al, The effects of iron and folate therapy on maximal exercise performance in female marathon runners with iron and folate deficiency, *Clin. Sci.,* 72, 415, 1987.

19. Lukaski, H.C., Hoverson, B. S., Milne, D. B., Bolonchok, W. W., Copper, zinc, and iron status of female swimmers, *Nutr. Res.*, 9, 493, 1989.
20. Powell, P.D., Tucker, A., Iron supplementation and running performance in female cross-country runners, *Int. J. Sports Med.*, 12, 462, 1991.
21. Lampe, J.W., Slavin, J.L., Apple, F.S., Iron status of active women and the effect of running a marathon on bowel function and gastrointestinal blood loss, *Int. J. Sports Med.*, 12, 173, 1991.
22. *Recommended Dietary Allowances (10th ed.)*, National Academy Press, Washington, D.C. 1989.
23. Hickson, J.F., Schrader, J., Trischler, L.C., Dietary intakes of female basketball and gymnastics athletes, *J. Am. Diet. Assoc.*, 86, 251, 1986.
24. Tilgner, S., Schiller, M.R., Dietary intakes of female college athletes: the need for nutrition education, *J. American Diet. Assoc.*, 89, 967, 1989.
25. Ersoy, G., Dietary status and anthropometric assesment of child gymnasts, *J. Sports Med. Phys. Fitness*, 31, 577, 1991.

Chapter 7

IRON STATUS IN ATHLETES INVOLVED IN ENDURANCE AND IN PREVALENTLY ANAEROBIC SPORTS

Federico Schena
Alberto Pattini
Sante Mantovanelli

CONTENTS

0-8493-7916-4/95/$0.00+$.50
© 1995 by CRC Press, Inc.

I. INTRODUCTION

Iron deficiency among endurance athletes has been reported by a large number of studies,[1-4] although the incidence of sideropenic anemia seems to be low.[5] Lower levels of serum ferritin, which have been recognized as a good index of bodily iron stores,[6-9] were reported in endurance athletes in comparison to sedentary subjects.[1,2,10] Reduced dietetic iron intake,[11] poor intestinal absorption,[10] gastro-intestinal bleeding during heavy efforts, and increased iron concentration in the stools after endurance races[12-14] have been reported as important causes of iron deficiency. Furthermore, iron losses may be increased by profuse sweating during prolonged training and racing.[14-16] Finally, muscle stress and mild intravascular hemolysis, resulting in hemoglobinuria and myoglobinuria after exercise, have been reported in athletes, particularly in runners. This fact was suggested as the primary source of iron store reduction in runners.[14,17-19]

Iron deficiency seems to be widespread among middle- and long-distance runners, whereas its incidence among subjects practicing different sport activities is still uncertain.[11,20-22] Clement and Sawchuck[11] reported low levels of serum ferritin but no deficiency in hemoglobin concentration in the 29% of the males and the 82% of the females in a group of elite Canadian runners. Ehn et al.,[10] Wishnitzer et al.,[23] measuring the iron marrow stores of elite marathon runners with normal hemoglobin, observed a complete depletion of hemosiderin in about 60% of the athletes and a decreased level in the remaining 40%.

Moreover, a reduction of iron stores has been found in three different groups of cross-country skiers,[9,24,25] while normal iron status has been reported for cyclists, rowers, and swimmers.[21,22] Adequate data regarding other sports are not available.

The purpose of this study was the evaluation of hematological parameters of the iron status in a large group of well-trained athletes. They were involved either in prevalently aerobic (running, cross-country skiing, roller skiing, cycling), or in prevalently anaerobic (ice hockey, alpine-skiing, soccer) sports. Data were compared with those of sedentary age-matched subjects.

II. METHODS

326 athletes and 85 sedentary subjects were studied. All were young, healthy males and many of the athletes were members of the respective Italian National Teams. Informed, written consent was obtained from each subject before starting the study.

Athletes were divided on the basis of sport practiced and, in those sport groups where young athletes were present, by age: junior (jr.) 16 to 18 years and senior (sr.) >18 years (considering the shorter training period generally undertaken by younger athletes). In order to allow comparisons, sedentary subjects were divided in the same way. Data concerning age, body weight, height, and training frequency (only for the athletes) of all the groups are given in Table 1.

TABLE 1 Physical and Training Data of Athletes and Controls (Means ± Standard Deviations)

GROUP	n	Age (years)	Weight (kg)	Height (cm)	Training (h/week)
Controls sr.	67	27.4 ± 5.1	75.4 ± 8.3	176.1 ± 7.7	—
Country sk. sr.	73	26.9 ± 4.4	67.5 ± 5.1	178.4 ± 4.8	11.5 ± 1.1
Roller skiers	33	25.6 ± 4.1	69.8 ± 3.9	177.2 ± 4.7	7.0 ± 1.3
Runners	35	26.8 ± 3.7	62.7 ± 4.1	174.8 ± 6.8	6.5 ± 0.8
Cyclists sr.	18	30.1 ± 5.1	68.6 ± 4.7	173.9 ± 7.4	19.5 ± 4.5
Ice hockey pl.	20	23.9 ± 4.4	73.1 ± 6.6	174.4 ± 5.4	7.2 ± 0.4
Soccer pl. sr.	16	25.5 ± 4.4	74.4 ± 5.7	175.2 ± 6.5	7.4 ± 1.2
Alpine skiers	17	22.8 ± 1.7	75.3 ± 6.4	177.7 ± 5.4	6.9 ± 2.1
Controls jr.	18	16.6 ± 2.3	67.6 ± 6.5	176.3 ± 6.9	—
Cyclists jr.	66	17.3 ± 1.9	70.9 ± 3.4	181.0 ± 6.4	15.2 ± 2.4
Country sk. jr.	28	17.1 ± 2.4	64.6 ± 5.1	174.7 ± 4.8	8.5 ± 0.9
Soccer pl. jr.	20	16.8 ± 2.1	65.2 ± 3.2	176.0 ± 14.2	3.5 ± 0.4

Note: sk. = skiers, pl. = players

All the athletes were examined during the training period, just before the start of their respective racing season. None of the subjects received iron supplementation or donated blood in the four months preceding the investigation.

The subjects were instructed to accurately report, on a food diary, their dietary intakes for seven consecutive days. The food diaries were subsequently analyzed by a dietitian and the average values of the nutritional intake, diet composition and iron intake were calculated by a computerized program.[26]

A venous blood sample was taken from each subject after a rest period of at least 48 hours for the athletes in order to avoid alterations in the level of serum ferritin and other hematologic parameters due to acute response to exercise.[27,28]

Blood samples were assayed for the determination of the following parameters: red blood cells (RBC), hematocrit (Hct), hemoglobin concentration (Hb), mean corpuscular volume (MCV), mean corpuscular concentration (MCH) and mean corpuscular hemoglobin concentration (MCHC) by an automatic Coulter S Plus 40 analyser; serum iron concentration (SI) by the guanidin-ferrozin method (FZ iron test Roche), total iron binding capacity (TIBC) by the same method, after complete saturation with ferric chloride and removal of the iron excess with magnesium carbonate, serum ferritin (FERR) by radio-immuno assay (SPAC Ferritin, BYK). The percentage of saturation of transferrin (%SAT) was calculated according to the formula %SAT = SI/TIBC*100.

A level of serum ferritin <20 µg/l, corresponding to trace amounts, or complete absence of, hemosiderin in the bone marrow was accepted as a marker for latent iron deficiency.[11,29] Overall statistical significance was evaluated by one-way analysis of variance (ANOVA). When statistically significant differences among groups were found, a post-hoc Bonferroni t-test was used to determine the significance between groups. The comparison between endurance and anaerobic athletes was performed by an unpaired Student t-test. A significance level of $p < 0.05$ was accepted.

III. RESULTS

Average data and overall statistic evaluation obtained from the athletes, grouped according to their respective sport disciplines, and from sedentary subjects are shown in Tables 2-4.

A. NUTRITIONAL INTAKE

All the athlete groups showed a statistically higher total energy intake than sedentary subjects. This difference was also present for the single nutrient components, but the proportion (calculated as the percentage of total energy) of each nutrient was similar in all the groups (Table 2). Iron intake differed significantly over all the groups (ANOVA $p = 0.04$), while no statistically significant difference was found in the direct comparison among the groups (all post-hoc comparisons $p > 0.05$).

B. HEMATOLOGICAL PARAMETERS

Hemoglobin concentration was the most suitable parameter in order to estimate differences between sedentary and sport-active subjects. Overall differences among athlete and control mean values were statistically significant (Table 3). Among the senior groups (Figure 1), Hb was significantly lower in runners, roller skiers, and soccer players, compared to age matched controls (-3.6%, -4.9%, and -5.4% respectively — $p < 0.01$). On the other hand, alpine skiers had significantly higher Hb (16.4 g/dl), whereas hockey players and cyclists were not significantly different from the controls. However, among younger athletes (Figure 1), cross- country skiers showed higher values than the other age matched groups (+3.25% vs. controls jr. — $p < 0.01$).

The influence of age on Hb may be appreciated in Figure 2. Younger controls had a significant reduction in Hb levels compared to older ones, while among athletes there were no significant differences.

The values of hemoglobin indexes MCH and MCHC (Table 3) followed the Hb level, but MCHC seemed to be less sensitive than MCH in showing different cell hemoglobinization. Moreover, the values of RBC and Hct were within the normal range according to the respective Hb levels.

C. IRON STATUS PARAMETERS

Iron status evaluation was performed through measurement of SI, TIBC, FERR, and calculation of %SAT. According to the recent literature[6,12,30,31] we considered serum ferritin as the principal parameter for estimation of the iron status in our subjects.

Figure 3 reports the difference in FERR level among controls and athletes. Cross-country skiers and runners showed a significantly lower level in FERR compared to controls (-46.8% and -61.5%, respectively, $p < 0.01$) and other athletic groups. The lowest average value was found in cross-country skiers jr. (21.6 µg/l) where it was less than 50% of the value of age-matched sedentary subjects. However,

TABLE 2   Nutitional Data from Four Day Recording (Mean ± Standard Deviation)

GROUP	n	Total intake (KCal/d)	Carbohydrate (g/d)	%	Protein (g/d)	%	Fat (g/d)	%	Iron (mg/d)
Controls sr.	67	2970 ± 251	396 ± 41	51	90 ± 15	21	98 ± 9	28	15.8 ± 3.9
Country sk. sr.	73	3450 ± 452	499 ± 38	58	93 ± 20	19	89 ± 9	23	19.1 ± 4.2
Roller skiers	33	3322 ± 294	488 ± 51	58	84 ± 18	18	88 ± 8	24	18.2 ± 4.5
Runners	35	3350 ± 223	502 ± 36	60	90 ± 12	18	85 ± 6	22	16.4 ± 3.0
Cyclists sr.	18	3880 ± 450	562 ± 48	59	94 ± 14	17	98 ± 12	24	17.1 ± 3.4
Ice hockey pl.	20	3400 ± 268	456 ± 38	53	112 ± 15	23	96 ± 11	24	19.5 ± 4.2
Soccer pl. sr.	16	3207 ± 354	454 ± 32	57	86 ± 16	19	90 ± 14	24	15.6 ± 2.7
Alpine skiers	17	3524 ± 352	475 ± 31	54	105 ± 10	21	99 ± 13	25	18.0 ± 1.4
Controls jr.	18	2851 ± 301	378 ± 40	53	93 ± 12	23	83 ± 10	24	15.2 ± 2.1
Country sk. jr.	28	3370 ± 249	495 ± 38	58	100 ± 15	20	82 ± 12	22	15.7 ± 3.4
Cyclists jr.	66	3452 ± 352	489 ± 50	57	106 ± 11	22	85 ± 7	21	16.6 ± 2.0
Soccer pl. jr.	20	3221 ± 328	437 ± 29	54	108 ± 18	24	78 ± 14	22	15.4 ± 1.6
ANOVA		**	**	ns	**	ns	*	ns	*

Note: Sk. = skiers, Pl. = players, % = relative percentage of total energy intake.
ANOVA = one-way analysis of variance: * = $p < 0.05$, ** = $p < 0.01$, ns = $p > 0.05$.

TABLE 3   Hematologic Parameters (Mean ± Standard Deviation)

Group	n	RBC (10^9/l)	Hb(g/l)	Hct (%)	MCV(fl)	MCH (pg)	MCHC
Controls sr.	67	4.96 ± 0.03	156 ± 9	45.0 ± 1.3	90.7 ± 1.2	31.4 ± 0.8	34.6 ± 0.8
Country sk. sr.	73	5.41 ± 0.04	154 ± 12	44.7 ± 0.5	92.0 ± 0.6	30.5 ± 0.3	33.2 ± 0.5
Roller skiers	33	4.88 ± 0.06	148 ± 14	44.4 ± 0.4	91.0 ± 1.5	30.4 ± 0.7	33.4 ± 0.6
Runners	35	4.95 ± 0.06	151 ± 17	45.1 ± 0.5	91.0 ± 1.8	30.4 ± 0.7	33.6 ± 0.9
Cyclists sr.	18	5.01 ± 0.04	152 ± 15	45.1 ± 0.2	90.1 ± 1.8	30.4 ± 0.5	33.7 ± 0.7
Ice hockey players	20	4.91 ± 0.05	153 ± 17	44.6 ± 0.4	90.9 ± 1.9	31.1 ± 0.9	34.3 ± 0.7
Soccer pl. sr.	16	5.00 ± 0.02	148 ± 26	45.4 ± 0.7	87.4 ± 1.5	29.6 ± 0.7	32.6 ± 0.7
Alpine skiers	17	5.41 ± 0.07	164 ± 14	48.9 ± 0.6	90.4 ± 1.8	30.3 ± 0.9	33.5 ± 0.8
Controls jr.	18	4.90 ± 0.07	150 ± 33	43.3 ± 0.9	88.4 ± 1.6	30.8 ± 0.5	34.7 ± 0.9
Country sk. jr.	28	4.98 ± 0.05	155 ± 14	46.3 ± 0.4	89.9 ± 1.2	30.1 ± 0.7	33.6 ± 0.5
Cyclists jr.	66	4.98 ± 0.03	149 ± 25	44.7 ± 0.3	89.8 ± 1.2	29.9 ± 0.5	33.4 ± 0.8
Soccer pl. jr.	20	5.19 ± 0.02	151 ± 23	44.5 ± 0.7	85.9 ± 1.5	29.1 ± 0.7	33.8 ± 0.7
ANOVA		*	*	**	*	ns	ns

Note: RBC = red blood cells, Hb = hemoglobin concentration, Hct = hematocrit, MCV = mean cellular volume, MCH = mean corpuscular hemoglobin, MCHC = mean corpuscular hemoglobin concentration, sk. = skiers, pl. = players.
ANOVA = one-way analysis of variance: * = p <0.05, ** = p <0.01, ns = p >0.05.

TABLE 4 Iron Status Parameters (Means ± Standard Deviations).

Group	n	SI (mg/l)	TIBC (mg(l)	%SAT (%)	FERR (μg/l)
Controls sr.	67	100.6 ± 2.6	277.1 ± 1.9	36.1 ± 0.9	74.2 ± 4.6
Country sk. sr.	73	91.5 ± 3.1	304.4 ± 4.3	29.9 ± 0.5	39.5 ± 2.7
Roller skiers	33	108.7 ± 5.5	315.2 ± 11.0	34.4 ± 0.5	78.8 ± 8.5
Runners	35	92.5 ± 5.5	339.4 ± 4.8	27.2 ± 0.6	28.6 ± 3.7
Cyclists sr.	18	88.7 ± 8.1	289.1 ± 10.1	30.1 ± 0.6	86.4 ± 14.9
Ice hockey players	20	85.9 ± 4.9	297.1 ± 6.3	28.9 ± 0.5	65.8 ± 10.6
Soccer pl. sr.	16	107.8 ± 7.14	291.1 ± 19.3	32.5 ± 0.6	80.6 ± 5.3
Alpine skiers	17	93.4 ± 7.7	329.2 ± 12.6	28.4 ± 0.5	82.4 ± 12.2
Controls jr.	18	87.3 ± 10.5	299.5 ± 4.81	29.5 ± 0.5	46.1 ± 71
Country sk. jr.	28	94.3 ± 6.3	324.3 ± 9.4	29.1 ± 0.2	21.6 ± 3.3
Cyclists jr.	66	91.8 ± 3.2	314.9 ± 4.9	29.1 ± 0.5	47.1 ± 3.7
Soccer pl. jr.	20	98.4 ± 7.1	322.7 ± 19.3	30.5 ± 0.6	33.0 ± 5.2
ANOVA		ns	*	*	**

Note: SI = serum iron concentration, TIBC = total iron binding capacity, %SAT = percentage of TIBC saturation, FERR = serum ferritin, sk. = skiers, pl. = players.
ANOVA = one-way analysis of variance: * = $p < 0.05$, ** = $p < 0.01$, ns = $p > 0.05$.

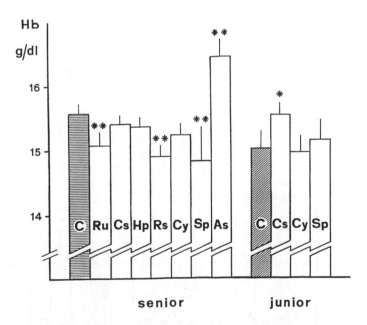

FIGURE 1. Average values of hemoglobin concentration (Hb) in athlete and control groups. Senior = age >18 years, junior = age 16 to 18 years. C = controls, CS = cross-country skiers, RU = runners, RS = roller skiers, HP = ice-hockey players, CY = cyclists, AS = alpine skiers, and SP = soccer players. Statistical significance between control and athlete groups: * = $p < 0.05$ ** = $p < 0.01$.

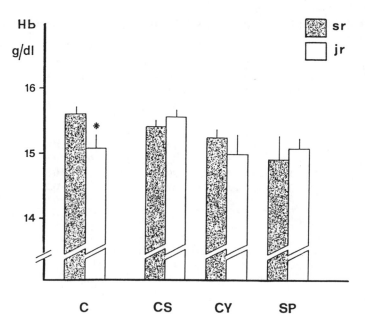

FIGURE 2. Influence of age on hemoglobin concentration (Hb) of athletes and controls. sr. = senior jr. = junior. Statistical significance between senior and junior groups: * = $p < 0.05$ ** = $p < 0.01$. For the abbreviations, see Figure 1.

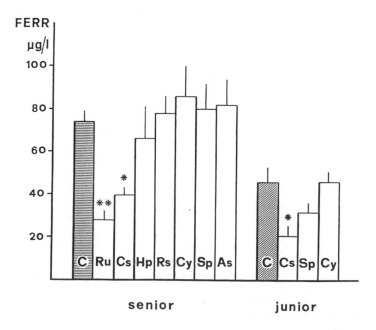

FIGURE 3. Average values of serum ferritin (FERR) in athlete and control groups. For the abbreviations see Figure 1.

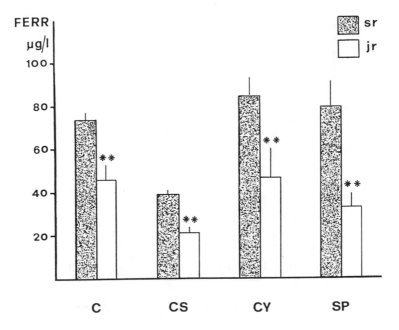

FIGURE 4. Influence of age on serum ferritin concentration (FERR) of athletes and controls. For the abbreviations see Figure 1.

roller skiers, cyclists sr., and soccer players sr. had FERR values slightly higher than controls.

The comparison of FERR levels between athletes of the same sport discipline, but different ages is shown in Figure 4. We found significantly lower FERR levels in junior compared to senior groups in sport active as well as in sedentary subjects. Despite these large variations in FERR, serum iron values were not significantly different among groups (Table 4) and correlated poorly with iron stores. On the contrary, TIBC constantly showed increased levels in subjects with reduced FERR value, with only the exception of alpine skiers (Table 4). Therefore, percentage of saturation is an inefficient index for the estimation of iron deficiency among groups.

D. IRON DEFICIENCY AND ANEMIA

After choosing a level of FERR <20 µg/l as a screening criterion for iron store reduction, we estimated the percent incidence of latent iron deficiency within each group (Figure 5). Decreased iron stores were globally found in 77 of the 411 subjects tested, 8 of 85 controls (9.4%), and 69 of 326 athletes (21.1%). According to their low average FERR, junior groups showed a higher percentage of iron deficiency. The maximum percentage was found in cross-country skiers jr. (67% vs. 19.2% of corresponding sr. group); a high incidence was also found in runners and in soccer players jr. (37.1% and 35% respectively), whereas none of the alpine skiers had FERR <20 µg/l. Endurance athletes seemed to be more prone to iron store reduction (57 on 253 = 22.5%), whereas athletes involved in prevalently anaerobic sports were

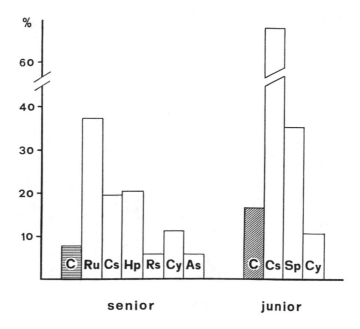

FIGURE 5. Percentage of latent iron deficiency (FERR <20 µg/l) in athlete and control groups. For the abbreviations see Figure 1.

less affected (12 on 73 = 16.4%). This difference was also reflected by the average FERR that is significantly lower in the former group (50.5 ± 3.4 vs. 72.8 ± 4.1 µg/l — p <0.001). Slight hemoglobin reduction (Hb <14 g/dl) was observed in 18 athletes (5.5%), without a close correlation to the iron status. However, in four athletes with Hb values below normal range (Hb <13 g/dl), the iron status indicated a complete depletion of iron stores: FERR <10 µg/l, %SAT <15%.

IV. DISCUSSION

This study was aimed at investigating the influence of different sport activities on iron status and the role of specific training modalities (endurance vs. anaerobic sports) on the development of iron deficiency.

The amount of nutritional intakes differentiated all the athletes from the sedentary subjects, while no specific deficiencies were detected in any group with regard to the percentage of nutrients. Relative higher energy intake was reported in high-trained runners and cross-country skiers,[12,32] derived from the considerably larger amount of fat in a typical western diet. On the contrary, our athletes assumed higher doses of carbohydrates and they reduced fat intake to less than 25% of the total energy intake. This was probably influenced by the typical "mediterranean" diet that is very popular among Italian athletes.

Total iron intake was similar in all the groups and closely related to the amount of protein ingestion. It was in the range of the amount recommended for training people, but slightly lower than that reported by others.[32]

The results obtained in our study confirm that the Hb concentration in male adult athletes (with the exception of alpine skiers) is slightly lower than in sedentary subjects, as previously reported by several investigators.[1,2,20,28,33] Reduction in Hb and Hct values, at least in endurance sports, has been attributed to plasma volume expansion resulting from training, rather than to a real decrease in the total body content of hemoglobin.[33-35] However, it has been recently proposed that increased levels of 2,3 DPG, resulting from endurance training, could determine a real reduction in the erythropoietic activity.[36]

The significantly higher Hb levels found in alpine skiers must be ascribed to recurring altitude exposures. It must be recognized that both alpine and cross-country skiers are frequently submitted to altitude stress; however their Hb levels are different. This discrepancy suggests that run training generally used by cross-country skiers could produce higher rate of RBC catabolism and decrease HB blood levels.[37] On the contrary, in alpine skiers, who generally are trained by specific anaerobic exercises, altitude, rather than training, may influence the Hb concentration. Nevertheless, altitude stimulation on Hb production is also effective, even if to a lower extent, in cross-country skiers, since among endurance athletes, cross-country skiers show the highest Hb levels which can result from an erythropoietic altitude stimulation.

Average FERR values indicate reduced iron stores in athletes involved in some endurance sports such as running and cross-country skiing. On the contrary, cyclists and roller skiers have FERR values similar to those of non-endurance athletes such as alpine skiers, soccer, and ice hockey players.

Our data on runners and cross-country skiers are in agreement with other studies,[1,2,20,24,25] whereas the results on cyclists show some difference.

Haymes et al.[24] measured the iron status of the U.S.A. cross-country ski team year round. The FERR values recorded at the beginning of the training period was higher than those reported in the present paper (56.1μg/l vs. 39.5 μg/l), but the values recorded at the end of the "dry-land training" are quite similar to ours.

Dufaux et al.[21] reported high levels of FERR in professional cyclists who participated in the Tour de France. Our data, taken from a large population of cyclists, confirm the high FERR and the low incidence of iron deficiency in these athletes. However their FERR values were almost twice as large as our values, but they could not avoid simultaneous or preceding iron supplementation by the athletes. This impairs a quantitative comparison between our data and theirs.

It is rather surprising that roller skiers have normal FERR values. In fact, roller skiing is an endurance sport and its bio-mechanics is quite similar to cross-country skiing. We think that the evident disparity in FERR between roller and cross-country skiers should be due to lack of running as a training method in the former group. Indeed, cross-country skiing is performed by the athletes of both the groups in winter, for training and for racing, however only cross-country skiers are involved in running for training in summer.[37]

It is well demostrated in runners that increased amounts of iron-containing substances are lost in the urine, and this becomes a primary source of iron store depletion. Myoglobinuria due to myofibrillar stress, and hemoglobinuria due to intravascular hemolysis, are also reported as frequent causes of iron losses in runners.[17-19] Iron losses through bladder trauma and renal hematuria have also been described.[38] It must be stressed that some intravascular hemolysis regularly occurs in all sport activities, but it may lead to iron store reduction only in running. Several studies investigated the pathophysiology of intravascular hemolysis: increased body temperature, decreased pH, impared mechanical properties of RBC wall, increased blood flow velocity, traumatic injury of RBC in peripheral muscular vessels, and, most importantly, mechanical trauma on the capillaries of the feet are all reported causes of intravascular hemolysis.[19,39] Some of the factors reported above may explain the relative decreased FERR values (Figure 4) and higher incidence of iron deficiency (Figure 5) among ice hockey players in comparison with soccer players, the first group being usually exposed to repeated muscular injuries.

Furthermore, the normal iron stores in roller skiers, who are particularly subjected to prolonged heat exposure during training, suggest that iron loss through sweating is not a noticeable cause of iron deficiency.

In younger subjects we found that FERR values were about half as high as in the respective older colleagues. (Figure 4). It is well known that iron stores are decreased in young people and that FERR levels remain low until the age of 10 to 15 years; after this age FERR increases progressively towards adult values.[40] Among the different junior groups, cross-country skiers and soccer players showed lower FERR values compared to controls and to cyclists (Figure 3). However, the difference was significant only for cross-country skiers, who showed the lowest FERR values and the highest incidence of iron deficiency among all groups. Therefore, reduced FERR in these junior subjects should indicate a real imbalance in the iron status. It was suggested that the interaction between increased iron needs for body growth, blood expansion, and muscle iron-containing enzyme synthesis on one hand, and the insufficient nutritional iron intake on the other hand, might be the cause of iron store reduction in younger athletes.[41]

Our data show that latent iron deficiency, as indicated by a FERR level <20 µg/l, is more widespread among athletes than among sedentary subjects (Figure 5). Recently, Robertson et al.[12] reported the lack of higher iron deficiency in athletes than in sedentary subjects. Since the mean FERR value they measured in the athletes was not different from that generally reported by the literature, the discordant conclusion they met derived from very low FERR found in their control group.

Among different sports, a higher percentage of iron deficiency was found in the endurance disciplines, in comparison to those prevalently anaerobic, and both the athletic groups show increased percentage in comparison to controls. Despite this ample incidence of iron deficiency, only 18 athletes among 326 tested (5.5%) showed a certain degree of low level Hb (Hb <14g/dl). However, recent reports indicate that iron deficiency, even without anemia, may reduce mytocondrial iron-dependent enzymes, causing a decrease in the aerobic performance.[11,39,42,43]

In agreement with the more recent literature[6,12] we found that SI is not sensitive in identifying iron store deficiency, at least in the absence of manifest sideropenic anemia.

V. CONCLUSIONS

The results reported in this study suggest that certain sport activities effectively reduce the bodily iron stores, and our data indicate that running is the most risky physical exercise in producing a considerable wasting of iron store.

Even if inadequate iron nutritional intake was not detected in our athletic subjects, increasing iron intake, up to the highest recomended level, should be preferable in athletes in order to compensate for the losses.

Furthermore, if the sport practiced is running, or if running is commonly used for training, even an optimal food iron intake may prove insufficient to prevent a reduction in iron stores, and iron deficiency will develop in a considerable number of athletes.

Finally, considering the rising number of young people that are participating in sports activities, special attention must be devoted to their iron status in order to prevent a high incidence of iron deficiency among younger athletes.

REFERENCES

1. Casoni, I., Borsetto, C., Cavicchi, A., Martinelli, S. and Conconi, F. , Reduced hemoglobin concentration and red cell hemoglobinization in Italian marathon And ultramarathon runners, *Int. J. Sports Med.*, 6, 176, 1985.
2. Colt, E. and Heyman, B., Low ferritin levels in runners, *J. Sports Med.*, 24, 13, 1984.
3. Hunding, A., Jordal, R. and Paulev, P. E., Runner's anemia and iron deficiency, *Acta Med. Scand.*, 209, 315, 1981.
4. Lampe, J. W., Slavin, J. L. and Apple, F. S., Poor iron status of women runners training for a marathon, *Int. J. Sports Med.*, 7, 111, 1986.
5. De Wijn, J. F., De Jongste, J. L., Mosterd, W. and Willebrand, D., Haemoglobin, packed cell volume, serum iron and iron binding capacity of selected athletes during training, *J. Sports Med.*, 11, 42, 1971.
6. Cavill, I., Jacobs, A. and Worwood, M., Diagnostic methods for iron status, *Ann. Clin. Biochem.*, 23, 168, 1986.
7. Jacobs, A., Miller, F., Worwood, M., Beamish, M. R. and Wardrop, C. A., Ferritin in the serum of normal subjects and patients with iron deficiency and iron overload *Br. Med. J.*, 4, 206, 1972.
8. Lipschtz, D. A., Cook, J. D. and Finch, C. A., A clinical evaluation of serum ferritin as an index of iron stores, *N. Engl. J. Med.*, 290, 1213, 1974.
9. Pattini, A. and Schena, F., Incidenza della carenza di ferro in sciatori di fondo, *Med. Sport*, 41, 1, 1988.
10. Ehn, L., Carlmark, B. and Höglund, S., Iron status in athletes involved in intense physical activity, *Med. Sci. Sports Exercise*, 12:1, 61, 1980.
11. Clement, D. B. and Sawchuk, L. L., Iron status and sports performance, *Sports Med.*, 1, 65, 1984.
12. Robertson, J. D., Maughan, R. J., Milne, A. C. and Davidson, R. J. L., Hematological status of male runners in relation to the extent of physical training, *Int. J. Sport Nutr.*, 2, 366, 1992.

13. Sullivan, S. N., Gastrointestinal bleeding in distance runners, *Sports Med.*, 3, 1, 1986.
14. Seiler, D., Nagel, D., Franz, H., Hellstern, P., Leitzmann, C. and Jung, K., Effects of long-distance running on iron metabolism and hematological parameters, *Int. J. Sports Med.*, 10, 357, 1989.
15. Paulev, P. E., Jordal, R. and Pedersen, N. S., Dermal excretion of iron in intensely training athletes, *Clin. Chim. Acta*, 127, 19, 1983.
16. Lamanca, J. J., Haymes, E. M., Daly, J. A., Moffatt, R. J. and Waller, M. F., Sweat iron loss of male and female runners during exercise, *Int. J. Sports Med.*, 9, 52, 1988.
17. Bank, W. J., Myoglobinuria in marathon runners: possible relationship to carbohydrate and lipide metabolism, *Ann. N. Y. Acad. Sci.*, 301, 942, 1977.
18. Ben, B. T. and Motley, C. P., Myoglobinemia and endurance exercise: a study on 25 participants in a triathlon competition, *Am. J. Sports Med.*, 12, 113, 1984.
19. Miller, B. J., Pate, R. R. and Burgess, W., Foot impact force and intravascular hemolysis during distance running, *Int. J. Sports Med.*, 9, 56, 1988.
20. Diehl, D. M., Lohman, T. G., Smith, S. C. and Kertzer, R., Effects of physical training and competition on the iron status of female field hockey players, *Int. J. Sports Med.*, 7, 264, 1986.
21. Dufaux, B., Hoederath, A., Streitberger, I., Hollmann, W. and Assmann, G., Serum ferritin, transferrin, haptoglobin, and iron in middle- and long-distance runners, elite rowers,and professional racing cyclists, *Int. J. Sports Med.*, 2, 43, 1981.
22. Pelliccia, A. and Di Nucci, G. B., Anemia in swimmers: fact or fiction? Study of hematologic and iron status in male and female top-level swimmers, *Int. J. Sports Med.*, 8, 227, 1987.
23. Wishnitzer, R., Vorst, E. and Berrebi, A., bone marrow iron depression in competitive distance runners, *Int. J. Sports Med.*, 4, 27, 1983.
24. Haymes, E. M., Puhl, J. L. and Temples, T. E., Training for cross-country skiing and iron status, *Med. Sci. Sports Exercise*, 18: 2, 162, 1986.
25. Pattini, A., Di Salvo, V., Schena, F. and Le Grazie, C., Iron values and haematological parameters of cross-country skiers, *Clin. Tri. J.*, 25: 5, 296, 1988.
26. Basshorn, S., Fletcher, L. R. and Stanton, R. H. J., Dietary analysis with the aid of a microcomputer, *J. Microcomputer Appl.*, 7, 279, 1984.
27. Pattini, A., Schena, F. and Guidi, G. C., Serum ferritin and serum iron changes after cross-country and roller ski endurance races. *Eur. J. Appl. Physiol.*, 61, 55, 1990.
28. Dickson, D. N., Wilkinson, R. L. and Noakes, T. D., Effects of ultra-marathon training and racing on hematologic parameters and serum ferritin levels in well-trained athletes, *Int. J. Sports Med.*, 3, 111, 1982.
29. Magnusson, B., Hallberg, L., Rossander, L. and Swolin, B., Iron metabolism and "sports anemia". I. A study of several iron parameters in elite runners with differences in iron status, *Acta Med. Scand.*, 216, 149, 1984.
30. Dallman, P. R., Biochemical basis for the manifestation of iron deficiency, *Annu. Rev. Nutr.,* 6, 13, 1986.
31. Beaton, S., Corey, P. N. and Steele, C., Conceptual and methodological issues regarding the epidemiology of iron deficiency and their implications for studies of the functional consequences of iron deficiency, *Am. J. Clin. Nutr.*, 50, 575, 1989.
32. Fogelholm, M., Rehunen, S., Gref, C. -G., Laakso, J. T., Lehto, J., Ruokonen, O. and Himberg, J. -J., Dietary intake and thiamin, iron, and zinc status in elite nordic skiers during different training periods, *Int. J. Sport Nutrit.*, 2, 351, 1992.
33. Frederickson, L. A., Puhl, J. and Runyan, W. S., Effects of training on indices of iron status of young female cross-country runners, *Med. Sci. Sports Exercise*, 15:4, 271, 1983.
34. Puhl, J. and Runyan, W. S., Hematological variations during aerobic training of college women, *Res. Q. Exercise Sports*, 51, 533, 1980.
35. Convertino, V. A., Brock, P. J, Keil, L. C., Beronoer, E. M. and Greanleaf, J. E., Exercise training induced hypervolemia: role of plasma albumin, renin and vasopressin, *J. Appl. Physiol.*, 48, 665, 1980.
36. Hespel, P., Lijnen, P., Fagard, R., Van Hoff, R., Goosen, W. and Amery, A., Effect of training on erythrocyte 2-3 diphosphoglycerate in normal men *Eur. J. Appl. Physiol.*, 57, 456, 1988.

37. Pattini, A. and Schena, F., Effects of training and iron supplementation on iron status of cross-country skiers, *J. Sports Med. Phys. Fit.*, 38, 347, 1990.
38. Blacklock, N. J., Bladder trauma in the long-distance runner: 10,000 Metres Haematuria, *Br. J. Urol.*, 49, 129, 1977.
39. Schoene, R. B., Escourrou, P., Robertson, H. T., Nilson, K. L., Parsons, J. R. and Smith, N. J. , Iron repletion decreases maximal exercise lactate concentration in female athletes with minimal iron-deficiency anemia, *J. Lab. Clin. Med.*, 102:2, 306, 1983.
40. Siimes, M. A., Addiego, J. E. and Dallman, P. R., Ferritin in serum: diagnosis of iron deficiency and iron overload in infants and children, *Blood*, 43, 581, 1974.
41. Ehn, L., Carlmark, B., Höglund, S., Iron in young sportsmen, in *Swimming Medicine IV*, Erickson, B. and Furberg, B., Eds., University Park Press, Baltimore, 1977, 85.
42. Finch, C. A., Gollnick, P. D., Hlastala, M. P., Miller, L. R., Dillmann, E. and Mackler, B., Lactic acidosis as a result of iron deficiency, *J. Clin. Invest.*, 64, 129, 1979.
43. Lamanca, J. J. and Haymes, E. M., Effects of low ferritin concentration on endurance performance, *Int. J. Sport Nutrit.*, 2, 376, 1992.

Chapter **8**

INADEQUATE IRON STATUS IN ATHLETES: AN EXAGGERATED PROBLEM?

Mikael Fogelholm

CONTENTS

I. INTRODUCTION

Iron is one of the most popular dietary supplements used by athletes.[1] The reason for this is partly iron's important role in exercise metabolism, and partly a strong belief that iron status, particularly in female athletes, is not optimal for sports performance.[2] Being an integral part of hemoglobin, myoglobin, and of several mitochondrial enzymes, iron is undoubtedly important for physical work capacity. Nevertheless, a critical review of the literature does not support the hypothesis that athletes need supplementary iron to optimize their sports performance.

This review starts by describing how exercise may affect iron balance, that is, iron losses and intake. The second part of the review answers the question "Does physical activity, such as athletic training, affect indicators of iron status?" Finally, I will appraise the effects of iron supplementation on iron status and on physical performance.

II. EFFECTS OF EXERCISE ON IRON BALANCE

A. IRON LOSSES IN SWEAT, URINE, AND FECES

In temperate environments, daily water loss in a sedentary man rarely exceeds 1 l. During physical activity, however, more than a liter may be lost in 1 h. In a Tour de France simulation study (5 h cycling in a respiratory chamber), daily sweat loss reached 3 to 4 l.

During the past 20 years, seven groups have measured iron concentration in exercise-induced sweat.[4-10] In the above papers, the range for sweat iron concentration was 0.5 to 9.0 μmol/l (0.03 to 0.5 mg/l).

The Nordic dietary recommendation[11] for daily iron intake of males is 10 mg. In a European diet, the bioavailability of iron is approximately 10%.[12] Consequently, the daily iron need for a male is about 1 mg. Calculated from the iron concentration found in sweat analyses,[4-10] daily losses in 4 l of sweat might increase a male's iron need by 12 to 200%.

According to the above results, iron excretion through sweat might be considerable in athletes. We should, however, be cautious with the interpretation because of methodological problems in collecting sweat. Trace element analyses are particularly difficult due to contamination.[13] Composition of sweat varies with the collection site,[4,6] hence, single sampling points (e.g., arm or back) may not represent whole body sweat losses.[14] Finally, it is uncertain whether a short sampling period represents long-term conditions.[13] The large variation between different studies probably reflects the above mentioned methodological problems.

Homeostatic regulation of sweat composition is another factor making direct conclusions from short-term studies difficult. An inverse relationship between sweat rate and ionic concentration has indeed been found for iron.[7] Moreover, Nickerson et al.[8] reported 40% lower sweat iron concentration in iron-deficient vs. iron-sufficient female runners.

Following strenuous running, iron (from erythrocytes or hemoglobin) may be lost in urine.[10,15-17] This phenomenon, sometimes called athletic pseudonephritis, disappears rapidly after finishing the run.[16,17]

Feces may be yet another route for increased iron loss in athletes. After strenuous endurance running (e.g., a marathon), several investigators have found gastrointestinal blood loss in 10 to 83% of the subjects.[18-22] By this route, daily iron loss might reach 2.0 mg.[22] Further, aspirin or other analgesics may increase fecal blood content.[21]

Because a marathon is an extremely strenuous event, gastrointestinal bleeding might be less during routine training. Only Lampe et al.[19] have measured fecal hemoglobin concentration in female runners during normal training. The mean fecal iron loss was ca. 1.1 mg/d in athletes and only 0.2 mg/d in controls. However, because the athletes' fecal hemoglobin distribution was highly skewed to the right, the above arithmetic mean value may give too high an impression on average iron losses.

B. DIETARY INTAKE: A BALANCING FACTOR?

There are several factors possibly increasing iron losses in athletes. Unfortunately, quantitative analysis of these losses is difficult, if not impossible. In iron balance, losses are counterbalanced by dietary iron intake.

Mean iron intakes for male and female athletes, in relation to energy intake in studies published between 1980 and 1992, are presented in Figure 1.[1,2,19,23-67] The Nordic Nutritional Recommendation[11] for iron intake is also shown in the figures. All groups of male athletes have a mean intake above the recommended level of 10 mg/d. More than half of the groups ingested twice the recommended allowance. When group mean results for energy and iron intake are compared across all studies in Figure 1, the association for male athletes is strong and positive ($r = 0.82$, $p < 0.0001$).

The Nordic Recommendation[11] for females is presented as an interval (12 to 18 mg/d, reflecting the variation in menstrual iron losses). The intake was above this interval only in a few studies. Most athlete groups had an iron intake between 10 and 16 mg/d. The association between energy and iron intake is positive, albeit not as strong as for male athletes ($r = 0.52$, $p < 0.01$).

Interpretation of dietary data is difficult, both because of inaccurate estimates of usual intake and of uncertainties in the daily intake recommendations. For instance, it has been suggested that iron recommendations should be higher for athletes.[68] It might be realistic to conclude that a factorial estimation of athletes' iron balance (quantitative comparison of losses and dietary intake) does not elucidate whether iron status is adequate or suboptimal.[69]

III. IRON STATUS IN ATHLETES

A. NUTRITIONAL STATUS: SOME DEFINITIONS

Nutritional status means sufficiency of host nutriture to permit cells, tissues, organs, anatomical systems, or the host her/himself to perform optimally the intended,

IRON INTAKE/MALE ATHLETES

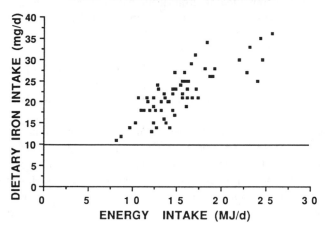

IRON INTAKE/FEMALE ATHLETES

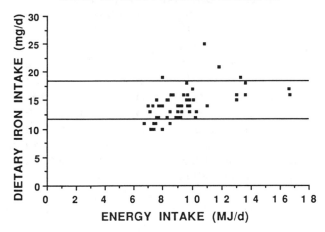

FIGURE 1. Male and female athletes' iron intake, in relation to daily energy intake. A summary from studies published from 1980 to 1992. The Nordic recommended iron intake for males (10 mg/d), and the recommendation interval for females (12 to 18 mg/d) are shown by horizontal lines. Each point represents the mean value for a group of athletes.

nutrient dependent function.[70] Hence, nutritional status affects work capacity, endurance, $\dot{V}O_2$ max, and submaximal $\dot{V}O_2$.

Nutritional adequacy means a state above which objective improvement of physical functions (e.g., health or fitness) no longer occurs.[71] In *marginal deficiency*, risk for severe deficiency is moderate.[72] In this stage, nutrient excretion decreases, as does nutrient content in some tissues and in stores (such as iron in bone marrow and liver). The term "deficiency" might even be too strong, and Brubacher[73] called this stage "marginal supply". In fact, marginal deficiency can be regarded as adaptation to suboptimal intake. People can stay in nutrient balance, despite decreased body content of one or more nutrients. In *subclinical deficiency,* risk for severe symptoms are high.[72] Functional changes occur in major metabolic pathways, impairing physical fitness.[70]

Detecting individuals at risk for nutritional deficiency is difficult and uncertain. Individual results are usually weighed against *reference intervals,* i.e., inner 95% in a well-defined group.[74] The lower or upper limit of the reference interval may also be called *decision limit* or *discrimination value.*

B. INDICES OF IRON STATUS IN ATHLETES

Iron status in athletes has been studied more than all other micronutrients together. Blood hemoglobin and serum ferritin concentrations are two of the most widely used chemical indicators. Only rarely has a significant difference between athletes' and controls' blood hemoglobin concentration[1,75] or transferrin saturation[76] been found.

Results from studies comparing serum ferritin concentration between athletes and untrained controls are presented in Table 1.[1,19,37,38,57,59,75-84] Only one study with female,[77] and three studies with male, runners[76,82,83] found lower serum ferritin concentration in athletes. Nevertheless, the mean serum ferritin concentration was generally low in females: the weighed means are 25 and 30 µg/l in athletes and controls, respectively.

As a decision limit for iron depletion, authors have used serum ferritin concentration 12, 15, 20, 25 or 30 µg/l (Table 2).[8,25,27,30,36,40,45,57,63,77-79,82,83,85-87] The highest percentage for athletes below the decision limit (89) was found in nine female runners consuming a lacto-vegetarian diet.[83] In male subjects, in contrast, the percentage of serum ferritin results <20 µg/l was only 0 to 11. Using 25 or 30 µg/l as the decision limit, three groups reported slightly higher prevalence (19 to 29%) in male runners.[25,76,87]

Six papers have presented the prevalence of marginal results for both athlete and control females.[40,58,77-80] The weighed mean prevalences are 37 and 23% in athletes (n = 329) and controls (n = 286), respectively. The 95% confidence interval for the difference (37 – 23 = 13) is 6 to 21. Hence, these studies, pooled together, support the hypothesis that marginal serum ferritin results are more frequently found in female athletes than in controls.

It has been suggested that runners are more prone to iron depletion than athletes participating in other events. However, the weighed mean serum ferritin concentration for female runners (n = 251; cf. Table 1) was 25 µg/l, precisely the same as for non-runner athletes (n = 179). The prevalence of serum ferritin results <12 µg/l was 35% for runners (n = 142, cf. Table 2) and 31% for non-runners (n = 120). Nevertheless, when <20 µg/l results are also considered, the prevalences are 42 and 25% in runners (n = 253) and non-runners (n = 195), respectively. The 95% confidence interval for the difference (42 – 25 = 17) is 8 to 26.

TABLE 1   Serum Ferritin as an Indicator of Iron Status in Athletes:
           Comparison of Population Mean Between Athletes and
           Sedentary Controls

S-ferritin, µg/l			Subjects				
Athletes		Controls	Sex	Sport	N/Ath	N/Con	Ref.
26	<	35	F	R	111	65	77
33	=	40	F	R	19	8	19
27	=	40	F	R	9	8	19
16	=	26	F	R	11	11	40
18	=	30	F	R	14	11	61
26	=	21	F	R	37	21	75
34	=	40	F	R	16	14	78
20	=	40	F	R	14	14	78
22	=	23	F	R	20	30	79
22	=	29	F	O	7	19	38
33	=	26	F	O	12	11	40
21	=	18	F	O	100	66	57
19	=	23	F	O	15	30	79
30	=	40	F	O	9	100	80
45	=	40	F	O	21	100	80
20	=	26	F	O	16	13	81
64	<	81	M	R	43	100	76
45	<	150	M	R	45	32	82
80	<	150	M	R	56	32	82
65	<	115	M	R	61	62	83
56	=	60	M	R	35	26	75
76	=	70	M	O	427	150	1
83	=	95	M	O	14	11	37
66	=	66	M	O	8	19	38
65	=	48	M	O	23	123	80
77	=	48	M	O	14	123	80
47	=	48	M	O	17	123	80
77	=	64	M	O	13	15	81
140	=	115	M	O	81	62	83
79	=	73	M	O	17	20	84

Note: M = male, F = female, R = running, O = other events. < significant difference. = no
significant difference. N/Ath = number of athletes, N/Con = number of controls.

Following increased physical exercise, significantly decreased blood hemoglobin (change 1 to 14 g/l) or serum ferritin (change 6 to 20 µg/l) concentration has been found in both sexes (Table 3).[37,49,79,81,88-97] Most of the other time trends reported for these two iron status indices were also negative, although nonsignificant, suggesting a weak biological gradient. Positive changes were rarely reported, and then for male subjects.[81,95-97]

Altogether, the cross-sectional and longitudinal studies suggest that particularly athletic training and running may affect serum ferritin concentration. Magnusson et al.[76] have suggested that the reason behind reduced ferritin would be a shift in iron storage from reticuloendothelial cells to hepatocytes, rather than diminished body iron supply. Unfortunately, this interesting hypothesis remains unproven. Because

TABLE 2   Serum Ferritin as an Indicator of Nutritional Status
in Athletes: Percentage of Subjects Outside the
Lower Decision Limit.

Percentage Outside			Subjects				
Limit	Athl	Contr	Sex	Sport	N/Ath	N/Con	Ref.
<12 µg/l	35	—	F	R	51	—	30
	45	9	F	R	11	11	40
	89	—	F	R	9	—	63
	22	—	F	R	9	—	63
	29	21	F	R	14	14	78
	25	21	F	R	16	14	78
	28	—	F	R	32	—	85
	17	9	F	O	12	11	40
	31	46	F	O	100	66	57
	43	27	F	O	15	30	79
	29	—	F	O	15	—	86
	12	—	M	R	25	—	8
	3	—	M	R	86	—	85
	6	—	M	O	31	—	27
	0	—	M	O	15	—	79
<20 µg/l	50	22	F	R	111	65	77
	13	10	F	O	21	100	80
	5	—	M	R	59	—	36
	32	—	M	R	75	—	45
	4	4	M	O	427	150	1
	4	2	M	O	23	123	80
<25 µg/l	19	2	M	R	43	81	76
<30 µg/l	82	—	F	R	17	—	25
	29	—	M	R	35	—	25
	8	0	M	R	81	62	83
	14	2	M	R	22	52	87
	0	0	M	O	61	62	83
	0	2	M	O	12	52	87

Note: M = male, F = female, R = running, O = other events.

lowered blood hemoglobin concentration appears without any other signs of iron deficiency, increased plasma volume is an apparent explanation for this phenomenon.[98]

IV. EFFECTS OF IRON SUPPLEMENTATION IN ATHLETES

A. CHANGES IN BLOOD HEMOGLOBIN AND SERUM FERRITIN

Iron supplementation does not increase blood hemoglobin concentration in athletes without iron deficiency anemia.[92,95,99-103] In anemic subjects, iron treatment effectively normalizes decreased hemoglobin concentration.[104]

**TABLE 3   Blood Chemistry as an Indicator of Iron Status
During Lower and Higher Physical Activity**

Interval (wk)	Activity Low	Activity High	Change	n	Sex	Sport	Ref.
			B-hemoglobin, g/l				
14	142	> 141	-1	24	F	R	88
9	138	= 131	-7	10	F	R	49
24	134	= 131	-3	21	F	R	93
8	143	= 138	-5	8	F	R	94
26	139	> 132	-7	12	F	O	48
?	141	> 135	-6	13	F	O	89
26	134	= 132	-2	16	F	O	81
7	133	= 126	-7	8	F	O	91
35	140	= 139	-1	5	F	O	95
3	154	> 140	-14	15	M	R	90
7	157	> 148	-9	11	M	O	91
65	155	> 145	-10	40	M	O	92
35	166	= 158	-8	5	M	O	95
26	153	= 155	+2	13	M	O	81
17	149	< 155	+6	16	M	O	96
			S-ferritin, μg/l				
?	27	> 14	-13	20	F	R	79
14	31	> 25	-6	24	F	R	88
9	30	= 22	-8	10	F	R	49
24	16	= 14	-2	21	F	R	93
78	36	= 32	-4	18	F	R	97
?	24	> 16	-8	13	F	O	89
7	12	> 5	-7	8	F	O	91
26	27	= 20	-7	16	F	O	81
35	38	= 30	-8	5	F	O	95
3	61	= 59	-2	15	M	R	90
78	113	= 193	-10	60	M	R	97
7	48	> 28	-20	11	M	O	91
3	83	= 83	0	14	M	O	37
26	50	= 77	+27	13	M	O	81
35	50	= 65	+15	5	M	O	95
17	24	= 21	-3	16	M	O	96

Note: M = male, F = female, R = running, O = other events, ? = unknown.

Serum ferritin increases after iron treatment (Table 4).[99-103,105,106] The response is evident (57 to 100%)[96,99-101] after high-dose (≥10 × dietary recommendation), but smaller (13 to 32%)[66,95] after low-dose (1 × recommendation) supplementation.

B. IRON SUPPLEMENTATION AND PERFORMANCE

A majority of the interest on mineral supplementation and fitness has been focused on iron. Because iron regulates oxygen delivery and utilization, hence

TABLE 4   Effects of Iron Supplementation on Iron
Depleted Women: Studies Showing Either No
Association or an Association Between
Increased Serum Ferritin Concentration and
Aerobic Fitness

Duration Wk	B-hemoglobin g/l		S-ferritin µg/l		Fitness	Ref.
	Pre	Post	Pre	Post		
No association						
8	137	139	14	26	B-LA (ns) $\dot{V}O_2$ max (ns)	99
8	134	135	12	38	AnT (ns) $\dot{V}O_2$ max (ns)	100
2	147	146	29	52	RQ (ns) $\dot{V}O_2$ max (ns)	101
8	141	144	16	23	B-LA (ns) $\dot{V}O_2$ max (ns)	102
10	131	140	30	60	AnT (ns) $\dot{V}O_2$ max (ns)	103
Association						
14	120	126	6	10	RQ(–) $\dot{V}O_2$ max (ns)	47
8	131	134	14	27	endurance (+) $\dot{V}O_2$ max (ns)	105
2	122	127	10	22	B-LA (–) $\dot{V}O_2$ max (ns)	106

Note: (+) = increase, (-) = decrease, (ns) = no significant changes. B-LA = blood lactate concentration; $\dot{V}O_2$ max = maximal oxygen uptake; Ant = anaerobic threshold; RQ = respiratory quotient.

aerobic fitness, the attention on iron is not surprising. Because of greater iron loss through menstruation, female athletes have been studied more than males.

Functional consequences of iron deficiency anemia have been extensively reviewed by Dallman[107] and Scrimshaw.[108] Decreased blood hemoglobin affects voluntary activity, work productivity, and exercise-induced heart rate and blood lactate. Both decreased blood hemoglobin concentration and decreased activity in mitochondrial enzymes in the muscle affect fitness in anemic subjects.[109,110]

Even mild anemia impairs submaximal aerobic fitness.[111] Although the World Health Organization (WHO)[112] recognizes a 20 g/l decrease in blood hemoglobin indicative for anemia, Margolis et al.[113] suggested 10 g/l as a meaningful change. Mainly because of improved dissociation of O_2 from hemoglobin in mild iron deficiency, a decrease in $\dot{V}O_2$ max is only evident in severe anemia.[110]

In anemic subjects, iron supplementation raises blood hemoglobin concentration and improves fitness.[107,108] Fitness is enhanced even before changes in blood hemoglobin probably because of improved mitochondrial enzyme activity.[114,115]

During the last few years several studies have clarified the effects of iron depletion indicated by low serum ferritin and normal blood hemoglobin concentration (Table 4). Most investigators have not found an association between increased serum ferritin and aerobic fitness.[99-103] In these studies the initial mean serum ferritin and blood hemoglobin concentrations were 12 to 30 µg/l and 131 to 147 g/l, respectively.

In contrast to the above findings, three studies have suggested that treatment of iron depletion improves fitness.[47,105,106] Improved fitness was shown by decreased blood lactate concentration[47,106] and by increased exercise time-to-exhaustion.[105] In all three reports, the authors suggested that enhanced intramuscular oxidative metabolism was the reason for improved fitness.

Before supplementation, the mean serum ferritin and blood hemoglobin concentration in the above three studies varied from 6 to 14 µg/l and from 120 to 131 g/l, respectively. In two of these studies,[47,106] blood hemoglobin concentration increased significantly, although the mean change was not more than 6 g/l. Hence, it seems that at least some subjects were mildly anemic, not only iron depleted. This might be the most evident contrast to studies[99-103] with no association between increased serum ferritin and physical fitness.

V. IS IRON SUPPLEMENTATION FOR ATHLETES WARRANTED?

Physical exercise seems to cause a slight decrease in serum ferritin concentration in female athletes, and a simultaneous increase in the prevalence of marginal serum ferritin results. It is possible, although not conclusively shown, that marginal ferritin results occur more often in runners than in other athletes.

The reason for decreased serum ferritin concentration remains to be solved. Magnusson et al.[76] have suggested a shift in iron storage. However, because the mean iron intake for several groups of female athletes is low (cf. Figure 1), one cannot overlook the possibility of inadequate dietary iron intake. Moreover, there is an increasing popularity for vegetarianism, particularly among female runners and gymnasts. This may reduce the amount of bioavailable iron. Indeed, the highest prevalence of iron depletion (89%) has been found in a group of female vegetarian runners.[63]

Lower hemoglobin concentrations, occasionally found in athletes, are most likely caused by plasma dilution. Iron deficiency anemia is not more prevalent in athletes than in the general population.[98] Even female athletes are in iron balance, although with slightly smaller iron stores than found normally. Because iron absorption is inversely related to the amount of iron stored, enhanced absorption might well explain the lack of manifest anemia.

Another viewpoint worth considering is that iron depletion should in fact be accepted only when at least two of the common indicators (serum ferritin concentration, red blood cell protoporphyrin, and/or percentage transferrin saturation) are below the decision limit.[98] Because most investigators have determined only serum ferritin, the prevalence of truly iron-depleted (decreased body iron content, but normal blood hemoglobin concentration) athletes is probably lower than indicated in Table 2.

Iron stores can easily be enlarged by an 8 to 10 week iron supplementation. Nevertheless, if an athlete does not have anemia due to iron deficiency, increased stores will not improve sports performance. Moreover, it has not been shown that taking supplementary iron is needed to prevent iron deficiency anemia in athletes. Therefore, there are no physiological reasons for iron supplementation. A real "iron problem" in athletes remains unproven.

REFERENCES

1. Fogelholm, G. M., Himberg, J.-J., Alopaeus, K., Gref, C.-G., Laakso, J. T., Lehto, J. J., Mussalo-Rauhamaa H., Dietary and biochemical indices of nutritional status in male athletes and controls, *J. Am. Coll. Nutr.*, 11, 181, 1992.
2. Burke, L. M., Read, R.S.D., Diet pattern of elite Australian male triathletes, *Phys. Sportsmed.*, 15, 140, 1987.
3. Brouns, F., Saris, W. H. M., Stroecken, J., Beckers, E., Thissen, R., Rehrer, N. J., Ten Hoor, F., Eating, drinking, and cycling. A controlled Tour de France simulation study, part I, *Int. J. Sports Med.*, 10, S32, 1989.
4. Aruoma, O. I., Reilly, T., MacLaren, D., Halliwell, B., Iron, copper and zinc concentrations in human sweat and plasma: the effects of exercise, *Clin. Chim. Acta*, 177, 81, 1988.
5. Beller, G. A., Maher, J. T., Hartley, L. H., Bass, D. E., Wacker, W. E. C., Changes in serum and sweat magnesium levels during work in the heat, *Aviat. Space Environ. Med.*, 46, 709, 1975.
6. Gutteridge, J. M. C., Rowley, D. A., Halliwell, B., Cooper, D. F., Heeley, D. M., Copper and iron complexes catalytic for oxygen radical reactions in sweat from human athletes, *Clin. Chim. Acta*, 145, 267, 1985.
7. Lamanca, J. J., Haymes, E. M., Daly, J. A., Moffat, R. J., Waller, M. F., Sweat iron loss of male and female runners during exercise, *Int. J. Sports Med.*, 9, 52, 1987.
8. Nickerson, H. J., Holubets, M. C., Weiler, B. R., Haas, R. G., Schwartz, S., Ellefson, M. E., Causes of iron deficiency in adolescent athletes, *J. Pediatr.*, 114, 657, 1989.
9. Paulev, P.-E., Jordal, R., Standberg-Pedersen N., Dermal excretion of iron in intensely training athletes, *Clin. Chim. Acta*, 127, 19, 1983.
10. Seiler, D., Nagel, D., Franz, H., Hellstern, P., Leitzman, C., Jung, K., Effects of long-distance running on iron metabolism and hematological parameters, *Int. J. Sports Med.*, 10, 357, 1989.
11. Nordisk Ministerråd, *Nordiska Näringsrekommendationer*, Rapport 1989:2, Statens Livsmedelsverk, Uppsala, 1989.
12. Anonymous, Recommended daily amounts of vitamins & minerals in Europe, *Nutr. Abstr. Rev.*, (Series A), 60, 827, 1990.
13. Brune, M., Magnusson, B., Persson, H., Hallberg, L., Iron losses in sweat, *Am. J. Clin. Nutr.*, 43, 438, 1986.
14. Jacob, R. A., Sandstead, H. H., Munoz, J. M., Klevay, L. M., Milne, D. B., Whole body surface loss of trace metals in normal males, *Am. J. Clin. Nutr.*, 34, 1379, 1981.
15. Halvorsen, F. A., Lyng, J., Ritland, S., Gastrointestinal bleeding in marathon runners, *Scand. J. Gastroenterol.*, 21, 493, 1986.
16. Riess, R. W., Athletic hematuria and related phenomena, *J. Sports Med.*, 19, 381, 1979.
17. Siegel, A. J., Hennekens, C. H., Solomon, H. S., van Boeckel, B., Exercise-related hematuria. Finding in a group of marathon runners, *J. Am. Med. Assoc.*, 241, 391, 1979.

18. Baska, R. S., Moses, F. M., Graeber, G., Kearney, G., Gastrointestinal bleeding during an ultramarathon, *Dig. Dis. Sci.*, 35, 276, 1990.
19. Lampe, J. W., Slavin, J. L., Apple, F. S., Iron status of active women and the effect of running a marathon on bowel function and gastrointestinal blood loss, *Int. J. Sports Med.*, 12, 173, 1991.
20. McMahon, L. F., Ryan, M. J., Larson, D., Fisher, R. L., Occult gastrointestinal blood loss in marathon runners, *Ann. Intern. Med.*, 100, 846, 1984.
21. Robertson, J. D., Maughan, R. J., Davidson, R. J. L., Faecal blood loss in response to exercise, *Br. Med. J.*, 295, 303, 1987.
22. Steward, J. G., Ahlquist, D. A., McGill, D. B., Ilstrup, D. M., Schwartz, S., Owen, R. A., Gastrointestinal blood loss and anemia in runners, *Ann. Intern. Med.*, 100, 843, 1984.
23. Barr, S. I., Energy and nutrient intakes of elite adolescent swimmers, *J. Can. Diet. Assoc.*, 50, 20, 1989.
24. Barr, S. I., Relationship of eating attitudes to anthropometric variables and dietary intakes of female collegiate swimmers, *J. Am. Diet. Assoc.*, 91, 976, 1991.
25. Clement, D. B., Asmundson, R. C., Nutritional intake and hematological parameters in endurance runners, *Phys. Sportsmed.*, 10, 37, 1982.
26. Dahlström, M., Jansson, E., Nordevang, E., Kaiser, L. Discrepancy between estimated energy intake and requirement in female dancers, *Clin. Physiol.*, 10, 11, 1990.
27. Dallongeville, J., Ledoux, M., Brisson, G., Iron deficiency among active men, *J. Am. Coll. Nutr.*, 8, 195, 1989.
28. Deuster, P. A., Day, B. A., Singh, A., Douglass, L., Moser-Veillon, P. B., Zinc status of highly trained women runners and untrained women, *Am. J. Clin. Nutr.*, 49, 1295, 1989.
29. Deuster, P. A., Kyle, S. B., Moser, P. B., Vigersky, R. A., Singh, A., Schoomaker, E. B., Nutritional intake and status of highly trained amenorrheic and eumenorrheic women runners, *Fertil. Steril.*, 46, 636, 1986.
30. Deuster, P. A., Kyle, S. B., Moser, P. B., Vigersky, R. A., Singh, A., Schoomaker, E. B., Nutritional survey of highly trained woman runners, *Am. J. Clin. Nutr.*, 45, 954, 1986.
31. Dreon, D. M., Butterfield, G. E., Vitamin B$_6$ utilization in active and inactive young men, *Am. J. Clin. Nutr.*, 43, 816, 1986.
32. Ellsworth, N. M., Hewitt, B. F., Haskell, W. L., Nutrient intake of elite male and female nordic skiers, *Phys. Sportsmed.*, 13, 78, 1985.
33. van Erp-Baart, A. M. J., Saris, W. H. M., Binkhorst, R. A., Vos, J. A., Elvers, J. W. H., Nationwide survey on nutritional habits in elite athletes. Part I and II, *Int. J. Sports Med.*, 10, S3, 1989.
34. Faber, M., Spinnler Benadé, A.-J., Nutrient intake and dietary supplementation in body-builders, *S. Afr. Med. J.*, 72, 831, 1987.
35. Faber, M., Spinnler Benadé, A.-J., Mineral and vitamin intake in field athletes (discus-, hammer-, javelin-throwers and shotputters), *Int. J. Sports Med.*, 12, 324, 1991.
36. Fogelholm, M., Estimated energy expenditure, diet and iron status of male Finnish endurance athletes, *Scand. J. Sports Sci.*, 11, 59, 1989.
37. Fogelholm, M., Lahtinen, P., Nutritional evaluation of a sailing crew during a transatlantic race, *Scand. J. Med. Sci. Sports*, 1, 99, 1991.
38. Fogelholm, M., Rehunen, S., Gref, C.-G., Laakso, J. T., Lehto, J. J., Ruokonen, I., Himberg, J.-J., Dietary intake and thiamin, iron and zinc status in elite Nordic skiers during different training periods, *Int. J. Sports Nutr.*, 2, 351, 1991.
39. Guilland, J.-C., Penaranda, T., Gallet, C., Boggio, V., Fuchs, F., Klepping, J., Vitamin status of young athletes including the effects of supplementation, *Med. Sci. Sports Exercise*, 21, 441, 1989.
40. Haymes, E. M., Spillman, D. M., Iron status of women distance runners, sprinters, and control women, *Int. J. Sports Med.*, 10, 430, 1989.
41. Hickson J. F., Schrader, J., Cunningham-Trischler, L., Dietary intakes of female basketball and gymnastic athletes, *J. Am. Diet. Assoc.*, 86, 251, 1986.
42. Holland, A., Dietary intake and nitrogen balance in athletes with and without consumption of a protein supplement, *Hum. Nutr.: Appl. Nutr.*, 41A, 367, 1987.

43. Kaiserauer, S., Snyder, A. C., Sleeper, M., Zierath, J., Nutritional, physiological, and menstrual status of distance runners, *Med. Sci. Sports Exercise*, 21, 120, 1989.

44. Keith, R. E., O'Keeffe, K. A., Alt, L. A., Young, K. L., Dietary status of trained female cyclists, *J. Am. Diet. Assoc.*, 89, 1620, 1989.

45. Lampe, J. W., Slavin, J. L., Apple, F. S., Effects of moderate iron supplementation on the iron status of runners with low serum ferritin, *Nutr. Rep. Int.*, 34, 959, 1986.

46. Lampe, J. W., Slavin, J. L., Apple, F. S., Poor iron status of women runners training for a marathon, *Int. J. Sports Med.*, 7, 111, 1986.

47. Lukaski, H. C., Hall, C. B., Siders, W. A., Altered metabolic response of iron-deficient women during graded, maximal exercise, *Eur. J. Appl. Physiol.*, 63, 140, 1991.

48. Lukaski, H. C., Hoverson, B. S., Milne, D. B., Bolonchuk, W. W., Copper, zinc, and iron status of female swimmers, *Nutr. Res.*, 9, 493, 1989.

49. Manore, M. M., Besenfelder, P. D., Wells, C. L., Carroll, S. S., Hooker, S. P., Nutrient intakes and iron status in female long-distance runners during training, *J. Am. Diet. Assoc.*, 89, 257, 1989.

50. Miyamura, J. B., McNutt, S. W., Lichton, I. J., Wenkam, N. S., Altered zinc status of soldiers under field conditions, *J. Am. Diet. Assoc.*, 87, 595, 1987.

51. Moffat, R. J., Dietary status of elite female high school gymnasts: inadequacy of vitamin and mineral intake, *J. Am. Diet. Assoc.*, 84, 1361, 1984.

52. Myerson, M., Gutin, B., Warren, M. P., May, M. T., Contento, I., Lee, M., Pi-Sunyer, F. X., Pierson, R. N., Brooks-Gunn, J., Resting metabolic rate and energy balance in amenorrheic and eumenorrheic runners, *Med. Sci. Sports Exercise*, 23, 15, 1991.

53. Nieman, D. C., Butler, J. V., Pollet, L. M., Dietrich, S. J., Lutz, R. D., Nutrient intake of marathon runners, *J. Am. Diet. Assoc.*, 89, 1273, 1989.

54. Nowak, R. K., Knudsen, K. S., Olmstea Schultz, L., Body composition and nutrient intakes of college men and women basketball players, *J. Am. Diet. Assoc.*, 88, 575, 1988.

55. Pate, R. R., Sargent, R. G., Burgess, M. L., Dietary intake of women runners, *Int. J. Sports Med.*, 11, 461, 1990.

56. Perron, M., Endres, J., Knowledge, attitudes, and dietary practices of female athletes, *J. Am. Diet. Assoc.*, 85, 573, 1985.

57. Read, M. H., McGuffin, S. L., The effects of B-complex supplementation on endurance performance, *J. Sports Med.*, 23, 178, 1983.

58. Risser, W. L., Lee, E. V., Poindexter, H. B. W., Steward West, M., Pivarnik, J. M., Risser, J. M. H., Hickson, J. F., Iron deficiency in female athletes: its prevalence and impact on performance, *Med. Sci. Sports Exercise*, 20, 116, 1988.

59. Short, S. H., Short, W. S., Four-year study of university athletes' dietary intake, *J. Am. Diet. Assoc.*, 82, 632, 1983.

60. Singh, A., Day, B. A., DeBolt, J. E., Trostmann, U. H., Bernier, L. L., Deuster, P. A., Magnesium, zinc, and copper status of US Navy SEAL trainees, *Am. J. Clin. Nutr.*, 49, 695, 1989.

61. Singh, A., Deuster, P. A., Day, B. A., Moser-Veillon, P. B., Dietary intakes and biochemical markers of selected minerals: comparison of highly trained runners and untrained women, *J. Am. Coll. Nutr.*, 9, 65, 1990.

62. Smoak, B. L., Singh, A., Day, B. A., Norton, J. P., Kyle, S. B., Pepper, S. J., Deuster, P. A., Changes in nutrient intakes of conditioned men during a 5-day period of increased physical activity and other stresses, *Eur. J. Appl. Physiol.*, 58, 245, 1988.

63. Snyder, A. C., Dvorak, L. L., Roepke, J. B., Influence of dietary iron source on measures of iron status among female runners, *Med. Sci. Sports Exercise*, 21, 7, 1989.

64. Valliéres, F., Tremblay, A., St-Jean, L., Study of the energy balance and the nutritional status of highly trained female swimmers, *Nutr. Res.*, 9, 699, 1989.

65. Watkin, V. A., Myburgh, K. H., Noakes, T. D., Low nutrient intake does not cause the menstrual cycle interval disturbances seen in some ultramarathon runner, *Clin. J. Sports Med.*, 1, 154, 1991.

66. Weight, L. M., Noakes, T. D., Labadarios, D., Graves, J., Jacobs, P., Berman, P. A., Vitamin and mineral status of trained athletes including the effects of supplementation, *Am. J. Clin. Nutr.*, 47, 186, 1988.

67. Worme, J. D., Doubt, T. J., Singh, A., Ryan, C. J., Moses, F. M., Deuster, P. A., Dietary patterns, gastrointestinal complaints, and nutrition knowledge of recreational triathletes, *Am. J. Clin. Nutr.*, 51, 690, 1990.
68. Haymes, E. M., Lamanca, J. J., Iron loss in runners during exercise: implications and recommendations, *Sports Med.*, 7, 277, 1989.
69. Aggett, P., Scientific considerations in the formulation of RDI, *Eur. J. Clin. Nutr.*, 44, 37, 1990.
70. Solomons, N. W., Allen, L. H., The functional assessment of nutritional status: principles, practice and potential, *Nutr. Rev.*, 41, 33, 1983.
71. Piertzik, K., Vitamin defiency-aetiology and terminology, in *B Vitamins in Medicine. Proceedings of a Symposium held in Helsinki, October 1985.*, Himberg, J.-J., Tackmann, W., Bonke, D. and Karppanen, H., Eds., Friedr. Wieweg & Sohn, Wiesbaden, 1986, 31.
72. Wood, B., Thiamin status in Australia, *World Rev. Nutr. Diet.*, 46, 148, 1985.
73. Brubacher, G. B., Scientific basis for the estimation of the daily requirements for vitamins, in *Elevated Dosages of Vitamins*, Walter, P., Stähelin, H. and Brubacher, G., Eds., Hans Huber Publishers, Stuttgart, 1989, 3.
74. Solberg, H. E., International Federation of Clinical Chemistry and International Committee for Standardization in Haematology: approved recommendation (1986) on the theory of reference values. Part 1. The concept of reference values, *J. Clin. Chem. Clin. Biochem.*, 25, 337, 1987.
75. Balaban, E. P., Cox, J. V., Snell, P., Vaughan, R. H., Frenkel, E. P., The frequency of anemia and iron deficiency in the runner, *Med. Sci. Sports Exercise* 21, 643, 1989.
76. Magnusson, B., Hallberg, L., Rossander, L., Swolin B., Iron metabolism and "sports anemia". II. A hematological comparison of elite runners and control subjects, *Acta Med. Scand.*, 216, 157, 1984.
77. Pate, R. R., Miller, B. J., Davis, J. M., Slentz, C. A., Klingshirn, L. A., Iron status of female runners, *Int. J. Sport Nutr.*, 3, 222, 1993.
78. Durstine, J. L., Pate, R. R., Sparling, P. B., Wilson, G. E., Senn, M. D., Bartoli, W. P., Lipid, lipoprotein, and iron status of elite woman distance runners, *Int. J. Sports Med.*, 8, S119, 1987.
79. Rowland, T. W., Stagg, L., Kelleher, J. F., Iron deficiency in adolescent girls. Are athletes at increased risk?, *J. Adol. Health*, 12, 22, 1991.
80. Hemmingson, P., Bauer, M., Birgegård, G., Iron status in elite skiers, *Scand. J. Med. Sci. Sports*, 1, 174, 1991.
81. Lukaski, H. C., Hoverson, B. S., Gallagher, S. K., Bolonchuk, W. W., Physical training and copper, iron, and zinc status of swimmers, *Am. J. Clin. Nutr.*, 51, 1093, 1990.
82. Casoni, I., Borsetto, C., Cavicchi, A., Martinelli, S., Conconi, F., Reduced hemoglobin concentration and red cell hemoglobinization in Italian marathon and ultramarathon runners, *Int. J. Sports Med.*, 6, 176, 1985.
83. Dufaux, B., Hoederath, A., Streitberger, I., Hollman, W., Assman, G., Serum ferritin, transferrin, haptoglobin, and iron in middle- and long-distance runners, elite rowers, and professional cyclists, *Int. J. Sports Med.*, 2, 43, 1981.
84. Resina, A., Gatteschi, L., Giamberardino, M. A., Imreh, F., Rubenni, M. G., Vecchiet, L., Hematological comparison of iron status in trained top-level soccer players and control subjects, *Int. J. Sports Med.*, 12, 453, 1991.
85. Colt, E., Heyman, B., Low ferritin levels in runners, *J. Sports Med.*, 24, 13, 1984.
86. Rowland, T. W., Kelleher, J. F., Iron deficiency in athletes, *Am. J. Dis. Child.*, 143, 197, 1989.
87. Dickson, D. N., Wilkinson, R. L., Noakes, T. D., Effects of ultra-marathon training and racing on hematologic parameters and serum ferritin levels in well-trained athletes, *Int. J. Sports Med.*, 3, 111, 1982.
88. Blum, S., Rothman Sherman, A., Boileau, R. A., The effects of fitness-type exercise on iron status in adult women, *Am. J. Clin. Nutr.*, 43, 456, 1986.
89. Diehl, D. M., Lohman, T. G., Smith, S. C., Kertzer, R., Effects of physical training and competition on the iron status of female field hockey players, *Int. J. Sports Med.*, 7, 264, 1986.
90. Dressendorfer, R. H., Keen, C. L., Wade, C. E., Claybaugh, J. R., Timmis, G. C., Development of runner's anemia during a 20-day road race: effect of iron supplements, *Int. J. Sports Med.*, 12, 332 1991.

91. Magazanic, A., Weinstein, Y., Dlin, R. A., Derin, M., Schwartzman, S., Allalouf, D., Iron deficiency caused by 7 weeks of intensive physical exercise, *Eur. J. Appl. Physiol.*, 57, 198, 1988.

92. Guglielmini, C., Casoni, I., Patracchini, M., Manfredini, F., Grazzi, G., Ferrari, M., Conconi, F., Reduction of Hb levels during the racing season in nonsideropenic professional cyclists, *Int. J. Sports Med.*, 10, 352, 1989.

93. Fogelholm, M., Micronutrient status in females during a 24-week fitness-type exercise program, *Ann. Nutr. Metab.*, 36, 209, 1992.

94. Frederickson, L. A., Puhl, J. L., Runyan, W. S., Effects of training on indices of iron status of young female cross-country runners, *Med. Sci. Sports Exercise*, 15, 271, 1983.

95. Haymes, E. M., Puhl, J. L., Temples, T. E., Training for cross-country skiing and iron status, *Med. Sci. Sports Exercise*, 18, 162, 1986.

96. Pattini, A., Schena, F., Effects of training and iron supplementation on iron status of cross-country skiers, *J. Sports Med. Phys. Fitness*, 30, 347, 1990.

97. Kaiser, V., Janssen, G. M. E., van Wersch, J. W. J., Effect of training on red blood cell parameters and plasma ferritin: a transverse and a longitudinal approach, *Int. J. Sports Med.*, 10, S169, 1989.

98. Weight, L. M., "Sports anemia." Does it exist?, *Sports Med.*, 16, 1, 1993.

99. Fogelholm M., Jaakkola, L., Lampisjärvi, T., Effects of iron supplementation in female athletes with low serum ferritin concentration, *Int. J. Sports Med.*, 13, 158, 1992.

100. Newhouse, I. J., Clement, D. B., Taunton, J. E., McKenzie, D. C., The effects of prelatent/latent iron deficiency on physical work capacity, *Med. Sci. Sports Exercise*, 21, 263, 1989.

101. Powell, P. D., Tucker, A., Iron supplementation and running performance in female cross-country runners, *Int. J. Sports Med.*, 12, 462, 1991.

102. Klingshirn, L. A., Pate, R. R., Bourque, S. P., Davis, J. M., Sargent, R. G., Effect of supplementation on endurance capacity in iron-depleted women, *Med. Sci. Sports Exercise*, 24, 819, 1992.

103. Matter, M., Stittfall, T., Graves, J., Myburgh, K., Adams, B., Jacobs, P., Noakes, T. D., The effect of iron and folate therapy on maximal exercise performance in female marathon runners with iron and folate deficiency, *Clin. Sci.*, 72, 415, 1987.

104. Hunding, A., Jordal, R., Paulev, P-E., Runner's anemia and iron deficiency, *Acta Med. Scand.*, 209, 315, 1981.

105. Rowland, T. W., Deisroth, M. B., Green, G. M., Kelleher, J. F., The effect of iron therapy on the exercise capacity of nonanemic iron-deficient adolescent runners, *Am. J. Dis. Child.*, 142, 165, 1988.

106. Schoene, R. B., Escourrou, P., Robertson, H. T., Nilson, K. L., Robinson Parsons, J., Smith, N. J., Iron repletion decreases maximal exercise lactate concentrations in female athletes with minimal iron-deficiency anemia, *J. Lab. Clin. Med.*, 102, 306, 1983.

107. Dallman, P. R., Manifestations of iron deficiency, *Semin. Hematol.*, 19, 19, 1982.

108. Scrimshaw, N. S., Functional consequences of iron deficiency in human populations, *J. Nutr. Sci. Vitaminol.*, 30, 47, 1984.

109. McLane, J. A., Fell, R. D., McKay, R. H., Winder, W. W., Brown, E. B., Holloszy, J. O., Physiological and biochemical effects of iron deficiency on rat skeletal muscle, *Am. J. Physiol.*, 241, C47, 1981.

110. Perkkiö, M. V., Jansson, L. T., Brooks, G. A., Refino, C. J., Dallman, P. R., Work performance in iron deficiency of increasing severity, *J. Appl. Physiol.*, 58, 1477, 1985.

111. Viteri, F. E., Torun, B., Anaemia and physical work capacity, *Clin. Haematol.*, 3, 609, 1974.

112. World Health Organization, Nutritional anemias, *WHO Techn. Rept. Series*, 503, 1972.

113. Margolis, H. S., Hardison, H. H., Bender, T. R., Dallman, P. R., Iron deficiency in children: the relationship between pretreatment laboratory tests and subsequent hemoglobin response to iron therapy, *Am. J. Clin. Nutr.*, 34, 2158, 1981.

114. Ohira, Y., Edgerton, V. R., Gardner, G. W., Gunawardena, K. A., Senewiratne, B., Ikawa, S., Work capacity after iron treatment as a function of hemoglobin and iron deficiency, *J. Nutr. Sci. Vitaminol.*, 27, 87, 1981.

115. Ohira, Y., Edgerton, V. R., Gardner, G. W., Senewiratne, B., Barnard, R. J., Simpson, D. R., Work capacity, heart rate and blood lactate responses to iron treatment, *Br. J. Haematol.*, 41, 365, 1979.

Chapter 9

CALCIUM AND IRON INTAKES OF DISABLED ELITE ATHLETES

Jayanthi Kandiah

CONTENTS

0-8493-7916-4/95/$0.00+$.50
© 1995 by CRC Press, Inc.

I. INTRODUCTION

In recent years, the role of nutrition in athletic performance has gained increased recognition. Calcium and iron are among numerous other nutrients that are of great concern among athletes, especially female athletes. Since iron is an important component of hemoglobin, myoglobin, cytochrome, and various enzymes, iron deficiency caused by sports and/or dietary shortages can affect several metabolic functions which are related to various athletic performances.[1-5] Though the recommended dietary allowances (RDA) for males between the age of 19 to 25 years is 10 mg/d, and for females in the same age category is 15 mg/d, research has indicated, unlike female athletes, most male athletes are able to meet their recommendations.[6-11]

Calcium, like iron, is an important mineral and a major component of the human skeleton. It plays a significant role in neural transmission, blood coagulation, and other cellular functions.[12] Research has revealed that athletes between the age of 19 to 25 years are prone to having calcium deficiency due to a decreased intake of calcium in their diet, i.e., less than 800 mg /d.[11,13-14]

Cerebral Palsy (CP) is a group of neuromuscular conditions caused by damage to the neurons in the brain that control and coordinate muscle tone, reflexes, and action. These disorders might be unilateral or bilateral, associated with spasticity, athetosis, rigidity, or ataxia, commonly referred to by medical classification, or by the areas in which the body is affected, called functional classification.[15-19] CP occurs either during the prenatal (premature, maternal illness, or blood incompatibilities), natal (trauma), and postnatal (infections, poisoning, malnutrition) stage of life.

Athletes with CP who participate in athletic performances are frequently classified functionally. There are eight classifications ranging from Class I (severe involvement in all four limbs, limited trunk control, poor functional strength in upper extremities — in need of electric wheelchair) to Class VIII (minimally affected hemiplegic, with or without minimal coordination problems, able to run and jump freely with a good balance).[16,19]

Few comprehensive studies address the nutritional status of children with CP.[19-29] Results of these studies indicate that children with CP have low intake of calories,[19,21,24-26] calcium,[19,22,24-26] iron,[19,22-25,27-29] vitamin C,[19,28] vitamin A,[27] and thiamin.[19,24] The increased susceptibility to nutrient deficiencies is attributed to low nutritional intake and drug nutrient interaction, in addition to type and severity of physical disability. Very limited research has been conducted on adults with CP.[30]

The dietary needs of athletes are not significantly different from those recommended for all healthy individuals. Though there are no specific Recommended Dietary Allowances and no minimum requirements for athletes in training, the distribution of nutrients composing the athlete's diet should be about 15% protein, 25 to 30% fat, and 55 to 60% carbohydrate.[31]

Diet is an integral part of athletic training and it is essential that both normal and disabled athletes are aware of the different nutrients present in foods and the contributions made by various nutrients to athletic performance.[32-35] With increased participation of disabled athletes in local, state, and international competitions, it is essential that greater emphasis be stressed in the dissemination of nutrition education. Thus, the objective of the study is to investigate the dietary intake of calcium and iron in athletes with cerebral palsy (CP) and athletes who are vision impaired (VI).

II. MATERIALS AND METHODS

One hundred and eight athletes, throughout the United States with CP or who were VI, attended a 5 d training camp at Ball State University in the summer of 1992. Athletes were recruited by word of mouth and through their coaches. Thirty-three athletes, 19 (3 females and 16 males) with CP and 14 (1 female and 13 males) VI athletes volunteered in this research. These athletes were considered "elite" because they were the best in their segment of the population and were selected to attend the Special Olympics in Barcelona, Spain in September of 1992.

Part I of the study involved gathering anthropometric measurements (height and weight), which were obtained by an athletic trainer. A personal and general information questionnaire, which inquired about the type of disability, classification of the disability, age, sex, education level, use of medication, number of years an athlete was involved in competitive athletics, and the type of competition participated in by an athlete, was collected. Nutrition students were available for athletes who needed assistance in filling out the questionnaire (i.e. either writing or reading). These forms were then reviewed with each athlete to reconfirm that accurate information was documented.

In Part II of the study athletes were requested to maintain their normal dietary habits and were instructed to record dietary intakes for 3 d. Since the athletes were not in their home environment and their eating habits were different than in the training camp, athletes took the 3 d diet forms to their respective homes and mailed them upon completion. The athletes were contacted weekly by telephone, by a registered dietitian, to answer any questions that the athletes had. Dietary data were obtained from 3 d (2 weekdays, 1 weekend day) of weighed food intakes. The diets were analyzed using the West Diet Program (version 1; 1990. ESHA Research and West Publishing Company, St. Paul, Minneapolis), Calcium and iron intakes were compared with the Recommended Dietary Allowances.[36] The statistical analysis was done using release 4.1 of SPSS, the statistical package for the social science, to compute the mean calcium and iron intake over the 3 d, and the percentage of calcium and iron coming from the different food groups. Experimental procedures were in accord with Ball State University ethical standards of the Institutional Committee on Investigations Involving Human Subjects.

III. RESULTS AND DISCUSSION

Nineteen athletes with CP (8 track, 9 field and 2 swimming) and 14 VI athletes (7 track, 4 field, and 3 swimming) participated in this research. The mean subject age was 27 ± 6.4 (SD) years, mean height was 67.5 ± 5.0 (SD) inches and mean weight was 153 ± 35.1 (SD) lbs. All the athletes had some kind of formal education, 88%

TABLE 1   Percent of Calcium Contributed by
the Different Food Groups from
the Three Day Dietary Intake of
Athletes with VI and CP

Dis.[1]	Milk & Dairy	Bread & Grain	Fruit	Veg.	Meat & Alter.	Misc.[2]
VI	41.09	31.08	3.83	6.44	11.03	5.81
CP	44.19	22.41	3.96	6.15	9.52	13.45

[1] Disability of the athletes: VI = vision impaired, CP = cerebral palsy.
[2] Miscellaneous food group comprises calcium found in mixed foods.

TABLE 2   Percent of Iron Contributed by the
Different Food Groups from the
Three Day Dietary Intake of
Athletes with VI and CP

Dis.[1]	Milk & Dairy	Bread & Grain	Fruit	Veg.	Meat & Alter.	Misc.[2]
VI	2.38	46.21	4.62	12.63	27.01	7.16
CP	2.42	47.11	8.62	10.36	21.05	9.45

[1] Disability of the athletes: VI = vision impaired, CP = cerebral palsy.
[2] Miscellaneous food group comprises iron found in mixed foods.

had college while 22% had high school education. Mean number of years that CP and VI athletes had participated in competitive events was 8 ± 4.8 years. Thirty-three athletes (100%) participated regularly in athletic activities. Of the 32 athletes who were classified, 6 were non-ambulatory (19%). None of the subjects were on any kind of vitamin, mineral, or protein supplement. During the study, three subjects were on medication prescribed by their respective physicians.

Complete 3-d dietary data were obtained from all the participants. According to the 1989 RDA, an adult male or female between the age of 25 to 50 years should receive 800 mg of calcium/d. In this study, 64% VI and 53% CP athletes consumed an average of less than 800 mg calcium/d. Similar findings were reported in other studies that looked at children and adults with CP.[20,22,24,25,30] Three VI athletes approached the recommendation (range of 713 to 750 mg calcium/d). As shown in Table I, milk and dairy products provided the highest amount of calcium for all subjects (41.09% for VI and 44.19% for CP). Unlike the female VI athlete who had an average intake of 919 mg of calcium/d, the three female CP athletes did not meet

**TABLE 3. Percent of Athletes that Met the RDA
for Calcium and Iron**

Type of Disability	RDA for Calcium	RDA for Iron
Vision Impaired	36	93
Cerebral Palsy	51	63

the recommended intake for calcium. Their average intake of calcium was 446, 532, and 638 mg of calcium/day respectively. Evidence from previous research has also associated a low intake of calcium to be common among female athletes.[9,14,37] In the current study, if more female athletes had participated, it may have been possible to find a higher percentage of them not meeting the RDA for calcium.

Table 2 shows the two categories of athletes, the percent of iron obtained from the 3-d dietary intake, and the food groups that provide the various amounts of iron. From the diets of VI and CP athletes, an average of 20.8 mg of iron/d and 15.4 mg of iron/d respectively, were contributed through milk and dairy products, breads and enriched grains, fruits, vegetables, meat and meat alternatives, and miscellaneous foods. The RDA of iron for males is 10 mg/d (25 to 50 years), and for females 15 mg/d (25 to 50 years). Some of the reasons why the RDA is higher for females than males are because of the loss of iron through menstruation, higher incidence of iron deficiency anemia, and decreased intake of calories among women.

Ninety-three percent of the VI and 63% of the CP athletes met the RDA for iron (Table 3). As observed in Table 2, on an average, breads and enriched grains (VI-46.21%, CP-47.11%) were the major contributors of iron, followed by meat and meat alternatives (VI-27.01%, CP-21.05%). Among the VI athletes, only the female subject had low dietary iron (12 mg/d). Four males and all the female CP athletes failed to meet the RDA. The female athletes had a mean intake of 11 mg of iron/d. Keith et al.[38] found that normal female cyclists between the age of 19 to 34 years failed to consume less than 67% of the RDA for iron. Athletes in their study had low intake of red meats and legumes. Similar observations have also been reported by Short and Short[9] and others.[10,37,39]

Research has revealed that an average American diet provides 6 to 7 mg of iron per 1000 calories.[40] The low intake of iron among CP and VI athletes in this study could be attributed to low calorie consumption brought about by their concern about weight gain. None of the athletes with decreased dietary iron had any eating difficulties.

In the future, with increased participation of disabled athletes in various competitions, it is of utmost importance that the nutritional status of these athletes be closely monitored. Dietitians who will be working with these athletes need to be aware of the dietary problems, and appropriate nutrition education must be made available to alleviate the onset of chronic diseases in this population. Dietary counseling must be made available for these athletes, particularly with respect to the type of foods eaten daily, the nutritive value of these foods, and their importance in athletic performance.

Calcium and iron are one of the many nutrients that is frequently lacking in the diet of athletes. Perhaps the reason why athletes have low intake of iron and calcium is because of the hectic training schedules. This limitation in time prevents them from eating three well balanced meals per day. Instead, they rely heavily on snacking and eating on the run with foods that are less nutrient dense.

Nutrition educators, health professionals, coaches, and care givers should encourage CP and VI athletes to consume a varied diet that provides calcium and iron. Lean meats, including beef, pork, lamb, veal, and poultry are the best sources of bioavailable iron. Whole grains, fruits and vegetables, and other plant foods contain considerable amounts of iron, but are poorly absorbed in the absence of enhancing factors. To obtain adequate calcium, dairy products such as lowfat or nonfat milk, yogurt, cheese, broccoli, and tofu could be eaten.

In conclusion, this study demonstrated that CP and VI athletes, like normal athletes, are at risk of having iron or calcium deficiency. Female athletes are at a greater risk for both iron and calcium deficiency. The poor dietary habits of athletes with CP and VI could be corrected by nutrition education made available through training camps, colleges, and universities at both the local and national level.

ACKNOWLEDGMENT

This research was supported by United Cerebral Palsy of Central Indiana, Inc.

REFERENCES

1. Gardner, G.W., Edgerton, U.R., Senewiratne, B., Physical work capacity and metabolic stress in subjects with iron deficiency anemia, *Am. J. Clin. Nutr.*, 30, 910, 1977.
2. Viteri, F.E., Torun, B., Anemia and physical capacity, *Clin., Haematol.*, 3, 609, 1974.
3. Davies, K.J.A., Magurie, J.J., Brooks, G.A., Muscle mitochondrial biogenetics, oxygen supply, and work capacity during dietary iron deficiency and repletion, *Am. J. Physiol.*, 242, E418, 1982.
4. Pate, R.R., Magurie, M., Wyk, J.V., Dietary iron supplementation in women athletes, *Phys. Sportsmed.*, 7, 81, 1979.
5. Rowland, T.W., Iron deficiency in the young athlete, *Pediatr. Clin. North. Am.*, 37, 1153, 1990.
6. Risser, W.L., Lee, E.J. Poindexter, H.B., Iron deficiency in female athletes: its prevalence and impact on performance, *Med. Sci. Sports Exercise*, 20, 116, 1988.
7. Frederickson, L.A., Puhl, J.L., Runyan, W.S., Effects of training on indices of iron status of young female cross-country runners, *Med. Sci. Sports Exercise*, 15, 271, 1983.
8. Weaver, C.M., Rajaram, S., Exercise and iron status, *J. Nutr.*, 122, 782, 1992.
9. Short, S.H., Short, W.R., Four-year study of university athletes dietary intake, *J. Am. Diet. Assoc.*, 82, 632, 1983.
10. Ellsworth, N.M., Hewitt, B.F., Haskell, W.L., Nutrient intake of elite male and female nordic skiers, *Phys. Sport Med.*, 13, 84, 1985.
11. Snyder, A.C., Schulz, L.O., Foster, C., Voluntary consumption of a carbohydrate supplement by elite speed skaters, *J. Am. Diet. Assoc.*, 89, 1125, 1989.
12. Whitney, E.N., Rolfes, S.R., *Understanding Nutrition*, 6th ed., West Publishing, Minneapolis, 1993, chap. 11.
13. Myburgh, K.H., Grobler, N., Noakes, T.D., Factors associated with shin soreness in athletes, *Phys. Sports Med.*, 16, 129, 1988.
14. Barr, S.I., Realationship of eating attitudes to anthropometric variables and dietary intakes of female collegiate swimmers, *J. Am. Diet. Assoc.*, 91, 976, 1991.
15. Seskin, L., Nutrition and the cerebral palsied child, *Jr. Dent. Guid Council Handicap*, 14, 2, 1975.

16. Sherrill, C., Mushett, C., Jomes, J.A., Cerebral palsy and the CP athlete, in *Training Guide to Cerebral Palsy Sports*, 3rd ed., Jones, J.A., Ed., Human Kinetics Books, Champaign, Illinois, 1988, 9.

17. Mecham, M.J., *Cerebral Palsy*, 1st ed., Pro-Ed, Austin, Texas, 1986, chap. 1.

18. Palmer, S., Cerebral palsy, in *Pediatric Nutrition in Developmental Disorders*, 1st ed., Palmer, S., Ekvall, S., Eds., Charles C Thomas, Illinois, 1978, chap. 4.

19. Phelps, W.M., Dietary requirements in cerebral palsy, *J. Am. Diet. Assoc.*, 27, 869, 1950.

20. Eddy, T.P., Nicholson, A.L., Wheeler, E.F., Energy expenditures and dietary intakes in cerebral palsy, *Dev. Med. Child Neurol.*, 7, 377, 1965.

21. Evers, S., Munoz, M.A., Vanderkooy, P., Jackson, S., Lawton, M.S., Nutrition rehabilitation of the developmentally disabled residents in a long-term-care facility, *J. Am. Diet. Assoc.*, 91, 471, 1991.

22. Thommessen, M., Riis, G., Kase, B.F., Larsen, S., Heiberg, A., Energy and nutrient intake of disabled children: do feeding problems make a difference?, *J. Am. Diet. Assoc.*, 91, 1522, 1991.

23. Karle, I.P., Bleiler, R.E., Ohlson, M.A., Nutritional status of cerebral-palsied children, *J. Am. Diet. Assoc.*, 38, 22, 1961.

24. Hammond, M.I., Lewis, M.N., Johnson, E.W., A nutritional study of cerebral palsied children, *J. Am. Diet. Assoc.*, 49, 196, 1966.

25. Berg, K., Effect of physical activation and of improved nutrition on the body composition of school children with cerebral palsy, *Acta P. Diat. Scand.*, 204, 53, 1970.

26. Aliakbari, J., Webb, Y., Nutrient intakes of cerebral palsied children, *J. Am. Diet. Assoc.*, 86, 144, 1986.

27. Berg, K., Isaksson, B., Body composition and nutrition of school children with cerebral palsy, *Acta P. Diat. Scand.*, 204, 41, 1970.

28. Gouge, A.L., Ekvall, S.W., Diets of handicapped children: physical, psychological, and socioeconomic correlations, *Am. J. Ment. Defic*, 80, 1975.

29. Berg, K., Nutrition of children with reduced physical activity due to cerebral palsy, *Nutr. Diet.*, 19, 12, 1973.

30. Ferrang, T.M., Johnson, R.K., Ferrara, M.S., Dietary and anthropometric assessment of adults with cerebral palsy, *J. Am. Diet. Assoc.*, 92, 1083, 1992.

31. Marcus, J.B., *Sports and Cardiovascular Nutritionists (SCAN)*, The American Dietetic Association, Chicago, Illinois, 1986, 50.

32. Smith, M., Nutrition and physical fitness and athletic performance for adults, *J. Am. Diet. Assoc.*, 87, 934, 1987.

33. O'Neal, F.T., Hankinson-Hynak, M.T., Gorman, J., Research and current topics in sports nutrition, *J. Am. Diet. Assoc.*, 86, 1007, 1986.

34. Hoffman, C.J., Coleman, E., An eating plan and update on recommended dietary practices for the endurance athlete, *J. Am. Diet. Assoc.*, 91, 325, 1991.

35. Leaf, A., Frisa, K.B., Eating for health or athletic performance?, *Am. J. Clin. Nutr.* 49, 1066, 1989.

36. Food and Nutrition Board, *Recommended Dietary Allowances*, 10, National Academy of Sciences, Washington, D.C., 1989, chaps. 9, 10.

37. Perron, M., Endres, J., Knowledge, attitudes, and dietary practices of female athletes, *J. Am. Diet. Assoc.*, 85, 573, 1985.

38. Keith, R.E., O'Keeffe, K.A., Alt, L.A., Dietary status of trained female cyclists, *J. Am. Diet. Assoc.*, 89, 1620, 1989.

39. Risser, W.L., Lee, E.J., Poindexter, H.B., West, M.S., Pivarnik, J.M., Risser, J.M., Hickson, J.F., Iron deficiency in female athletes: its prevalence and impact on performance, *Med. Sci. Sports Exercise*, 20, 116, 1988.

40. Finch, C.A., Huebers, H., Perspectives in iron metabolism, *N. Engl. J. Med.*, 306, 1520, 1982.

Chapter **10**

DIETARY CALCIUM AND THE BIOAVAILABILITY OF IRON IN PHYSICALLY ACTIVE ADULTS

Yibo Zhu-Wood
Constance V. Kies

CONTENTS

I. INTRODUCTION

The nutritional virtue of meat is its iron content and availability. Most dietary iron is poorly absorbed but the iron in meat is not only relatively well absorbed, it appears to assist in the absorption of iron from other foods. Red meats are by far the richest source of heme iron, the form most easily and effectively absorbed across the intestinal mucosa of humans. High meat-containing diets have been demonstrated to increase urinary and bone losses of calcium thus increasing the risk of developing osteoporosis. It would seem logical, therefore, to make sure that meat-containing diets also contain adequate amounts of calcium, or to enrich these diets with a calcium supplement. However, calcium may inhibit the absorption of nonheme iron by decreasing stomach and intestinal acidity. Heme iron absorption is less affected than nonheme iron by gastrointestinal track pH. Whether or not heme iron absorption is affected by dietary calcium has not been extensively investigated.

The most common nutritional deficiencies currently affecting adult women involve iron and calcium. The daily use of a calcium supplement by women in their childbearing years and beyond is believed to reduce the risk of postmenopausal osteoporosis. Iron supplementation is also widely recommended in adult women, particularly when iron requirements are increased because of pregnancy, lactation, and/or endurance training. However, research and clinical observations suggest that iron absorption is adversely affected by other minerals, such as calcium,[1] because calcium supplementation reduces the absorption of dietary iron.

II. DIETARY IRON ABSORPTION

Iron homeostasis is maintained, primarily, by the body adjusting iron absorption to its needs. Iron absorption is affected by age, iron status, and state of health, conditions within the gastrointestinal tract, the amount and chemical form of the ingested iron, and the amounts and proportions of various other components of the diet, both organic and inorganic.

Because of the separate pathways into intestinal mucosal cells, dietary iron can be considered as being composed of two distinct pools: a heme iron pool and a nonheme iron pool.[2-5] Heme provides 10 to 15 percent of the food iron consumed in industrialized countries.[6] Heme iron is highly available and may account for as much as one-fourth of the iron absorbed from diets high in meat content.[7] Heme iron absorption is relatively unaffected by the combination of food items, and only slightly influenced by the individual's iron status.

Nonheme iron, on the other hand, is found in cereals, fruits, vegetables, and dairy products. It comprises the major source of dietary iron. In developing countries, it is frequently the only source of dietary iron.[8] The absorption of nonheme iron is highly variable depending on the nature of the meal. Radioisotope studies of single meals have demonstrated that meal composition has a major impact on determining how much of the nonheme iron is absorbed. Using the extrinsic-tag method absorption, studies were performed in rats and humans in order to compare the effects of known dietary enhancers (ascorbic acid and meat) and inhibitors (tea and bran) on nonheme iron absorption.[9] The results showed that meat and tea had a marked effect on the absorption of nonheme iron in humans, but did not influence its absorption in rats. Depending upon the balance between enhancers and inhibitors, the percentage of nonheme iron absorption may range from 1 to 40% and can vary as much as 20-fold in the same individual.[10,11]

Iron absorption from diets consisting almost entirely of cereals may be as low as 1 to 2%, whereas in diets containing large quantities of meat, fish, or poultry, iron absorption may approach 20 to 25%.[12] Absorption of nonheme iron also is significantly affected by the individual's iron status. As the amount of iron storage in the body increases, there is a progressive decrease in the intestinal absorption of nonheme iron and, to a lesser extent, of heme iron. Conversely, a decrease in body iron is associated with an increase in iron absorption.[13]

Although knowledge of the mechanisms by which food components influence nonheme iron absorption is far from complete, it is possible to identify a number of dietary factors that have a significant effect.

A. ANIMAL TISSUES

Population studies regarding iron status have identified meat as the important dietary factor.[14] Meat, fish, and poultry improve iron absorption by providing highly available heme, as well as by increasing nonheme iron absorption two- to fourfold. When iron bioavailability of veal muscle was tested with corn or black beans, the absorption of the veal muscle iron was slightly decreased, but the vegetable iron absorption was almost doubled.[15] The mechanism involved in the enhancement of nonheme iron absorption by heme iron has not been well defined.

B. ASCORBIC ACID

Ascorbic acid as an enhancer of nonheme iron absorption has been studied in great detail. Relatively small quantities, for example, a glass of orange juice containing 40 to 50 mg ascorbic acid with a breakfast of bread, egg, and tea or coffee, markedly increased iron absorption from 3.7 to 10.4%.[16]

The increase in absorption of nonheme iron has been found to be directly proportional to the quantity of ascorbic acid present, and this effect has been seen both with naturally occurring and synthetic ascorbic acid.[17] However, ascorbic acid may undergo oxidative degradation during food processing or storage. The absorption of nonheme iron was significantly higher in 20 different Western-type vegetarian lunch and dinner meals high in ascorbic acid content when analyzed immediately following preparation, than in similar type meals that were warmed at 75°C for 4 h.[18] The ascorbic acid content decreased after warming, as did nonheme iron absorption. The enhancer effect of ascorbic acid is luminal and occurs only when the sources of ascorbic acid and iron are taken together. In one study, when 500 mg of ascorbic acid was added to the meal, absorption increased about sixfold, whereas the same 500 mg had little effect when taken 4 to 8 h prior to the meal.[19]

C. TEA AND COFFEE

Tea and coffee are two commonly consumed beverages that can inhibit iron absorption. Disler et al.[20,21] demonstrated that iron absorption from a meal was reduced by as much as 87% when tea was included. Fairweather et al.[22] conducted a study to examine the effect of tea on iron metabolism in weanling rats. Study rats were fed a semisynthetic diet containing normal (38 μg/g) or low (9 μg/g) levels of iron for 28 d. They were given water or tea infusion (20 g leaves/1 cup of water) to drink. At the end of the study period, all rats given the low iron diet were severely anemic, and those given tea showed a greater degree of iron depletion. However, the influence of green tea on iron absorption has not yet been recognized.[23]

Coffee's effect on iron absorption has not been studied in detail. However, dual isotope studies were performed in iron-replete human subjects to evaluate the effect of coffee on nonheme iron absorption.[24] Results showed that when a cup of drip coffee or instant coffee was ingested with a meal composed of semipurified ingredients, iron absorption was reduced from 5.88% to 1.64 and 0.94%, respectively. When the strength of the instant coffee was doubled, the percentage of iron absorption fell from 0.94 to 0.53%. The same degree of inhibition was found when coffee was taken up to 1 h after a meal. However, no decrease in iron absorption occurred when coffee was consumed 1 h before a meal. These studies showed that coffee inhibited iron absorption in a concentration-dependent fashion. Tea and coffee are thought to influence iron absorption at a luminal level by the formation of insoluble iron tannates.[20,24]

D. CALCIUM

Animal studies have shown that calcium interferes with the absorption of iron.[25] Calcium had an inhibitory effect on iron absorption in rats and mice fed an iron-replete diet. Rats and mice also developed iron deficiency anemia when increasing amounts of calcium were added to their diet.[13] It has been suggested that calcium probably either induces iron deficiency by delaying the uptake of iron into the intestinal mucosal cells, or by influencing the further transfer of iron from these cells into the circulation.[13]

Human studies have been done on the effect of calcium on iron absorption.[13] One study involved 34 healthy volunteers in which the extrinsic-tag technique was used to label nonheme iron. The administration of 180 mg of labeled calcium to a semisynthetic meal containing meat reduced iron absorption by 50%. Meals without meat reduced iron absorption by 70%.[26] Similar results were seen in another study reported by Cook et al.[1] The influence of calcium supplements on the absorption of dietary nonheme iron was evaluated in 61 normal, volunteer subjects using a double radioisotope technique. The results suggested that taking regular calcium supplements with meals makes it more difficult for women to meet their daily iron requirement.[1] Using the extrinsic-tag technique to label the nonheme iron in a composite hamburger meal, Hallberg and Rossander[27] found that serving the meal with milk (250 ml containing 273 mg Ca) instead of water reduced the absorption of iron by 14%. In the same laboratory,[28] calcium also was found to have a direct, dose-related, inhibiting effect on iron absorption. The ingestion of 300 mg of calcium with an experimental meal, which contained no known enhancers or inhibitors of iron absorption, significantly reduced iron absorption by 50 to 60%.

These findings, that calcium directly inhibits iron absorption, have important nutritional implications. Diets in both developing and industrialized countries often contain only marginal amounts of the bioavailable iron and calcium, particularly in regard to premenopausal women.[28] Since high calcium intakes, especially with main meals, will impair iron absorption, use of calcium supplements or high calcium foods to improve calcium status might impair iron status. Although the mechanism for the direct effect of calcium on iron absorption is unknown, changes in intestinal PH are thought to be involved.[1]

III. BEEF HEME IRON/CALCIUM CARBONATE INTERACTION AFFECTING NUTRITIONAL STATUS OF PHYSICALLY ACTIVE ADULTS

Some groups of athletes should be added to the list of anemia "at risk" populations. It is obvious that physical performance, endurance capacity, and resistance to fatigue in humans are dependent upon many different factors.[29] Based upon the results of several surveys, 50 to 80% of all females that seriously participate in running-type aerobic exercise, and 5 to 30% of all males undertaking similar exercise programs, develop an iron-deficiency anemia, called runner's anemia. Among many possible causes which may bring about the development of sports anemia, the most commonly recognized are poor dietary choices and destruction of red blood cells during physical exercise.[29] Due to the false or erroneous interpretation of nutritional messages, many athletes have reduced consumption of beef and other meats, which are important sources of heme iron, in response to concern over the connection between dietary fat and heart disease. Athletes and very active women may also ingest less than adequate amounts of highly available iron due to extreme emphasis on carbonate intake. In results presented at a national American Dietetic Association meeting, female runners who practiced red meat eating had a lower incidence of anemia than did those who avoided eating red meat no matter whether or not they were taking iron supplements.

Osteoporosis is four times more prevalent and severe in women than in men. It becomes more common, and its onset is more rapid in women after menopause. Although researchers have not found a consistent relationship between the incidence of osteoporosis and calcium intake, low calcium intake is a suspected risk factor. Female marathon runners tend to develop osteoporosis, called brittle bone disease, at ages far younger than those of the general population. Higher incidence occurs in those who have stopped menstruating, or who menstruate only occasionally in association with strenuous training. The primary causes of bone loss in these physically active young women are certainly, in part, due to a deficiency of estrogen levels

TABLE 1   Contents of Iron and Calcium (mg/serving)
in Different Kinds of Food

Food Items	Total Iron	Calcium	Heme Iron*
		Contents (mg/serving)	
Oreo cookies		0.25	2.60
Carrots		0.11	5.31
Beef salami	0.62	1.00	4.00
Whole wheat bread		0.39	45.00
Apple juice		0.41	21.57
Hot chocolate milk		0.27	62.41
Raisins		0.82	9.62
Green beans		1.20	44.18
Peaches		0.50	12.45
Orange juice		0.83	37.60
Breakfast granola bar		0.59	16.99
Beef frankfurter	0.71	1.16	5.60
Turkey	0.27	0.90	2.18
Tuna	0.40	1.20	3.13
Grape juice		0.41	29.07
Potato chips		0.35	7.00
Rice		1.00	5.32
Pudding		0.46	48.36

*   Data for heme iron calculated from Monson et al., 1978[36] and Schrecker et al., 1982.[37]

because of low body fat stores and physical stress. Dietary lack of calcium is probably a contributing factor as well. Consequently, women athletes are being encouraged to increase their dietary calcium. Calcium carbonate is the most commonly used supplemental calcium, but it reduces the acidity in the gastrointestinal tract which adversely affects the absorption of nonheme iron.

In an attempt to further identify the relationship between calcium intake and iron absorption, a human study was conducted in our laboratory to examine the effects on iron status of physically active young women consuming laboratory diets containing high and low amounts of heme iron with and without calcium carbonate supplementation. Thirteen adult female subjects participated in this 56-d study, which was divided into four experimental periods of 14 d each. Beef was used as the dietary source of heme iron and was fed at 165 g/subject/day during the high heme iron periods. During the low heme iron periods, 165 g of turkey breast and tuna fish were substituted for the beef. During the low calcium periods, the ordinary foods composing the basal diet supplied 400 mg of calcium. During the high calcium periods, 800 mg of calcium carbonate supplements divided among the three daily meals were fed to each subject each day, in addition to the 400 mg of calcium supplied by the food. The contents (mg/serving) of iron and calcium in different kinds food during the study are given in Table 1.

As shown in Table 2, mean iron intakes from the turkey/tuna diet with calcium supplementation was 12.24 mg/d, the turkey/tuna diet without calcium supplementation was 11.84 mg/d, the beef diet with calcium supplementation was 13.78 mg/d,

TABLE 2 **Iron Utilization of Subjects Fed Diets Varied in Heme Iron and Calcium**

Parameter	Mean Values While Received*			
	T + Ca	T	B + Ca	B
Fe intake (mg/d)	12.24 b	11.84 c	13.78 a	12.26 b
Fecal excretion (mg/d)	11.88 b	10.83 c	12.45 a	11.11 c
Urinary excretion (mg/d)	0.74 a	0.65 ab	0.68 a	0.59 b
Fe balance (mg/d)	–0.40 c	0.37 b	0.65 ab	0.98 a
Apparent Fe absorption %	2.78 c	8.53 b	9.65 b	12.38

* Mean values with no repeated letter superscripts are significantly different from one another ($p < 0.05$).

and the beef diet without calcium supplementation was 12.68 mg/d. Iron intake was slightly higher with calcium supplementation than without calcium supplementation in both the beef and turkey diet because each supplemental calcium tablet contained 0.4 mg of iron, and three tablets per day were fed during calcium supplementation periods.

Fecal iron excretions were significantly affected by the heme iron levels and calcium levels designed in the study ($p < 0.05$ and 0.01, respectively). More iron was lost in feces when calcium supplements were used with the feeding of the beef and turkey/tuna than without calcium supplementation. According to Gosztonyi,[30] total iron in feces of normal human adults can reach 6 to 16 mg/d depending upon the amount of iron ingested. Statistic tests showed that feeding the beef diet resulted in excretion of more iron than when the turkey diet was fed ($p < 0.05$). This is not surprising since iron intakes were higher when the beef diet was fed.

Urinary iron losses were not significantly affected by the heme iron intake levels, but were significantly ($p < 0.05$) affected by calcium intake. Mean iron losses in urine of subjects when consuming the turkey/tuna and beef diets without calcium supplementations were 0.65 and 0.59 mg/d, respectively, lower than with additional calcium supplements, 0.74 and 0.68 mg/d respectively ($p < 0.01$).

Iron balances of subjects consuming four different combinations of the test diet were calculated by adding fecal and urinary iron losses and subtracting these losses from iron intakes. Both intake levels of heme iron and calcium significantly ($p < 0.01$) affected the iron balances. The mean iron balance was negative with feeding of the turkey diet with calcium supplements, –0.40 mg/d. Greatest apparent iron retention occurred with feeding of the beef diet without calcium supplementation, 0.98 mg/d. Iron retentions of subjects were higher when the beef-containing diets were fed than when the turkey/tuna diets were given. Apparent absorption of iron was calculated by subtracting fecal losses from intakes, dividing by intakes and multiplying by 100. The percentage of apparent iron absorption was significantly ($p < 0.05$) higher when

TABLE 3   Serum Iron Status of Subjects Fed Diets Varied in Heme Iron and Calcium

Parameter	Mean Values While Receiving*				
	pre-	T + Ca	T	B + Ca	B
Total iron (µg/ml)	100.1 a	97.1 ab	94.4 b	82.2 c	85.5
Iron % saturation	31.2 a	33.2 a	33.4 a	29.5 a	30.4
IBC	318.3 a	290.0 b	281.9 c	293.0 b	279.5 bc
Hb (g)	12.9 a	13.2 a	13.2 a	13.3 a	13.2 a
HCT %	37.6 a	37.7 a	37.8 a	37.9 a	37.4 a
MCV (fL)	89.9 a	91.3 a	91.5 a	91.4 a	91.5 a
MCH (pg)	30.3 b	32.1 a	31.9 a	32.0 a	32.2 a
MCHC (g/dL)	34.1 b	35.1 a	35.0 a	35.0 a	35.1 a

Note: IBC = Iron binding capacity, Hct = Volume packed red cells, MCV = Mean corpuscular volume, MCH = Mean corpuscular hemoglobin, MCHC = Mean corpuscular hemoglobin concentration.

* Mean values with no repeated letter superscript are significantly different from one another ($p < 0.05$).

the beef diet was fed without calcium supplement than when the beef diet was fed with calcium supplements. Similar directional responses occurred with feeding of the turkey/tuna diet with and without calcium supplementations.

Our results indicated that beef, as a red meat, improved iron absorption by providing higher amounts of bioavailable heme iron (62% of total iron) than white-meat turkey, which mainly contains nonheme iron (70% of total iron). Our results also showed that calcium acts as an inhibiting factor on nonheme iron absorption. The subjects' apparent iron absorption significantly ($p < 0.05$) decreased during the calcium carbonate supplementation period.

Calcium carbonate is one of the most commonly used dietary supplemental calciums.[25] It reduces the acidity of the gastrointestinal tract and, although heme iron absorption is relatively unaffected by the combination of food items, the absorbability of nonheme iron is adversely affected by a decrease in acidity of the stomach and upper intestinal tract. Thus, for individuals using calcium carbonate as a nutritional supplement, it is preferable to use them in combination with heme-rich diets rather than with diets which are poorly supplied with heme iron.

As shown in Table 3, mean hemoglobin, serum iron, total iron binding capacity, serum iron saturation (%), and hematocrit (HCT) levels of the subjects during the study were in the normal range.

Because of the relatively short length of experimental periods used in this study, it is not surprising that few significant differences in these parameters of iron status were found which could be related to dietary treatment. The significantly lower total blood serum iron levels observed during both beef-feeding periods, in comparison to

TABLE 4   Calcium (Ca) Utilization of
Subjects Fed Diets Varied in
Heme Iron and Calcium

Parameter	Mean Values While Receiving*			
	T + Ca	T	B + Ca	B
Ca intake (mg/d)	1226 a	441 b	1240 a	459 b
Fecal Ca (mg/d)	844 a	295 b	831 a	307 b
Urinary Ca (mg/d)	260 b	102 c	304.6 a	102 c
Ca balance (mg/d)	121 a	42.9 b	101 a	50.4 b
Apparent Ca absorption %	31.1 a	33.0 a	32.7 a	33.1 a

*   Mean values with no repeated letter superscripts are
significantly different from one another ($p < 0.05$).

values during the turkey/tuna periods, seem surprising considering the higher iron
balances achieved during the beef-feeding periods. However, these are concentrations in subjects following an over-night fast (approximately 10 h); hence, they do
not represent peak levels, but rather lowest levels. Since heme iron is absorbed, not
only more completely, but also more quickly than nonheme iron, peak and trough
levels may well have occurred more quickly with the feeding of the beef diets than
with the feeding of the turkey/tuna diets.

Results also showed that iron binding capacity values tended to be increased
with the feeding of calcium carbonate supplements, regardless of level of heme iron.
Under conditions of adequacy of dietary protein, which was the case in the present
study, iron binding capacity values change very rapidly with changes in iron status.
Thus, when iron absorption is inhibited (as was the situation with calcium carbonate
supplementation of the experimental diets), body mechanism respond quickly to
compensate by increasing iron binding capacity.[31]

As shown in Table 4, urinary calcium losses were significantly affected by both
intakes of heme iron and calcium ($p < 0.05$ and 0.01), respectively. Results indicated
that more calcium was excreted in urine during the high calcium period with the beef-
feeding diet than with turkey/tuna-feeding diet ($p < 0.05$). Similar results have been
shown in Robertson's study[32] indicating that high animal protein intake, especially
red meat, increases urinary excretion of calcium with increased urinary sulfur excretion. This reduces the ability of urine to inhibit the agglomeration of calcium oxalate
crystals, and provides a possible physiochemical explanation for renal stone formation.

Fecal calcium excretions were not significantly affected by heme iron levels but
were significantly ($p < 0.05$) affected by calcium levels. Similar results were seen in
calcium balances. Results indicated that use of calcium carbonate supplementation
resulted in improved calcium retention.

TABLE 5   Serum Calcium (Ca) and Phosphorous (P) Status of Subjects Fed Diets Varied in Heme Iron and Calcium

Parameter	Pre-	T + Ca	T	B + Ca	B
		Mean Values While Receiving*			
Blood serum Calcium (mg/dl)	9.4 a	9.4 a	9.4 a	9.2 c	9.3
Blood serum Phosphorus (mg/dl)	4.0 a	3.9 a	3.8 b	3.9 a	4.0

* Mean values with no repeated letter superscripts are significantly different from one another (*p* <0.05).

Statistical analysis showed that blood calcium levels were significantly (*p* <0.05) lower when the beef diet was fed, regardless of whether or not calcium supplementation was employed (Table 5). Although the blood calcium levels during the study were within the normal range, 8.5 to 10.6 mg/dl, urinary test results indicated a significant (*p* <0.05) increase in urinary calcium loss resulting with the feeding of the beef diet. The negative relationship between blood serum calcium concentrations and urinary calcium losses are readily seen and explained. Using calcium supplementation may also be necessary to maintain proper calcium status in those individuals consuming a high amount of meat, especially red meat.[33]

In conjunction with the 56 d human feeding study, a survey was conducted to learn more about the dietary practices of physically active young adults. Forty-three students at the University of Nebraska-Lincoln volunteered to fill out a questionnaire. The exercise level of these students varied from 5 to 10 min per day up to more than 1 h per day.

Mean subject information, dietary practices/self perceptions, and frequencies of various food intakes grouped by three levels of exercise are listed in Tables 6–8.

There were no significant differences in mean ages of male and female participants among three levels of exercise groups. Male participants were significantly (*p* <0.05) taller and heavier than female participants in medium and high levels of exercise groups. However, no significant differences of height and weight between male and female participants in low exercise group were found.

As shown on Tables 7 and 8, significant differences were found among groups in dietary practices/self-perception and in frequency of intake of various kinds of food. While turkey/chicken was indicated as being the best liked meat by all three groups, numerically, a lower percentage of the members of the high exercise group indicated that this was their favorite in comparison to the other groups. Conversely, more members of the high exercise group indicated that beef was their favorite meat than did members of the other groups (*p* <0.05). Considering the assumption that beef is "America's best liked meat", these figures were surprising. There were no vegetarians

TABLE 6   Subject Information Grouped by Three Levels of Exercise and Sex

		Low ex.	Med ex.	High ex.
Sex	M	2	6	5
	F	13	15	2
Age (year)		22.2	22.5	21.1
	M	25.5	22.2	20.8
	F	21.7	22.7	22.0
Ht (cm)		166.2	169.3	178.2
	M	176.2	178.9	186.6
	F	164.7	165.4	157.5
Wt (kg)		60.1	67.5	85.1
	M	69.3	86.1	97.1
	F	58.7	60.0	55.3

Note: Low ex. = less than 30 minutes of exercise per day.
Med. ex. = 30 to 60 minutes of exercise per day.
High ex. = more than 60 minutes of exercise per day.

in the high exercise group; however, there were three lacto-ovo vegetarians in the moderate exercise group and two lacto-ovo vegetarians in the low exercise group.

Estimations of weekly intakes of red and white meats also numerically suggested higher intakes of white meats than of red meats by members of the high and moderate exercise groups. The reverse result was found for the low exercise group. Total meat consumption appeared to be higher for the high exercise group than for the other two groups ($p < 0.05$). More surprising was the significant difference in estimation of serving sizes of meat as estimated by the three groups ($p < 0.05$). As exercise level decreased, so too did the estimation of serving size of meat. Since the high exercise group already estimated a larger number of servings of meat, the larger serving sizes would result in even greater amounts of meat consumption.

Estimated milk consumption was low for all three groups, estimated at approximately five cups per week, and did not vary among groups. These intakes would make it very difficult for these individuals to meet their calcium needs from bioavailable food sources.

According to the American Dietetic Association Statement,[34] when caloric expenditure increases, additional caloric consumption will usually provide adequate amounts of both macro- and micronutrients. But, some research has shown that many athletes develop food aversions and restrict their energy intakes in order to maintain a certain body size.[35] Such caloric restrictions might compromise mineral intakes and energy balances.

When asked whether or not they were currently on a special diet, 28.6% in the high exercise group said yes, 52.4% in the medium exercise group said yes, and only 13.3% in the low exercise group said that they were dieting ($p < 0.01$). For those on a special diet, 100% of those in the high exercise group, and 63.6% in the medium exercise group indicated losing weight as the chief reason for dieting. Only 9%

TABLE 7   Dietary Practices/Self-Perception Grouped by Three Levesl of Exercise (Mean %)*

Items Ex.	High Ex.	Med. Ex.	Low Ex.
Like the best[a]			
Beef	28.6 a	19.0 b	13.3 c
Turkey/chicken	42.9 a	61.9 b	66.7 b
Others[b]	28.6	19.0	20.0
Cholesterol screening			
Within a year	28.6	47.6	26.7
More than a year	71.4	52.4	73.3
Overall health situation			
Excellent	14.3	19.0	13.3
Good	71.4	61.9	66.7
Fair	14.3	19.0	13.3
On a special diet			
Yes	28.6 a	52.4 b	13.3 c
No	71.4	47.6	86.7
Weight gain	0.0	9.1	0.0
Weight loss	100.0 a	63.6 b	100.0 a
Sports Performance	0.0	27.3	0.0
Nutrition Suppl.			
Yes	28.6	28.6	20.0
No	71.4	71.4	80.0
Life satisfaction			
Most satisfied	71.4	71.4	80.0
Partially satisfied	14.3	23.8	20.0
Disappointed	14.3 a	4.8 b	0.0 c
Sports drink			
Yes	42.9	14.3	13.3
No	57.1	85.7	86.7

*   Mean values with no repeated superscripts are significantly different from one another, $p < 0.05$.

a   Among 17 women in high and medium levels of exercise group, 9 of them like turkey the best, 3 of them like beef the best, 2 like fish the best, and 3 are lacto-ova vegetarians.

b   Others includes seafood/fish or meat substitute.

indicated that gaining weight was their reason and 27.3% indicated enhancement of sports performances was the prime objective. The high percentage of participants involved in weight loss programs coupled with their high activity levels could very easily cause those athletes energy imbalances and a result in macronutrient as well as micronutrient intake insufficiency.

When asked how satisfied in general they were with their life, surprisingly, no one in low exercise level group indicated dissatisfaction compared to 14.3% in the high exercise group and 4.8% in the medium exercise group ($p < 0.01$). Stress and

TABLE 8 Frequency of Various Food Intakes Grouped by Three Levels of Exercise*

	High Ex.	Med. Ex.	Low Ex.
Red meat (times/wk)	2.86 a	2.00 b	3.07 a
White meat (times/wk)	3.71 a	2.81 b	2.60 b
Total meat (times/wk)	6.57 a	4.81 c	5.67 b
Serving size of meat (oz/serving)	3.71 a	3.33 b	3.13 b
Milk (times/wk)	5.00	4.76	5.13
Vit. C rich fruit/veg (times/wk)	4.59 a	4.81 a	3.37 b
Colored vegetables (times/wk)	4.21 a	3.55 b	3.10 b
Bread/roll/pasta (times/wk)	6.21 b	5.86 b	6.87 a

* Mean values with no repeated superscripts are significantly different from one another, $p < 0.05$.

depression may indeed be a considerable psychological factor contributing to food aversion, and even eating disorders, in athletes resulting in severe nutritional problems.[35]

Research has shown that women athletes easily develop iron deficiency and iron deficiency anemia with improper diets. Results in our study indicated that, among 43 participants, 17 (40%) were women involved in high and medium levels of exercise. The three vegetarians in the medium exercise level group were all women. Nine out of the 17 women (52%), participating in high and medium levels of exercise, consumed turkey/chicken as their major meat source. Only 18% consumed beef as their main meat source ($p < 0.01$). There were 4 out of 17 highly active women taking multi-vitamin and mineral supplements on a regular basis.

IV. CONCLUSIONS

Human study results show that there is a trade-off. To achieve the best iron absorption by eating a high heme iron diet without calcium supplementation results in a poor calcium balance. To achieve the best calcium absorption by eating a low heme iron diet with calcium supplementation results in a poor iron balance. Taking all of these results into consideration, the best overall outcome should occur with the feeding of a calcium supplemented, high heme iron diet. This diet promoted good (if not the best) apparent iron absorption and good (if not the best) calcium retention. Thus, for physically active women at risk for development of anemia and osteoporosis, the best advice might be to eat diets containing moderate amounts of red meat if they plan to meet their calcium needs via use of calcium supplements.

Although no definitive conclusions can be drawn from the survey study, some interesting tendencies, by exercise levels, can be seen.

The tendency to misunderstand nutritional messages in medium and high exercise level women may have caused them to favor eating white-meated turkey and chicken, jeopardizing their iron intake and increasing the potential of developing iron deficiency and iron deficiency anemia (a trend which has been observed in several studies nationwide). Even in well-conditioned athletes, one of the motivations for special dietary practices is losing weight, as opposed to sensible, balanced dietary practices in order to maintain ideal body weight and human well-being. And finally, with regard to the question of satisfaction with life, the more exercise the participants have, the more they realize how far they have to go to reach their goals and are consequently more susceptible to the psychological downsides of striving than are those people who either choose not to strive at all or choose to strive very little.

REFERENCES

1. Cook, J. D., Dassenko, S. A., and Whittaker, L. K., Calcium supplementation: effect on iron absorption, *Am. J. Clin. Nutr.,* 53, 106, 1991.
2. Cook, J. D., Layrisse, M., Martinez-Torres, C., Walker, R., and Monsen, E., Food iron absorption measured by an extrinsic tag, *J. Clin. Invest.,* 51, 805, 1972.
3. Bjorn-Rasmussen, E., Hallberg, L., and Walker, R. B., Food iron absorption in man. I. Isotopic exchange between food iron and inorganic iron salts added to food: studies on maize, wheat, and eggs, *Am. J. Clin. Nutr.,* 25, 317, 1972.
4. Bjorn-Rasmussen, E., Hallberg, L., and Walker, R. B., Food iron absorption in man. II. Isotopic exchange of iron between labelled foods and between a food and an iron salts, *Am. J. Clin. Nutr.,* 26, 1311, 1973.
5. Bjorn-Rasmussen, E., Hallberg, L., Magnusson, B., and Svanberg, B., Measurement of iron absorption from composite meal, *Am. J. Clin. Nutr.,* 29, 772, 1976.
6. Hallberg, L. and Rossander, L., Absorption of iron from Western-type lunch and dinner meals, *Am. J. Clin. Nutr.,* 35, 502, 1982a.
7. Bothwell, T. H., Baynes, R. D., MacFarlane, B. J., and MacPhail, A. P., Nutritional iron requirements and food iron absorption, *J. Intern. Med.,* 226, 357, 1989.
8. Hallberg, L., Iron absorption from some Asian meals containing contamination iron, *Am. J. Clin. Nutr.,* 37, 272, 1983.
9. Reedy, M. B. and Cook, J. D., Assessment of dietary determinants of nonheme-iron absorption in humans and rats, *Am. J. Clin. Nutr.,* 54, 723, 1991.
10. Hallberg, L., Bioavailability of dietary iron in man, *Annu. Rev. Nutr.,* 1, 123, 1981.
11. Hunt, J. R., Mullen, L. M., Lykken, G. I., and Gallagher, S. K., Ascorbic acid: effect on ongoing iron absorption and status in iron-depleted young women, *Am. J. Clin. Nutr.,* 51, 649, 1990.
12. FAO/WHO Expert Consultation, Requirements of vitamin A, iron, folate and vitamin B_{12}, Food and Agriculture Organization of the United Nations, Rome, 1988.
13. Mertz, W., *Trace Elements in Human and Animal Nutrition,* Academic Press, California, 1986.
14. Bothwell, T. H., Charlton, R. W., and Cook, J. D., *Iron Metabolism in Man,* Blackwell, London, 1979.
15. Layrisse, M., Cook, J. D., and Martinez, D., Food iron absorption: a comparison of vegetable and animal foods, *Blood,* 33, 430, 1969.
16. Hallberg, L., Brune, M., and Rossander, L., The role of vitamin C in iron absorption, *Int. J. Vitam. Nutr. Res. Suppl.,* 30, 103, 1989.
17. Lynch, S. R. and Cook, J. D., Interaction of vitamin C and iron, *Ann. N.Y. Acad. Sci.,* 355, 32, 1982.

18. Hallberg, L. and Rossander, L., Bioavailability of iron from Western-type whole meals, *Scand. J. Gastroenterol.,* 17, 151, 1982b.
19. Cook, J. D. and Monsen, E. R., Vitamin C, the common cold, and iron absorption, *Am. J. Clin. Nutr.,* 30, 235, 1977.
20. Disler, P. B., Lynch, S. R., Charlton, R. W., and Bothwell, T. H., The effect of tea on iron absorption, *Gut,* 16, 193, 1975.
21. Disler, P. B., Lynch, S. R., and Sayers, M. H., The mechanism of the inhibition of iron absorption by tea, *S. Afr. J. Med. Sci.,* 40, 109, 1975.
22. Fairweather, S. J., Piper, Z., and Moore, G. R., The effect of tea on iron and aluminum metabolism in the rat, *Br. J. Nutr.,* 65, 61, 1991.
23. Kubota, K., Sakurai, T., and Nakazato, K., Effect of green tea on iron absorption in elderly patients with iron deficiency anemia, *Nippon-Ronen-Igakkai-Zasshi,* 27, 555, 1990.
24. Morck, T. A., Lynch, S. R., and Cook, J. D., Inhibition of food iron absorption by coffee, *Am. J. Clin. Nutr.,* 37, 416, 1983.
25. Solomons, N. W. and Rosenberg, I. H., *Current Topics in Nutrition and Disease: Absorption and Malabsorption of Mineral Nutrients,* Alan R. Liss, New York, 1984.
26. Monsen, E. R. and Cook, J. D., Food iron absorption in human, *Am. J. Clin. Nutr.,* 29, 1142, 1976.
27. Hallberg, L. and Rossander, L., Effect of different drinks on the absorption of nonheme iron from composite meals, *Hum. Nutr. Appl. Nutr.,* 36A, 116, 1982c.
28. Hallberg, L., Brune, M., and Erlandson, M., Calcium: of different amounts on nonheme and heme iron absorption in human, *Am. J. Clin. Nutr.,* 53, 112, 1991.
29. Szygula, Z., Erythrocytic system under the influence of physical exercise and training, *Sports Med.,* 10, 181, 1990.
30. Gosztonyi, T., *Iron Metabolism,* Plenum Press, New York, 1983.
31. Kies, C., Nutritional bioavailability of iron, *Am. Chem. Soc.,* Washington, D.C., 1982.
32. Robertson, W. G., Diet and calcium stones, *Miner-Electrolyte-Metab.,* 13, 228, 1987.
33. Kaneko, K., Masaki, U., Aikyo, M., and Yubuki, K., Urinary calcium and calcium balance in young women affected by high protein diet of soy protein isolate and adding sulfur-containing amino acids and/or potassium, *J. Nutr. Sci. Vitaminol. Tokyo,* 36, 105, 1990.
34. American Dietetic Association Statement, Nutrition and physical fitness, *J. Am. Diet. Assoc.,* 76, 437, 1985.
35. Smith, N. J., Excessive weight loss and food aversion in athletes simulating anorexia nervosa, *Pediatrics,* 66, 139, 1980.
36. Monsen, E. R., Hallberg, L., and Layrisse, M., Estimation of available dietary iron, *Am. J. Clin. Nutr.,* 11, 117, 1978.
37. Schrecker, B. R., Miller, D. D., and Stouffer, J. R., Measurement and content of nonheme and total iron in muscle, *J. Food Sci.,* 47, 740, 1982.

Chapter 11

FERROUS FUMARATE/CALCIUM CARBONATE INTERACTIONS AFFECTING ELECTROLYTE BALANCES OF PHYSICALLY ACTIVE HUMANS

Mihye Kym
Constance V. Kies

CONTENTS

0-8493-7916-4/95/$0.00+$.50

I. LITERATURE REVIEW

A. ELECTROLYTES

Mineral supplements such as sodium, potassium, calcium, and iron are often recommended to the athletes, however, these have been, and continue to be, controversial. Since the maintenance of normal blood pressure is critical to life, the body has an effective regulatory feedback mechanism allowing for a wide range of dietary sodium intake. Excessive losses of sodium from the body, usually induced by prolonged sweating while exercising in the heat, may lead to short-term deficiencies that may be debilitating to the athletic individual. The major electrolytes found in sweat are sodium and chloride, and other minerals lost in small amounts include potassium, magnesium, calcium, iron, copper, and zinc.[1]

Rehrer et al.[2] reported that after ultra-endurance running, mean plasma volume decreased by 8.3%. No significant changes in plasma osmolality, sodium, or chloride were observed, but plasma potassium did increase by 5%.

In general, exercise raises the concentration of several electrolytes in the blood. Sodium and potassium concentrations are elevated; the sodium increase may be due to greater body water loss than sodium loss, so a concentration effect occurs. The potassium may leak from the muscle tissue to the blood. However, prolonged sweating has been shown to decrease the body content of sodium and chloride by 5 to 7%, while potassium levels dropped about 1% during the recovery period after excessive sweating.[1]

Excessive loss of body water by dehydration will decrease endurance capacity. In such cases, techniques that help minimize body water losses may help prevent this decline in performance. In a scientific review, Millard et al.[3] compared the effects of 7% carbohydrate - electrolyte drink (CE) and an artificially sweetened placebo (P) on performance and physiological functions during a 40 km run in the heat. Results indicated that CE replacement elicits similar thermoregulatory and physiological responses during prolonged running in the heat, but increases run performance when compared with P. The same results were observed by Deuster et al.[4] Barr et al.[5] indicated that a need for sodium replacement would be unexpected in exercise of less than 6 h duration, assuming plasma sodium is normal at the start of exercise. Moreover, the amount of sodium in commercial beverages is inadequate to prevent a decrease in plasma sodium.

An electrolyte deficiency could impair physical performance, but supplements above and beyond normal electrolyte nutrition have not been shown to enhance performance. Housh et al.[6] demonstrated that ammonium chloride and sodium bicarbonate ingestion had no significant effect on power working capacity at the fatigue threshold.

There are some potential adverse effects of hypohydration and electrolyte losses on physical performance and certain health conditions, such as hyponatremia.[7] A health problem, especially high blood pressure, may be aggravated by salt ingestion but ameliorated by proper exercise.[1] Salt tablets actually increase dehydration because these draw water from the cells into the intestine to dilute the concentrated salt and can cause high blood pressure.

B. CALCIUM

The major health problems associated with impaired calcium metabolism involve diseases of the bones. For the physically active individual, a low serum calcium could be serious because of the effects on muscular contraction. Concern about disturbed calcium metabolism in female athletes, particularly endurance athletes, is growing. While the primary causes of bone loss in physically active women are certainly, in part, due to physical stress, dietary lack of calcium is probably a contributing factor. The diets of many female athletes are low in both calcium and iron, thereby making these nutrients of special concern to athletes.[8] These dietary deficiencies can be corrected through proper food choices and by consuming a great variety of food.

Research relating to calcium supplementation and physical performance is almost nonexistent. Excessive amounts may contribute to abnormal heart contractions, constipation, and the development of kidney stones in susceptible individuals. Moreover, excessive dietary calcium may interfere with the absorption of other key minerals, notably iron and zinc. However, women with exercise-induced amenorrhea may require calcium supplementation.[11]

It is well known that an increase in sodium intake can result in an increased urinary calcium excretion.[12] The effect of an increased calcium intake on sodium excretion is less obvious. Calcium supplementation in rats resulted in an increased sodium and/or potassium excretion in animal study.[13] In humans with constant sodium and potassium intakes, a daily supplement of 1 to 2 g calcium did not influence sodium and potassium excretions.[14,15]

An animal study has shown that voluntary running exercise and high calcium intake are efficacious for bone calcium deposition in growing rats, without altering calcium homeostasis. Moreover, in situations of insufficient calcium intake, excess exercise might induce the decrease in bone calcium deposition in growing rats.[9]

A case-control study has been reported on whether or not low bone density and other risk factors for osteoporosis are associated with stress fractures in athletes. The authors indicated that athletes with fractures had lower calcium intakes and dairy product intakes than control athletes, and are more likely to have lower bone density.[10]

C. IRON

Iron-deficiency anemia, and likely marginal iron deficiency, impair athletic performance by reducing the oxygen carrying capacity of blood and inhibiting mitochondrial enzyme function. Iron needs appear to be higher in athletes because of increased iron losses, presumably from increased red blood cell destruction, gastrointestinal blood loss, iron loss in sweat, and decreased iron absorption.[11] Based upon the results of several studies, 50 to 80% of all females seriously participating in running-type aerobic exercise, and 5 to 30% of all males undertaking similar exercise programs, develop an iron deficiency anemia due to a decrease of iron availability for hemoglobin synthesis.[16]

Most research with iron-deficient, nonanemic subjects has shown that iron supplementation improves iron status, by decreasing serum ferritin, for example, but appears to have little effect upon maximal oxygen consumption. Klingshirn et al.[17] found that oral iron supplementation improved iron status in iron-depleted female distance runners, but did not enhance endurance capacity. Moreover, Weight et al.[18] suggest that athletes are at no greater risk for developing a frank anemia than the non-exercising population, and that the term "sports anemia" is misleading.

Intense training for long-distance running has been associated with reduced hemoglobin levels and low iron stores. Whether iron supplementation helps prevent this "runner's anemia" remains controversial.[19,20] Female athletes frequently have difficulty meeting their iron needs because of caloric restrictions, avoidance of meat, and an extreme emphasis on carbohydrate intake. Moreover, excessive dietary calcium or calcium supplements may interfere with the absorption of iron. Calcium and iron supplements are both of concern to athletes and interaction of these minerals and electrolytes remain unclear. Electrolyte balances in athletes are important in relationship to blood pressure and normal cardiac and renal function.

II. OBJECTIVES

In an attempt to further determine ferrous fumarate/calcium carbonate interactions affecting sodium, potassium, and chloride status of physically active humans, a human study was conducted in our laboratory.

III. METHODS

The 56 d study was divided into four experimental periods of 14 d each. Using a 2 * 2 factorial design, two levels (high and low) of ferrous fumarate, and two levels (high and low) of calcium carbonate, were fed.

During the low calcium and low iron periods, the ordinary foods composing the basal diet provided approximately 400 mg calcium and 10 mg iron per day. During the high calcium periods, 900 mg of calcium per subject per day from calcium carbonate, divided among the three daily meals, was fed, thus subjects received a total of 1300 mg of calcium per subject per day during the high calcium periods. During the high iron periods, 30 mg of iron per subject per day from ferrous fumarate was fed; thus, subjects received a total of 40 mg of iron per subject per day.

Other than for the supplement alterations, subjects received a constant, measured, laboratory-controlled diet composed of ordinary foods. This included apple juice, pineapple juice, orange juice, whole wheat bread, potatoes, green beans, peaches, corn, and ice cream (see Table 1). A vitamin supplement was given each day to assure adequacy of intakes of these nutrients.

The ten adult male subjects were all students or employees of the University of Nebraska and were in good health on the basis of medical exams/health history records, as evaluated by medical personal of the University of Nebraska Division of Medical Services. Information on past and current dietary and exercise practices of these individuals was collected by use of questionnaires. All were required to participate in an aerobic exercise class 3 d a week for 1 h/class during the course of the study in order to equalize exercise experiences. Signed subject consent forms were required from all subjects.

Subjects made complete collections of urine and stools throughout the study. Fecal collections were divided into lots representing food eaten during each experimental period via appearance of orally-given fecal dyes, given at the beginning and end of each experimental period. Feces for each period were weighed, mixed, sampled, and frozen for later analyses. Fasting blood samples were drawn prior to the start of the study, at the end of the study, and at the end of each experimental period.

Analyses include determination of sodium, potassium, and chloride in food, blood serum, feces, and urine. Blood pressure was also measured. Sodium and potassium ratios were calculated. Blood also was analyzed by SMAC-26 procedure, which gives values for 26 blood components used to monitor human health. The project was approved by the University of Nebraska Institutional Review Committee for Studies Involving Human Subjects.

IV. RESULTS

Mean age of subjects was 30 years. Both mean systolic blood pressure (118.9 mmHg) and diastolic blood pressure (73.6 mmHg) were within normal range of <140/90 mmHg.

Serum electrolyte concentrations of the subjects are given in Table 2. Serum sodium concentrations numerically were found to be lower in the calcium-supplemental treatment period (141 meq/l) than other treatment periods. However, there were no significant differences among these experimental treatment periods. In general, blood electrolytes are held in very tight check. However, blood potassium concentrations were significantly lower during the iron-supplemental (4.06 meq/l), and the combination of iron and calcium-supplemental treatment (4.06 meq/l), than those of pre-study (4.20 meq/l). Serum potassium concentrations during the calcium-supplemental treatment period and no supplemental treatment period tended to be lower than iron-supplemental treatment and the combination of iron and calcium-supplemental treatment. Serum chloride concentrations were not found to differ significantly among the experimental treatment periods. As with sodium, serum chloride concentrations are maintained with very narrow limits in the healthy men.

Urinary electrolyte excretion values of the subjects are given in Table 3. Urinary sodium excretions were not significantly different in the experimental treatments. However, the lowest value was found in the calcium-supplemental treatment (3550 mg/d). Urinary potassium excretions were significantly higher in the combination iron and calcium-supplemental treatment period (2528 mg/d) than the calcium-supplemental treatment period (2195 mg/d) and no supplemental treatment period (2159 mg/d). Urinary chloride excretions were significantly lower in the iron-supplemental treatment period (180.2 meq/l) than calcium-supplemental treatment period (194.2 meq/l).

Urinary sodium-to-potassium ratios are used as predictors of sodium-to-potassium intake ratios and an increase in the sodium-to-potassium ratio is generally interpreted as indicator of an increased risk for hypertension. In the present study, the highest ratio was found in the no supplemental treatment (1.703) and the lowest value was found in the combination of iron and calcium-supplemental treatment (1.509) (see Table 4). These ratios for calcium-supplemental treatment and iron-supplemental treatment were 1.617 and 1.600, respectively. Calcium supplementation resulted in decreased urinary sodium excretions. Conflicting results were reported by Ayachi.[13]

Certain studies have suggested that elevated serum total calcium levels contribute to high blood pressure, while others report that deficiency in serum calcium levels has the same effect. The point should be stressed that careful selection of foods and well-balanced diets will provide the nutrients people need from the daily diet, thus eliminating the need for supplements.

TABLE 1   Content of Iron and Calcium in
           Different Kinds of Food of the
           Laboratory Diet (mg/serving)

Food Items	Iron	Calcium
Oreo Cookies	0.25	2.60
Carrots	0.11	5.31
Whole Wheat Bread	0.39	45.00
Apple Juice	0.41	21.57
Hot Chocolate Milk	0.27	62.41
Raisins	0.82	9.62
Green Beans	1.20	44.18
Peaches	0.50	12.45
Orange Juice	0.83	37.60
Breakfast Granola Bar	0.59	16.99
Turkey Breast	0.90	2.18
Tuna	1.20	3.13
Grape Juice	0.41	29.07
Potato Chips	0.35	7.00
Rice	1.00	5.32
Vanilla Pudding	0.46	48.36

TABLE 2   **Blood Serum Electrolyte Concentrations as Affected by Use of Calcium and Iron Supplements**

Diet Type	Concentrations (meq/l)		
	Sodium	Potassium	Chloride
Pre-study	142[a]	4.20[a]	102[b]
No Supplements	142[a]	4.13[ab]	104[a]
+ Calcium	141[a]	4.15[ab]	103[a]
+ Iron	142[a]	4.06[b]	103[a]
+ Iron & Calcium	142[a]	4.06[b]	103[a]

Note: Mean values in each column with no repeated letter superscripts are significantly different from one another ($p < 0.05$).

TABLE 3   **Urinary Electrolyte Excretion as Affected by Use of Calcium and Iron Supplements**

Diet Type	Excretions		
	Sodium (mg/d)	Potassium (mg/d)	Chloride (meq/l)
No Supplements	3677[a]	2159[b]	190.2[ab]
+ Calcium	3550[a]	2195[b]	194.2[a]
+ Iron	3770[a]	2355[ab]	180.2[b]
+ Iron & Calcium	3817[a]	2528[a]	190.4[ab]

Note: Mean values in each columns with no repeated letter superscripts are significantly different from one another ($p < 0.05$).

TABLE 4   **Sodium and Potassium Urinary Excretion Ratios as Affected by Use of Calcium and Iron Supplements**

Diet Type	Na: *p* Ratios
No Supplements	1.703
+ Calcium	1.617
+ Iron	1.600
+ Iron & Calcium	1.509

REFERENCES

1. Williams, M. H., *Nutrition for Fitness and Sports*, Wm. C. Brown, Dubuque, 1992, chap. 7–8.
2. Rehrer, N. J., Brouns, F., Beckers, E. J., Frey, W. O., Villiger, B., Riddoch, C. J., and Saris, W. H. M., Physiological changes and gastro-intestinal symptoms as a result of ultra-endurance running. *Eur. J. Appl. Physiol. Occup. Physiol.*, 64(1), 1, 1992.
3. Millard, S. M. L., Sparling, P. B., Rosskopf, L. B., and Dicarlo, L. J., Carbohydrate-electrolyte replacement improves distance running performance in the heat, *Med. Sci. Sports Exercise*, 24(8), 934, 1992.
4. Deuster, P. A., Singh, A., Hofmann, A., Moses, F. M., and Chrousos, G. C., Hormonal responses to ingesting water or a carbohydrate beverages during a two hour run, *Med. Sci. Sports Exercise*, 24(1), 72, 1992
5. Barr, S. I., Costill, D. L., and Fink, W. J., Fluid replacement during prolonged exercise, *Med. Sci. Sports Exercise*, 23(7), 811, 1991.
6. Housh, T. J., DeVries, H. A., Johnson, G. O., Evans, S. A., and McDowells, S., The effect of ammonium chloride and sodium bicarbonate ingestion on the physical working capacity at the fatigue threshold, *Eur. J. Appl. Physiol. Occup. Physiol.*, 62(3), 189, 1991.
7. Noakes, T. D., Berlinski, N., Solomon, E., and Weight, L., Collapsed runners: blood biochemical changes after IV fluid therapy, *Phys. Sports Med.*, 19(7), 70, 1991.
8. Faber, M., and Banade, A. J. S., Mineral and vitamin intakes in field athletes, *Int. J. Sports Medicine*, 12(3), 324, 1991.
9. Sato, Y., and Okano, G., Effects voluntary running exercise or high calcium intakes on bone metabolism in growing male rats, *Bull. Phys. Fitness Res. Inst.*, 0(77), 52, 1991.
10. Myburgh, K. H., Hutchins, J., Fatarr, A.B., Hough, S.F., and Noakes, T. D., Low bone density is an etiologic factor for stress fractures in athletes, *Ann. Intern. Med.*, 113(10), 754, 1990.
11. Etherton, P. M. K., Nutrition and athletic performance, *Nutr. Today*, 35, 1990.
12. Aalberts, J. S., Weegels, P. L., Heijden, L. V., Borst, M. H., Burema, J., Hautrast, J., and Kouwenhoven, T., Calcium supplementation: effect on blood pressure and urinary mineral excretion, *Am. J. Clin. Nutr.*, 48, 131, 1988.
13. Ayachi, S., Increased dietary calcium lowers blood pressure in the spontaneously hypertensive rats, *Metabolism* 28, 1234, 1979.
14. Luft, F. C., Aronoff, G. R., Sloan, R. S., Fineberg, N. S., and Weinberger, H. H., Short-term augmented calcium intakes have no effect on sodium homeostasis, *Clin. Pharmacol. Ther.*, 39, 414, 1986.
15. Tabuchi, Y., Ogihara, T., Hashizume, K., Saito, H., Kumahara, Y., Hypotensive effect of long-term oral calcium supplementation, *J. Clin. Hyperten.*, 3, 254, 1986.
16. Resina, A., Gatteschi, L., Rubenni, M. G., and Vecchiet, L., Hematological comparison of iron status in trained top level soccer players, *Int. J. Sports Med.*, 12(5), 453, 1991.
17. Klinghsirn, L. A., Pate, R. R., Bourque, S. P., Davis, J. M., and Sargent, R. G., Effect of iron supplementation on endurance capacity in iron-depleted female runners, *Med. Sci. Sports Exercise*, 24(7), 819, 1992.
18. Weight, L. M., Klein, M., Noakes, T. D., and Jacobs, P., Sports anemia: a real or apparent phenomenon in endurance-trained athletes?, *Int. J. Sports Med.*, 13(4), 344, 1992.
19. Dressendorfer, R. H., Keen, C. L., Wade, C. E., Claybaugh, J. R., and Timmis, G. C., Development of runner's anemia during a 20-d road race: effect of iron supplements. *Int. J. Sports Med.*, 12(3), 332, 1991.
20. Rowland, T. W., Stagg, L., and Kelleher, J. F., Iron Deficiency: are athletes at increased risk, *J. Adolescent Health*, 12(1), 22, 1991.

Chapter 12

PHYSICAL EXERCISE AND ZINC METABOLISM

Hideki Ohno
Yuzo Sato
Takako Kizaki
Hitoshi Yamashita
Tomomi Ookawara
Yoshinobu Ohira

CONTENTS

0-8493-7916-4/95/$0.00+$.50

I. INTRODUCTION

Zinc is without doubt an essential trace element in all biological systems. For example, there are approximately 90 related metalloenzymes known for which zinc is needed, which participate in the metabolism of lipids and carbohydrates and the synthesis of protein and nucleic acids. As a consequence, zinc has a metabolic role under various physiological and pathological conditions.[1-5] Previous data have also shown the importance of zinc for muscle performance and resistance to fatigue in animals[6,7] and humans.[8] Richardson and Drake[7] suggested that this effect is due to the participation of the metal in the formation of several enzymes such as lactate dehydrogenase (LD). The observation by Apple and Tesch[9] that slow twitch fibers from endurance-trained athletes were the only fibers that contained substantial amounts of LD_1, the LD isoenzyme that predominates in the heart muscle of most vertebrates, may strengthen this hypothesis. Therefore, with prolonged suboptimal zinc status, it would be predicted that muscle zinc levels in vegetarians would decrease, with resulting reduced muscle strength and endurance.[10] On the other hand, Dressendorfer and Sockolov[11] indicated that long-distance runners had significantly lower average serum zinc concentrations compared to sedentary control (76 and 94 µg/100 ml, respectively), and that the serum zinc was inversely related to training distance. The presence of hypozincemia in trained athletes has since been reported by other laboratories.[12-14] In works by several investigators, however, plasma zinc concentrations were similar among athletes and control subjects.[15-17] Furthermore, no homogenous, acute, exercise-induced trends could be found in plasma zinc concentrations.[14,18-20]

Meanwhile, there are few reports on the effects of physical exercise on zinc levels in human erythrocytes,[15,16,19] although erythrocytes are rich in zinc. Thus, the present review will deal concisely with effects of acute and chronic physical exercise on zinc concentrations in human erythrocytes and plasma (or serum), with particular emphasis placed on our works. The relationships between zinc and several proteins, including zinc metalloenzymes under physical exercise, are also discussed.

II. ZINC DISTRIBUTION IN BLOOD

Erythrocyte zinc constitutes 75 to 88%, plasma zinc 12 to 20%, and leukocyte zinc 3% of whole blood zinc in normal human blood.[21] Keilin and Mann[22,23] first demonstrated that zinc is an integral and necessary component of carbonic anhydrase (CA). The enzyme in erythrocytes has two major types of isoenzymes designated as the I type (CA-I) and II type (CA-II).[24] Funakoshi and Deutsch[24] have reported that all zinc in human hemolysates can be accounted for by both these CA isoenzymes (97.2%) and CuZn superoxide dismutase (CuZn-SOD) (2.5%). It seems likely, however, that this finding should be tempered in view of the facts that zinc binds to hemoglobin,[25] that other various zinc metalloenzymes, such as LDH, alcohol dehydrogenase, and glyceraldehyde-3-phosphate dehydrogenase, occur in erythrocytes,[26] and that leukocytes and platelets might have been still present in the hemolysates.[27] In our work, therefore, sufficient care was taken to remove leukocytes and platelets and then the following values of zinc distribution were obtained: total zinc, 1114 ± 23 μg/100 ml (mean $\pm$ SEM); CA-I-derived zinc, 867 ± 26 μg/100 ml; CA-II-derived zinc, 99.9 ± 3.9 μg/100 ml; CuZn-SOD-derived zinc, 60.3 ± 1.9 μg/100 ml; the other zinc, 87.0 ± 12.6 μg/100 ml; that is, 7.6% of the zinc in human erythrocytes is not bound to the CA isoenzymes or CuZn-SOD, but present in available form or attached to other enzymes.[28]

The erythrocyte concentrations of total zinc and of zinc derived from CA-I, were significantly higher in winter than in summer, suggesting that CA-I-derived zinc would be a significant part of the mobilizable, or available, zinc in the human body in a cold environment.[29] Actually, CA-I-derived zinc concentration in erythrocytes of male students definitely declined during acute exposure to cold (10°C for 60 min).[30] It has been shown that CA-I concentration in erythrocytes fluctuates under certain pathological or physiological conditions, although CA-II and CuZn-SOD are relatively constant.[31-34] Because the specific activity of CA-I is about one-fifth that of CA-II in control erythrocytes, one may speculate that CA-I contributes less to the total CO_2 hydrase activity compared with CA-II.[35] In general, thus, CA isoenzymes, especially CA-I, correlate significantly with erythrocyte zinc.[36]

On the other hand, the zinc present in human serum is composed of two principal species: one fraction is firmly bound α_2-macroglobulin (α_2-MG), and a second fraction is more loosely associated with albumin.[1,3,5] Similarly, previous studies have produced several differences of opinion concerning the relative distribution of zinc in normal human sera. Parisi and Vallee[37] reported that α_2-MG constitutes the principal zinc metalloprotein of human serum, and that it accounts for 30 to 40% of the total zinc concentration of serum. Song and Adham[38] concluded that ~30% of total serum zinc is associated with α_2-MG fraction. On the other hand, other investigators have claimed that zinc-bound α_2-MG represents ~20% of the total serum zinc concentration.[12,39] The results of our previous studies were in good agreement with those of the last two groups.[29,30,40] One atom of zinc is bound to one molecule of α_2-MG in control serum.[21] Over a wide range of values, the concentrations of albumin-bound zinc and total serum zinc were highly correlated with each other ($r = 0.91$), as were concentrations of albumin and albumin-bound zinc ($r = 0.69$), whereas α_2-MG-bound zinc was not strongly correlated either with total serum zinc or with the serum concentration of α_2-MG.[39]

The changes in zinc observed in acutely stressful situations should be evaluated in relation to the slight, but definite, circadian periodicity of serum zinc; however, normal circadian periodicity does not generally cause zinc values to rise or fall more than 5 to 10% from baseline.[1,5,41] The variation in serum zinc concentration was associated with a circadian variation in the blood levels of 17-hydroxycorticosteroids[42] and ionized calcium.[43] It has also been reported that zinc distributions in human serum change in various states.[1,3,5,44-46]

III. EFFECTS OF EXERCISE ON BLOOD ZINC

A. ACUTE EXERCISE

Studies of the influences of brief physical exercise (bicycle ergometer, 200 W for 30 min) on the activities of CA isoenzymes and zinc concentration in erythrocytes were made on five untrained, healthy male students.[47] There were significant decreases in the levels of zinc, CA-I, total CA activity, and CA-I-dependent activity immediately after the exercise, but after 30 min of rest they all returned to their pre-exercise levels. No significant change in CA-II level or CA-II-dependent activity was found after exercise. Immediately after exercise, total CA activity and CA-I-dependent activity, following the addition of Zn^{2+}, showed significant increases as compared with their respective activities. However, no such effects were observed just before exercise or after rest; the addition of Zn^{2+} had no effect on CA-II-dependent activity at any time. A significant correlation was found between the changes in zinc concentration and CA-I-dependent activity after exercise (r = 0.71). These findings suggested that active CA-I enzymes are converted, in part, to inactive enzymes during acute physical exercise, possibly by decreased zinc binding.

Oelshlegel et al.[25] reported that zinc binding to erythrocyte 2,3-diphosphoglycerate (2,3-DPG), which plays a major role in modulating erythrocyte oxygen affinity through binding to hemoglobin, can cause an increase in erythrocyte oxygen affinity. 2,3-DPG level in erythrocytes is increased after acute exercise.[48-51] Meanwhile, Hořejši and Komárková[52] indicated that CA also shifts the oxygen dissociation curve to the right and causes a decrease in erythrocyte oxygen affinity. Our previous study showed that there are negative correlations between the changes in 2,3-DPG level on one hand, and those in CA-I level and total CA activity on the other, after acute exercise.[50] Under physical exercise, however, whether or not direct linkage is present among CA, zinc, 2,3-DPG, and hemoglobin in erythrocytes remains to be explained.

In the study on a 70 km cross-country skiing competition, Hetland et al.[19] demonstrated that zinc concentration in erythrocytes remained essentially unchanged, although serum zinc concentration rose significantly immediately after the race. It appears, however, that the result should be discounted because there were definite signs of hemolysis. Accordingly, we next examined zinc fractions in erythrocytes and plasma under acute physical exercise.[53] Cycle ergometer exercise (~75% $\dot{V}O_2$ max for 30 min) was done on 11 sedentary healthy male students. As a result, lower concentrations of total zinc and of zinc derived from CA-I in erythrocytes were observed immediately after exercise, but they disappeared after 30 min of rest. The change in total zinc concentration in erythrocytes correlated well with that in CA-I concentration immediately after exercise, and after 30 min of rest. The concentration of CA-II-derived zinc did not vary substantially at any time. In another study, likewise, erythrocyte CuZn-SOD concentration did not change significantly after exercise with the same load as the above study.[54]

Conversely, there were significant increases in the plasma concentrations of total zinc and of α_2-MG-bound zinc immediately after exercise, whereas no such effect was noted in albumin-bound zinc. A positive correlation was found between total zinc and α_2-MG concentrations in plasma immediately after exercise. In addition, the change in activity of alkaline phosphatase, a zinc metalloenzyme, correlated well with that in the total zinc concentration in plasma. These results suggested that a brief physical exercise induces the movement of zinc into plasma, in part, from erythrocytes (and probably from skeletal muscles).[19,55]

Because urinary zinc losses were elevated following acute exercise,[20] it seems likely that the increase in plasma zinc concentration would be greater than it appeared. Furthermore, we recently revealed that CuZn-SOD emerges into urine, in connection with the reduced plasma level of CuZn-SOD, during and after 2 h regular soccer training.[56]

B. CHRONIC EXERCISE

Effects of short-duration training on zinc and CA isoenzymes in erythrocytes were studied on five untrained male students.[57] The training protocol consisted of a 30 min ride on a bicycle ergometer with a load of 200 W, 6 times/week for 2 weeks. There were increases in the levels of zinc, CA-I, total CA activity, and CA-I-dependent activity after the training. The zinc concentration showed a decrease immediately after acute exercise, both before and after the training, the latter being apparently greater than the former. Since there was an upward trend in pH and PO_2 in venous blood after training, it may be that an adaptive increase in the levels of CA-I and CA-I-dependent activity in erythrocytes occurred with increased alkalosis during training; however, the HCO_3^- level remained unchanged.

We next investigated the effects of physical training on fasting erythrocyte and plasma zinc distributions in seven previously sedentary male students.[58] The training consisted of running over 5 km, 6 times/week for 10 weeks. The erythrocyte concentrations of total zinc and of zinc derived from CA-I rose significantly after training, while no such effects were noted in CA-II-derived zinc, CuZn-SOD-derived zinc, or other zinc. It has been shown that thyroxine preferentially inhibits the biosynthesis of CA-I in rabbit reticulocyte lysates without affecting that of CA-II,[59] and that patients with hypothyroidism have a high erythrocyte CA-I level.[60] Moreover, Balsam and Leppo[61] have demonstrated that there is a significant decrease in thyroxine level in human plasma after a 6 week program of running training. It cannot be denied, thus, that the increase in erythrocyte CA-I concentration after the 10 week running training would be due, in part, to decreased levels of thyroid hormones. Meanwhile, no significant relationships existed between $\dot{V}O_2$ max on one hand, and total zinc concentration, CA-I concentration, and CA-I-dependent activity in erythrocytes on the other, after training. This result on total zinc is in keeping with that of Lukaski et al.[15] Dennis et al.[62] showed that loosely bound erythrocyte zinc may form part of the pool of labile zinc, since, *in vitro*, there is a rapid exchange of zinc between erythrocytes and plasma. Assuming that CA-I-derived zinc corresponds to the loosely bound erythrocyte zinc, CA-I would be regarded as a significant part of the mobilizable or available zinc in the human body during physical training.

In addition, we revealed that CA-I concentration in erythrocytes from 13 Himalayan expedition members decreased strikingly on the day after reaching the summit of Mt. Z 1 (6,400 m after about 4 weeks of exposure to altitude over 3,800 m); so that of additional interest seem to be studies regarding a linkage among acclimation to high altitude and CA-I and zinc in erythrocytes.[63]

On the other hand, no effect of the 10-week training was found in total or α_2-MG-bound zinc in plasma, although albumin-bound zinc concentration declined slightly, but significantly. Because plasma albumin concentration was stable, the decreased albumin-bound zinc after training might imply a reduction in the zinc-binding capacity. As demonstrated after a $\dot{V}O_2$ max test in men fed a low-zinc diet by Lukaski et al.,[64] the response to a $\dot{V}O_2$ max test of the van Beaumont quotient[65] (which is calculated to minimize the effect of hemoconcentration on plasma trace element concentration) for total plasma zinc was also decreased significantly after training. The result suggested a relative reduction of the circulating exchangeable zinc, which reflected an alteration in some body zinc pools. Therefore, it seems probable that the decreased albumin-bound zinc portended zinc deficiency.

Falchuk[45] has reported that serum zinc values for nearly all categories of acute disease are significantly lower than normal individuals, and that adrenocorticotropic hormone (ACTH) administration reduces serum zinc from 10 to 60 µg/100 ml, the decrements being due to changes in the zinc content of fraction II when chromatographed on Sephadex G-100, including albumin and β-globulins but no α_2-MG. Indeed, 20 min of submaximal treadmill running was associated with an elevation in ACTH concentration in human plasma.[66] Accordingly, the possibility exists that each running training for 10 weeks produced an increase in plasma ACTH concentration, with resulting decreased levels of plasma albumin-bound zinc. Similar results were noted for interleukin 1.[67,68] However, one major question remains to be answered: why was there an increase in erythrocyte zinc level, despite a tendency for plasma zinc to decrease during physical training?

IV. CONCLUSIONS

Laboratory diagnosis of severe zinc deficiency is relatively simple, but marginal zinc deficiency is extremely difficult to confirm due to the lack of suitable methods of assessing zinc status.[69] The level of zinc in plasma (or serum) does not always reflect body zinc status.[69-71] From the studies presented here, however, it may be concluded as follows:

1. Acute, as well as chronic, exercise induces an alteration in zinc distribution in human blood
2. CA-I may be a significant part of the mobilizable or available zinc in the human body during physical training
3. An increase in erythrocyte CA-I-derived zinc concentration and/or a decrease in plasma albumin-bound zinc concentration may portend hypozincemia during physical training
4. It seems likely that the response to a $\dot{V}O_2$ max test of the van Beaumont quotient[65] provides a reliable index of zinc deficiency due to training

REFERENCES

1. Beisel, W.R., Pekarek, R.S., and Wannemacher, R.W., Jr., Homeostatic mechanisms affecting plasma zinc levels in acute stress, in *Trace Element in Human Health and Disease*, Vol.1, Prasad, A.S., Ed., Academic Press, New York, 1976, 87.
2. Prasad, A.S., Trace elements: biochemical and clinical effects of zinc and copper, *Am. J. Hematol.*, 6, 77, 1979.
3. Solomons, N.W., On the assessment of zinc and copper nutriture in man, *Am. J. Clin. Nutr.*, 32, 856, 1979.
4. Aggett, P.J. and Harries, J.T., Current status of zinc in health and disease states, *Arch. Dis. Child.*, 54, 909, 1979.
5. Bogden, J.D., Blood zinc in health and disease, in *Zinc in the Environment, Part II: Health Effects*, Nriagu, J.O., Ed., John Wiley & Sons, New York, 1980, 137.
6. Isaacson, A. and Sandow, A., Effect of zinc on responses of skeletal muscle, *J. Gen. Physiol.*, 46, 655, 1963.
7. Richardson, J.H. and Drake, P.D., The effects of zinc on fatigue of striated muscle, *J. Sports Med. Phys. Fit*, 19, 133, 1979.
8. Krotkiewski, M., Gudmundsson, M., Backström, P., and Mandroukas, K., Zinc and muscle strength and endurance, *Acta Physiol. Scand.*, 116, 309, 1982.
9. Apple, F.S. and Tesch, P.A., CK and LD isozymes in human single muscle fibers in trained athletes, *J. Appl. Physiol.*, 66, 2717, 1989.
10. Brooks, S.M., Sanborn, C.F., Albrecht, B.H., and Wagner, W.W., Diet in athletic amenorrhea, *Lancet*, vol. i, 559, 1984.
11. Dressendorfer, R.H. and Sockolov, R., Hypozincemia in runners, *Phys. Sportsmed.*, 8, 97, 1980.
12. Haralambie, G., Serum zinc in athletes in training, *Int. J. Sports Med.*, 2, 135, 1981.
13. Keen, C.L. and Hackman, R.M., Trace elements in athletic performance, in *Sport, Health, and Nutrition*, Katch, F.I., Ed., Human Kinetics Publishers, Champaign, 1986, 51.
14. Berg, A., Kieffer, F., and Keul, J., Acute and chronic effects of endurance exercise on serum zinc levels, in *Biochemical Aspects of Physical Exercise*, Benzi, G., Packer, L., and Siliprandi, N., Eds., Elsevier, Amsterdam, 1986, 207.
15. Lukaski, H.C., Bolonchuk, W.W., Klevay, L.M., Milne, D.B., and Sandstead, H.H., Maximal oxygen consumption as related to magnesium, copper, and zinc nutriture, *Am. J. Clin, Nutr.*, 37, 407, 1983.
16. Deuster, P.A., Day, B.A., Singh, A., Douglass, L., and Moser-Veillon, P.B., Zinc status of highly trained women runners and untrained women, *Am. J. Clin Nutr.*, 49, 1295, 1989.
17. Lukaski, H.C., Hoverson, B.S., Gallagher, S.K., and Bolonchuk, W.W., Physical training and copper, iron, and zinc status of swimmers, *Am. J. Clin, Nutr.*, 51, 1093, 1990.
18. Lichti E.L., Turner, M., Deweese, M.S., and Henzel, J.H., Zinc concentration in venous plasma before and after exercise in dogs, *J. Miss. State Med. Assoc.*, 67, 303, 1970.
19. Hetland, Ø., Bruback, E.A., Refsum, H.E., and Strømme, S.B., Serum and erythrocyte zinc concentrations after prolonged heavy exercise, in *Metabolic Adaptation to Prolonged Heavy Exercise*, Howald, H. and Poortmans, J., Eds., Birkhäuser, Basel, 1975, 367.
20. Anderson, R.A., Polansky, M.M., Bryden, N.A., and Guttman, H.N., Strenuous exercise may increase dietary needs for chromium and zinc, in *Sport, Health, and Nutrition*, Katch, F.I., Ed., Human Kinetics Publishers, Champaign, 1986, 83.
21. National Research Council, Subcommittee on Zinc, *Zinc*, University Park Press, Baltimore, 1979, 123.
22. Keilin, D. and Mann, T., Carbonic anlydrase, *Nature*, 144, 442, 1939.
23. Keilin, D. and Mann, T., Carbonic anhydrase. Purification and nature of the enzyme, *Biochem. J.*, 34, 1163, 1940.
24. Funakoshi, S. and Deutsch, H.F., Human carbonic anhydrase. III. Immunochemical studies, *J. Biol. Chem.*, 245, 2852, 1970.

25. Oelshlegel, F.J., Jr., Brewer, G.J., Prasad, A.S., Knutsen, C., and Schoomaker, E.B., Effect of zinc on increasing oxygen affinity of sickle and normal red blood cells, *Biochem. Biophys. Res. Commun.*, 53, 560, 1973.

26. Swaminathan, R., Segal, N.H., Chapman, C., and Morgan, D.B., Red-blood-cell composition in thyroid disease, *Lancet*, vol. ii, 1382, 1976.

27. Beutler, E., West, C., and Blume, K.G., The removal of leukocytes and platelets from whole blood, *J. Lab. Clin. Med.*, 88, 328, 1976.

28. Ohno, H., Doi, R., Yamamura, K., Yamashita, K., Iizuka, S., and Taniguchi, N., A study of zinc distribution in erythrocytes of normal humans, *Blut*, 50, 113, 1985.

29. Ohno, H., Yamashita, K., Yahata, T., Kondo, T., Taniguchi, N., and Kuroshima, A., Seasonal variations of zinc distribution in human blood, *Trace Elem. Med.*, 5, 72, 1988.

30. Ohno, H., Yahata, T., Yamashita, K., Doi, R., Taniguchi, N., and Kuroshima, A., Zinc metabolism in human blood during acute exposure to cold, *Res. Commun. Chem. Pathol. Pharmacol.*, 52, 251, 1986.

31. Shields, G.S., Markowitz, H., Klassen, W.H., Carwright, C.E., and Wintrobe, M.M., Studies on copper metabolism. XXX. Erythrocyte copper, *J. Clin. Invest.*, 40, 2007, 1961.

32. Funakoshi, S. and Deutsch, H.F., Human carbonic anhydrase. V. Levels in erythrocytes in various states, *J. Lab. Clin. Med.*, 77, 39, 1971.

33. Taniguchi, N., Kondo, T., Ishikawa, N., Ohno, H., Takakuwa, E., and Matsuda, I. A solid-phase radioimmunoassay for human carbonic anhydrase B, *Anal. Biochem.*, 72, 144, 1976.

34. Yamashita, K., Ohno, H., Doi, R., Mure, K., Ishikawa, M., Shimizu, T., Arai, K., and Taniguchi, N., Distribution of zinc and copper in maternal and cord blood at deliverry, *Biol. Neonate*, 48, 362, 1985.

35. Ohno, H., Taniguchi, N., Kondo, T., Takakuwa, E., Terayama, K., and Kawarabayashi, T., Effect of physical exercise on the specific activity of carbonic anhydrase isozyme in human erythrocytes, *Experientia*, 38, 830, 1982.

36. Prasad, A.S., Schoomaker, E.B., Ortega, J., Brewer, G.J., Oberleas, D., and Oelshlegel, F.J., Jr., Zinc deficiency in sickle cell disease, *Clin. Chem.*, 21, 582, 1975.

37. Parisi, A.F. and Vallee, B.L., Isolation of a zinc α_2-macroglobulin from human serum, *Biochemistry*, 9, 2421, 1970.

38. Song, M.K. and Adham, N.F., Determination of native zinc content of alpha-2-macroglobulin in normal, hyperzincemic and hypozincemic sera by sucrose density gradient centrifugation, *Clin. Chim. Acta*, 99, 13, 1979.

39. Giroux, E.L., Durieux, M., and Schechter, P.J., A study of zinc distribution in human serum, *Bioinorg. Chem.*, 5, 211, 1976.

40. Ohno, H., Yahata, T., Yamashita, K., and Kuroshima, A., Effect of acute cold exposure on ACTH and zinc concentrations in human plasma, *Jpn. J. Physiol.*, 37, 749, 1987.

41. Hetland, Ö. and Brubakk, E., Diurnal variation in serum zinc concentration, *Scand. J. Clin. Lab. Invest.*, 32, 225, 1973.

42. Henkin, R.I., Trace metals in endocrinology, *Med. Clin. N. Am.*, 60, 779, 1976.

43. Markowitz, M.E., Rosen, J.F., and Mizruchi, M., Circadian variations in serum zinc (Zn) concentrations: correlation with blood ionized calcium, serum total calcium and phosphate in humans, *Am. J. Clin, Nutr.*, 41, 689, 1985.

44. Schechter, P.J., Giroux, E.L., Schlienger, J.L., Hoenig, V., and Sjoerdsma, A., Distribution of serum zinc between albumin and α_2-macroglobulin in patients with decompensated hepatic cirrhosis, *Eur. J. Clin. Invest.*, 6, 147, 1976.

45. Falchuk, K.H., Effect of acute disease and ACTH on serum zinc proteins, *N. Engl. J. Med.*, 296, 1129, 1977.

46. Yamashita, K., Ohno, H., Kondo, T., Kawamura, M., Mure, K., Yorozu, Y., Ishikawa, M., Shimizu, T., and Taniguchi, N., Maternal blood distribution of zinc and copper during labor and after delivery, *Gynecol. Obstet. Invest.*, 24, 161, 1987.

47. Ohno, H., Hirata, F., Terayama, K., Kawarabayashi, T., Doi, R., Kondo, T., and Taniguchi, N., Effect of short physical exercise on the levels of zinc and carbonic anhydrase isoenzyme activities in human erythrocytes, *Eur. J. Appl. Physiol.*, 51, 257, 1983.

48. Eaton, J. W., Faulkner, J.A., and Brewer, G.J., Response of the human red cell to muscular activity, *Proc. Soc. Exp. Biol. Med.*, 132, 886, 1969.

49. Austin, P.L., Steglink, L.D., Gisolfi, C.V., and Leuer, R.M., The effect of exercise on red blood cell 2,3-diphosphoglycerate in children, *J. Pediatr.*, 83, 41, 1973.

50. Ohno, H., Taniguchi, N., Kondo, T., Terayama, K., Hirata, F., and Kawarabayashi, T., Effect of physical exercise on erythrocyte carbonic anhydrase isozymes and 2,3-diphosphoglycerate in men, *Int. J. Sports Med.*, 2, 231, 1981.

51. Ohno, H., Watanabe, H., Kishihara, C., Nishino, M., and Taniguchi, N., Effect of physical exercise on blood glycolytic intermediates in men: crossover plot analysis, in *Biochemistry of Exercise*, vol. IV-A, Poortmans, J. and Niset, G., Eds., University Park Press, Baltimore, 1981, 100.

52. Hořejši, J. and Komárková, A., The influence of some factors of the red blood cells on the oxygen-binding capacity of haemoglobin, *Clin. Chim. Acta*, 5, 392, 1960.

53. Ohno, H., Yamashita, K., Doi, R., Yamamura, K., Kondo, T., and Taniguchi, N., Exercise-induced changes in blood zinc and related proteins in humans, *J. Appl. Physiol.*, 58, 1453, 1985.

54. Ohno, H., Sato, Y., Yamashita, K., Doi, R., Arai, K., Kondo, T., and Taniguchi, N., The effect of brief physical exercise on free radical scavenging enzyme systems in human red blood cells, *Can. J. Physiol. Pharmacol.*, 64, 1263, 1986.

55. Takala, T.E.S., Rahkila, P., Hakala, E., Vuori, J., Puranen, J., and Väänänen, K., Serum carbonic anhydrase III, an enzyme of type I muscle fibres, and the intensity of physical exercise, *Pflügers Arch.*, 413, 447, 1989.

56. Ohno, H., Yamashita, H., Ookawara, T., Kizaki, T., Sato, Y., and Taniguchi, N., Effect of physical exercise on urinary excretion of CuZn-superoxide dismutase in male high school students, *Acta Physiol. Scand.*, 148, 353, 1993.

57. Ohno, H., Hirata, F., Terayama, K., Kawarabayashi, T., Doi, R., Kondo, T., and Taniguchi, N., Effects of training of short duration on the levels of zinc and carbonic anhydrase isoenzymes in human erythrocytes, *Ind. Health*, 20, 365, 1982.

58. Ohno, H., Sato, Y., Ishikawa, M., Yahata, T., Gasa, S., Doi, R., Yamamura, K., and Taniguchi, N., Training effects on blood zinc levels in humans, *J. Sports Med. Phys. Fit.*, 30, 247, 1990.

59. Taniguchi, N., Ishikawa, N., and Kondo, T., Inhibitory effect of thyroxine on the biosynthesis of carbonic anhydrase isozymes in rabbit reticulocyte lysates, *Biochem. Biophys. Res. Commun.*, 85, 952, 1978.

60. Ohno, H., Taniguchi, N., Kondo, T., Matsuura, N., Okuno, K., Terayama, K., Hirata, F., and Kawarabayashi, T., A simple mass-screening test for thyroid disease using the immunoassay of carbonic anhydrase B type in children, *Jpn. J. School Med.*, 25, 129, 1983.

61. Balsam, A., and Leppo, L.E., Effect of physical training on the metabolism of thyroid hormones in man, *J. Appl. Physiol.*, 38, 212, 1975.

62. Dennis, E., Tupper, R., and Wormall, A., Studies on zinc in blood, *Biochem. J.*, 82, 466, 1962.

63. Ohno, H., Kato, T., Yamashita, K., and Taniguchi, N., Effect of high altitude on carbonic anhydrase concentration in human erythrocytes, *Jpn. J. Mountain Med.*, 6, 95, 1986.

64. Lukaski, H.C., Bolonchuk, W.W., Klevay, L.M., Milne, B.B., and Sandstead, H.H., Changes in plasma zinc content after exercise in men fed a low-zinc diet, *Am. J. Physiol.*, 247, E88, 1984.

65. Beaumont, W. van, Strand, J.C., Petrofsky, J.C., Hipskind, S.G., and Greenleaf, J.E., Changes in total plasma content of electrolytes and proteins with maximal exercise, *J. Appl. Physiol.*, 34, 102, 1973.

66. Gambert, S.R., Garthwaite, T.L., Pontzer, C.H., Cook, E.E., Tristani, F.E., Duthie, E.H., Martinson, D.R., Hagen, T.C., and McCarty, D.J., Running elevates plasma β-endorphin immunoreactivity and ACTH in untrained human subjects, *Proc. Soc. Exp. Biol. Med.*, 168, 1, 1981.

67. Klasing, K.C., Effect of inflammatory agents and interleukin 1 on iron and zinc metabolism, *Am. J. Physiol.*, 247, R901, 1984.

68. Cannon, J.G., Evans, W.-J., Hughes, V.A., Meredith, C.N., and Dinarello, C.A., Physiological mechanisms contributing to increased interleukin-1 secretion, *J. Appl. Physiol*, 61, 1869, 1986.

69. Fairweather-Tait, S.J., Zinc in human nutrition, *Nutr. Res. Rev.*, 1, 23, 1988.

70. Harland, B.F., Dietary fibre and mineral bioavailability, *Nutr. Res. Rev.*, 2, 133, 1989.

71. Thomas, E.A., Bailey, L.B., Kauwell, G.A., Lee, D.-Y., and Cousins, R.J., Erythrocyte metallothionein response to dietary zinc in humans, *J. Nutr.*, 122, 2408, 1992.

Chapter **13**

MAGNESIUM IN SPORTS PHYSIOLOGY AND PERFORMANCE

Lorraine R. Brilla
V. Patteson Lombardi

CONTENTS

0-8493-7916-4/95/$0.00+$.50
© 1995 by CRC Press, Inc.
139

I. INTRODUCTION

Magnesium, a major mineral which occurs most naturally as a divalent cation, is the second most abundant intracellular ion in the body next to potassium. Magnesium is crucial to a number of physical and chemical processes which are essential for optimal growth, health, and life itself. Salient body processes affected by low magnesium are summarized in Table 1. The magnesium requirement and the role of magnesium metabolism in various body systems has been studied.[1,2] The etiology and symptomatology of magnesium depletion has been reviewed and described.[3-7]

Magnesium is an activator of many enzymes including phosphatases, pyrophosphatases, transphosphorylases, hexokinases, and carboxylases. Many of these biological catalysts ultimately lead to the production of adenosine triphosphate (ATP), the energy currency of the body, which is used to synthesize macromolecules, perform mechanical work, and develop and maintain ionic gradients for impulse conduction and muscle contraction. Magnesium is also critical for maintaining the shape and function of deoxyribonucleic acid (DNA), ribonucleic acid (RNA), and ribosomes.[8,9]

Thus, magnesium is essential for the production of energy by anaerobic and aerobic metabolism, the transcription of genes in the nucleus, the translation of messenger RNA at the ribosome, and the formation and regulation of proteins, including those that make up muscle. It can be argued that no other ion has such a pervasive role in the physiology of the human body, yet interestingly, is so poorly understood.

Given the ubiquitous role of magnesium in metabolism, energy transduction, membrane fluidity, modulation of neural and humoral activity, and the formation and regulation of muscle proteins, it is clear that its role in both aerobic and anaerobic exercise and sports performance is important. However, since the dynamics of magnesium homeostasis are rather poorly understood,[9] and there are relatively few studies which have examined the role of magnesium in exercise, the precise role of magnesium in sports performance remains unclear. The primary goal of this paper is to review research on dietary magnesium requirements and deficiencies and to examine the roles of magnesium in muscle function and energy production. Additionally, the limited studies dealing with magnesium's influence on anaerobic and aerobic exercise will be reviewed, and a model will be proposed outlining the potential effects of magnesium supplementation or deficiency on sports performance.

TABLE 1. Salient Body Processes Affected by Low Magnesium

Function

Protein synthesis
RNA and DNA synthesis
enzymatic reactions[a]
Membrane changes[b]
Actomyosin cross-bridge cycling
Lipolysis
Vasoactivity
Erythrocyte function
Nerve transmission
Renal concentration of ions
Catecholamine secretion
Homeostasis of hormones:
    Adrenal cortical hormones
    Anti-diuretic hormone
    Thyroid hormones
    Parathyroid hormone
    Insulin

[a] Involved in the production of ATP: both oxidative phosphorylation and glycolysis.
[b] Distribution of several ions: potassium, sodium, and calcium.

II. BODY STORES OF MAGNESIUM

Total body magnesium of an adult ranges between 20 to 30 grams, 50% of which is stored in bone. The remainder is dispersed throughout the body with at least 45% in the intracellular fluid and 1% to 5% in the extracellular fluid compartment.[9,10] Using atomic absorption, the serum reference range is 1.3 to 2.1 meq/l (0.7 to 1.1 mmol/l), although values may vary slightly depending upon the method of serum analysis. The day-to-day variation for magnesium is 3.8% in serum.[11] Although there are no extreme differences based on gender, females reportedly have slightly higher serum magnesium levels during menstruation.[9] Yet, premenstrual syndrome (PMS) is associated with lower levels of magnesium in erythrocytes.[12,13] Although studies dealing with PMS and menstruation may be difficult to interpret because dietary intake and drugs such as diuretics have not been controlled, the studies may support the contention that massive body compartmental shifts of magnesium may occur throughout the menstrual cycle.

Magnesium is stored in both slowly exchanging and rapidly exchanging pools, and the relationship is presented in Figure 1. When dietary intakes are adequate, magnesium slowly exchanges between bone, skeletal muscle, and red blood cells. Magnesium exhibits rapid turnover in heart, liver, intestine, connective tissue, and skin. In a state of magnesium deficiency, the rapidly exchanging pools are maintained at the expense of slowly exchanging pools. For example, in hypomagnesemia, the heart, a component of the primary survival core, appears to capture magnesium from

SLOWLY-EXCHANGING POOLS

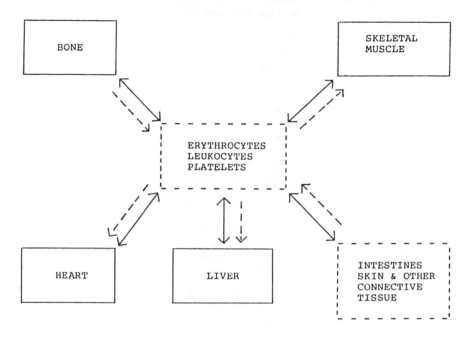

RAPIDLY-EXCHANGING POOLS

FIGURE 1.   Slowly and rapidly exchanging magnesium pools. (From Brilla, L.R., Fredrickson, J.H., and Lombardi, V.P., *Metabolism,* 38, 799.1989. With permission.)

the slowly exchanging bone store.[14] This is supported by the observation that rats on a diet moderately-deficient in magnesium have low magnesium levels in bone.[15]

Magnesium stores appear to be fairly mobile based on the specific and consistent demands placed upon a body system. Assuming that rapidly exchanged stores (heart, liver, intestines, skin, and other connective tissue) are maintained at the expense of those that are slowly-exchanged (bone and skeletal muscle), chronic swimming exercise appears to exert a protective effect on skeletal muscle magnesium, when a dietary magnesium deficiency exists.[14]

III. DIETARY REQUIREMENTS FOR MAGNESIUM

Magnesium is prevalent in many foods including legumes, dark green vegetables, seafoods, nuts, grains, and chocolate, with the most concentrated sources per serving found in spinach, oysters, sunflower seeds, and lima beans.[13] Despite widespread availability of magnesium, surveys demonstrate that the recommended daily allowance (RDA) of 400 mg/d is rarely achieved.[16] Based on the recently updated 1989 RDA data, the magnesium RDA for a 15 to 18 year old male is 400 mg/d, while that for a 15 to 18 year old female is 300 mg/d. For adults, the present values are 350 mg/d for males and 280 to 300 mg/d for females. It is recommended that a pregnant female acquire 320 mg/d; a lactating female, 355 mg/d during the first six months of lactation. Note the differences between the RDA and the U.S. RDA for labels. The RDA is based on the most recently updated data from 1989, while the U.S. RDA for food labels is based on the 1968 RDA data. There is no pressing need to update the food label values since they are considered generous by any standard and the cost of updating would be prohibitive. The U.S. RDA for food labels is given as the highest value from the 1968 research, that is 400 mg/d of magnesium is recommended.

The average daily dietary consumption of magnesium by adults in the U.S. is 76% of the RDA and has declined considerably from an estimated 410 mg/d since 1910.[17-21] In the survey, 36% of adults had diets in the suboptimal category of 70 to 99% of the magnesium RDA. Those participating in the survey showed that 39% of the population had dietary magnesium deficiency by the criterion of obtaining less than 70% of the magnesium RDA. These data indicate that 75% of the U.S. population has less than the magnesium RDA. Depending on heritability factors in magnesium metabolism, there is potentially 75% of the population which is susceptible to marginal to frank magnesium deficiency based on dietary assessment of magnesium alone. Magnesium, like other nutrients, is easily lost from foods during processing. The downward trend in the consumption of magnesium over the last century is likely due to our modern-day generation's greater reliance on processed foods. Since only about one-third of an adult's average daily magnesium intake is absorbed by the small intestine,[9] seemingly marginal dietary deficiencies may be compounded substantially.

A true dietary magnesium deficiency exists when less than 70% of the RDA for magnesium is obtained (equivalent to 210 mg/d or 280 mg/d). Average or marginal magnesium consumption may be further exaggerated in those who are extremely active or who are exposed to severe physical or psychological stress.[2,22-26]

Athletes who are most often weight-conscious, including gymnasts, ballerinas, and wrestlers, have an average consumption of magnesium that is about two-thirds of the RDA,[27-29] which is similar to that of young untrained subjects initiating an exercise program.[30] A lower than recommended magnesium intake (78% to 93% RDA) may occur even in physically active male subjects, despite a relatively high total food intake of 3000 kcal.[31] Elite female marathoners competing in the Olympic trials had less than the RDA in 23% of 51 subjects despite a mean value of 409 mg.[32] Additionally, there may be seasonal variations of magnesium intake with a high in the spring and summer, and a low in the winter months, likely induced by the availability of fresh vegetables, seafoods, legumes, nuts, and grains.[31]

Besides dietary practices, it is common for athletes to use supplements. In 50 male and 21 female triathletes, over 40% were below the RDA for magnesium.[33] In these athletes who supplemented, 23% still had magnesium intakes below the RDA. In a study of 91 athletes, those subjects who did not supplement were below the magnesium RDA; the average intakes were 91% of RDA for males and 75% of RDA for females.[34] Further research has shown that daily magnesium supplementation at

33% of RDA for three months did not alter blood magnesium values in athletes.[35] However, a magnesium saturation limit is demonstrated for strength training by urinary magnesium increases over 3.5 months of supplementation.[36] Acute magnesium supplementation during exercise did not ameliorate the decline in plasma magnesium with 120 min of exercise.[37] Magnesium-aspartate salts have been used to improve endurance performance with conflicting results.[38,39] No effect of this salt is seen on force production in humans.[40]

However, marginal magnesium intake may be offset because exercise may effect the absorption, and therefore the bioavailability, of magnesium. In rats, it has been demonstrated that exercise enhances magnesium absorption.[41] It still needs to be discerned what increased body magnesium needs may be for those who participate in regular, strenuous physical activity since it has been well documented that physical activity of certain types induces decreases in specific body pools of magnesium such as plasma and perhaps bone.[14,26]

In contrast to those who engage in restrictive dieting or rely on supplements, athletes who emphasize carbohydrate loading or vegetarianism may enhance their magnesium status. For example, marathon runners who consume a diet of approximately 3500 kcal, nearly two-thirds of which is carbohydrate, obtain almost double the RDA for magnesium.[42] Provided enough calories are consumed, a vegetarian diet can provide adequate to high levels of magnesium.[43]

A high-fat diet impedes the absorption of magnesium and may elevate body magnesium requirements to promote more efficient lipid metabolism.[44-46] Since dietary fat consumed by Americans averages an estimated 37% of total kilocalories ingested,[47] which is 7% higher than recommended by a number of national organizations,[47-50] it is likely that most Americans are predisposed to marginal magnesium deficiency.

While less is known about the effects of a high-protein diet on magnesium absorption in the small intestine, strength-trained, male athletes who consume well-over double the RDA for protein do have an adequate dietary intake of magnesium (about 135% RDA).[51] However, a high-protein diet may enhance the need for magnesium,[52] which is required for the synthesis of gastrointestinal enzymes and proteolytic activity. A diet high in protein is not only common to strength-event athletes, but is quite prevalent in the general U.S. population. Thus, despite daily intakes of magnesium meeting or exceeding the RDA, hyperproteinemia may make a large number of Americans, particularly strength-trained males, prone to minor magnesium deficiencies.

Together with carbohydrate, fat, and protein distributions in the diet, the ingestion of other minerals, particularly divalent cations, influences whole body magnesium and other mineral stores. Minerals are linked in a complex cascade, whereby an excess of one often depresses the absorption or bioavailability of another. For example, the ingestion of calcium reduces the bioavailability of magnesium[45] and iron.[13] Additionally, magnesium inhibits the absorption of calcium and iron, while other cations, such as zinc, hinder calcium and copper absorption.[13] Thus, a diet high in dairy products may act synergistically with other common dietary practices (e.g., low carbohydrate, high fat, high protein meals) to further reduce whole body magnesium stores. Furthermore, a diet high in magnesium and zinc (which is rare), or which is supplemented with these minerals, may accentuate a calcium deficiency unless additional calcium is ingested.

IV. CAUSES AND EFFECTS OF MAGNESIUM DEFICIENCY

Magnesium plays a vital role in maintaining the nervous, musculoskeletal and cardiovascular systems, yet hypomagnesemia is likely the most underdiagnosed electrolyte deficiency in hospital practice.[55-56] Serum magnesium is not included in routine patient screening and a deficit can mimic other electrolyte imbalances.[56] Even if it is measured, serum magnesium may be of limited prognostic value, since as little as 1% of the total body magnesium may be present in the extracellular fluid compartment.[10] Serum values may not reflect tissue levels, as patients with normal or marginal serum magnesium levels may have low whole body, muscle, or bone magnesium stores. While methods for measuring intracellular magnesium in muscle and leukocytes have been developed, their accuracy and usefulness require further verification.[10]

Magnesium infusion or loading may be the best way to determine true magnesium deficiency. For this procedure, magnesium sulfate is given intravenously and a 24 h urine sample is collected to assess differences between input and excretion. Patients with true magnesium deficiency retain abnormally large amounts of the intravenous load.[56] For example, patients with ischemic heart disease retain 31 to 57% of a magnesium load compared to only 5% in controls.[56] The magnesium load test and double-blinded supplementation crossover studies may yield the greatest benefit in trying to elucidate the effect of marginal magnesium deficiency vs. optimal body magnesium status, both for basic body functions and the implications for sports physiology and performance.

Deficiency of magnesium may occur due to inadequate dietary intake, protein malnutrition, malabsorption syndromes, alcoholism, vomiting, diarrhea, pancreatitis, diabetes, or kidney disease.[9] Patients who are given long-term intravenous feedings and/or thiazide diuretics may also develop magnesium deficiency.[13,58] It is likely that those who are exposed to physical or psychological stress also have a reduction in magnesium.[2,22-26,59,60-62]

Magnesium deficiencies may present without overt signs and symptoms, which do not appear until extracellular levels have dropped to 1 meq/l (0.5 mmol/l) or less.[9] Significant magnesium depletion can induce muscular weakness, irritability, tetany, bizarre facial and eye movements or twitches, difficulty in swallowing, confusion, hallucinations, convulsions, and cardiac arrhythmias.[5-7,9,13] Magnesium deficiency in infants and children can prevent normal growth and development. Along with phosphorus and calcium, magnesium is in great demand during pregnancy since it is needed to build the fetal skeleton.[63] These studies and others[1,2,64] show that using the clinical endpoints of overt signs and/or plasma magnesium values may not be appropriate where the magnesium deficiency is marginal vs. severe. Therefore caution must be exerted in declaring magnesium sufficiency even with apparently normal plasma magnesium or the absence of overt signs. Studies have also shown minimal relationship between serum and muscle magnesium: 47% of patients with low muscle Mg had normal serum values[65] and the researchers concluded that serum magnesium levels are of little value in the diagnosis of intracellular Mg deficits.

In contrast to magnesium deficiency, excess magnesium does not appear to induce symptoms of toxicity. Even large doses of magnesium ingested in the form of laxative Epsom salts have not been associated with ill effects, except diarrhea.[13] Persons who drink water with a high magnesium content experience a lower incidence of sudden death due to heart failure than those who drink water with normal levels of magnesium. A deficiency of magnesium appears to increase the likelihood of irreversible blood vessel or heart spasms.[10,13]

Given the pervasive role of magnesium in the production of energy in skeletal muscle and other body systems, it seems logical that both anaerobic and aerobic exercise performance could be altered dramatically by dietary practices and the subsequent availability of magnesium. Exercise itself may differentially affect magnesium absorption and metabolic magnesium requirement.

V. EARLY STUDIES ON MAGNESIUM AND DEFICIENCY

Researchers first examined the impact of magnesium withdrawal on growth during the early 1930s,[66] and later demonstrated that magnesium was essential for protein metabolism.[2,4,5,67,68] Since all enzymes are proteins, one would predict that a severe deficiency of magnesium would induce effects that are pervasive and detrimental to a number of biological systems. This is indeed the case, as low magnesium intake can adversely affect enzymes that regulate aerobic and anaerobic ATP production,[4,5] DNA and RNA synthesis,[4] and sodium, potassium, and calcium ion distribution.[5,67,69] The sodium-potassium ATPase enzyme that is present in nerve axons and all other cell membranes, requires the simultaneous presence of sodium, potassium, and magnesium.[8] Thus, magnesium is needed for the development of transmembrane electrical potentials and ultimately the conduction of nerve impulses.

Magnesium is also required for lipolysis[70–72] and the oxidation of fatty acids, and is used for the biosynthesis or inactivation of cholesterol, steroid,[8] adrenal catecholamine, thyroid, and parathyroid hormones.[3,44,68] Together with its function in muscle contraction and energy metabolism, magnesium's diverse lipolytic and neurohormonal actions make its potential role in exercise, sports, and performance more provocative.

Most studies have based their results on severe restriction of magnesium over a short time period. There have been some studies conducted over longer time periods to study the effects of chronic magnesium deficiency and to observe the effects of marginal magnesium deficiency rather than the radical deficiencies utilized in the early studies. Animals exposed to chronic suboptimal dietary magnesium for nearly two years do not demonstrate classic overt signs such as neuromuscular hyperexcitability, convulsions, or skin lesions, but do have less ability to cope with stress, greater heart and blood vessel damage, and shorter lifespans.[74] Magnesium deficiency may be present in spite of the absence of overt signs, and this marginal deficiency may result in impaired functions and perhaps contribute to the development of certain disease processes.[2] This marginal, or suboptimal, magnesium intake or body magnesium status can affect sports performance or the ability to participate in physical activity at the required level of intensity or duration.

Likewise, humans subjected to low magnesium up to 49 d demonstrate no overt signs of deficiency and have no significant changes in erythrocyte, plasma, or muscle magnesium, but do have a decreased renal clearance of magnesium.[75] Although bone levels were not measured, the authors postulated that body systems and functions requiring magnesium may have been maintained by mobilizing magnesium from bone.

A number of other researchers have verified that marginal magnesium deficiencies may exist without clinically overt signs or symptoms.[1,2,64] Additionally, a poor relationship has been demonstrated between serum and muscle magnesium, with almost half of the patients with low muscle magnesium having normal serum values.[65] It is apparent that rather than simply a routine plasma or serum magnesium test, a comprehensive and careful evaluation is necessary prior to classifying a patient as free of magnesium deficiency.

VI. MAGNESIUM AND ENERGY PRODUCTION

Physical activity requires greater absolute and relative energy production to meet the increased needs of working skeletal, cardiac, and smooth muscle. Additionally, during exercise, nearly all other body tissues and systems, except for the digestive system, have an increased metabolic activity. In maximal muscular exercise in well-trained athletes, overall metabolic rate (as measured in $kcal/m^2$ body surface area/h) and heat production can increase 20-fold above baseline during aerobic training and up to 50-fold above baseline during short bursts of anaerobic activity.[76,77]

Three overlapping and mutually supportive energy systems, (1) the immediate; (2) nonoxidative (glycolytic); and (3) oxidative pathways, provide the ATP needed for exercise.[78] The exercise mode, intensity, duration, frequency, and distribution of training sessions determine which energy system is most heavily activated. Activities which rely primarily upon the oxidative energy system, that is, the generation of ATP from mitochondrial electron transport chain and citric acid cycle reactions, are called *aerobic* exercises. These activities such as cross-country skiing, jogging, swimming, cycling, hiking, dancing, and stair climbing use over 50% of the body's muscle mass and are continuous in nature.[79,80] The energy nutrients used to fuel aerobic exercises include glucose, fatty acids and glycerol, and small amounts of amino acids.

In contrast, activities like sprinting and weight lifting, that are short-term, high-intensity, and/or intermittent are termed *anaerobic*. These last for sporadic periods of up to about 15 to 30 sec and rely heavily upon the immediate energy system, which includes (1) ATP that is already present in the muscle sarcoplasm; (2) ATP generated from ADP and inorganic phosphate by way of the myokinase reaction; and (3) ATP derived from creatine phosphate (CP), a short-term, high-energy phosphate compound that donates its phosphate to ADP by way of the creatine phosphokinase (CPK) reaction. The second and third components of the immediate energy system provide most of the ATP for high-intensity, extremely short-term exercises, since ATP already present in the muscle can sustain contractile activity for less than one second.[81] The creatine phosphate pool acts like a battery pack, which is depleted momentarily after a short burst of muscular activity, but is recharged by the generation of new ATP by oxidative metabolism when the muscle relaxes.[78,82] Resting muscles have 3 to 8 times as much creatine phosphate as ATP, enough for approximately 30 to 100 contractions.

Activities which are *transitional anaerobic*, that is, between pure anaerobic and aerobic exercises rely heavily upon *nonoxidative* metabolism for the generation of ATP. These activities, including short-distance running, circuit weight training, tennis, ballet, and boxing, use carbohydrates as the primary fuel for the glycolytic production of ATP in the cytosol. While some of these glycolytic, anaerobic activities may use over 50% of the body's muscle mass, they are maintained only periodically for no longer than 3 to 5 min.

All three energy systems, immediate, glycolytic, and oxidative, are involved in the bioenergetics, with each contributing according to the intensity and duration of the activity, and accounting for the physiological status of the individual embarking on the activity. Since many sports endeavors are interval in nature, creatine phosphate (immediate) and glycolysis provide most of the cellular energy required. However, even at short duration exercise, oxidative energy may contribute a portion of the energy needs. An overview of energy systems along with a proposed schematic for magnesium flux is presented in Figure 2. A caveat is that much research must be done on translocation and loss of magnesium in the various sporting activities before a definitive consensus can be generated. This is readily apparent in the darkened area on Figure 2 which indicates there is little insight into magnesium flux in the corresponding source.

Creatine phosphokinase (CPK, also called phosphocreatine kinase or creatine kinase) is a key enzyme in the formation of ATP by the immediate energy system. CPK is regulated by free magnesium and hydrogen ion concentrations.[83] The full enzyme-substrate-metal complex (CPK-ADP-CP-Mg^{2+}) including both magnesium and hydrogen ions is required for the reaction to proceed as follows:

$$\text{ADP + Creatine phosphate} \underset{Mg^{2+}, H^+}{\overset{\text{CPK}}{\rightleftharpoons}} \text{ATP + Creatine}$$

ATP is preferentially synthesized when magnesium levels are high, while creatine phosphate is synthesized when magnesium levels are low.[84,85]

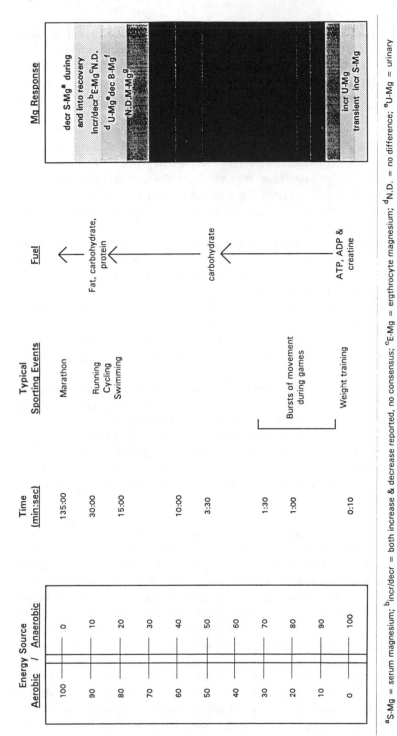

FIGURE 2. Putative magnesium responses to physical activity.

[a]S-Mg = serum magnesium; [b]incr/decr = both increase & decrease reported, no consensus; [c]E-Mg = ergthrocyte magnesium; [d]N.D. = no difference; [e]U-Mg = urinary magnesium; [f]B-Mg = bone magnesium; [g]M-Mg = skeletal muscle magnesium

Magnesium participates in many high-energy phosphate transfer reactions. Magnesium and magnesium chelates act as cofactors in the regulation of the following enzymes of glycolysis (nonoxidative metabolism): glucokinase (hexokinase), glucose-6-phosphatase, phosphoglucose isomerase, phosphofructokinase, aldolase, phosphotriose isomerase, phosphoglycerate kinase, phosphoglyceromutase, and enolase.[8,83]

While it is beyond the scope of this paper to cover the details of each of these chemical reactions, a few major points regarding magnesium are highlighted. Glucokinase catalyzes an essentially irreversible reaction in the very first step of glycolysis, producing glucose 6-phosphate from glucose with the actual substrate being the Mg^{2+} chelate of ATP (Mg^{2+}-ATP^{4-}). If it were not for the positive effector activity of the magnesium chelate and inorganic phosphate, the glucokinase reaction would proceed at only 5% of V max.[8]

The addition of a second phosphate group to fructose 6-phosphate is catalyzed by the key regulatory enzyme, phosphofructokinase (PFK). Magnesium is intimately involved in the regulation of PFK. PFK catalyzes the committed step in glycolysis which is the most important control site. High levels of magnesium inhibit PFK.[84]

Aldolase is a cytoplasmic glycolytic enzyme which catalyzes the cleavage of fructose 1,6-bisphosphate, also called fructose 1,6-diphosphate, to two triose phosphates. Aldolase is inhibited competitively by several compounds which are not its normal substrates and products, which include the magnesium-binding ligands ATP and inorganic phosphate.[85]

Enolase catalyzes the dehydration of 2-phosphoglycerate to phosphoenol-pyruvate (PEP), which substantially elevates the phosphoryl-transfer potential.[81] Magnesium is the only alkaline-earth metal that reacts with enolase.[86]

Additionally, magnesium has a dual kinetic role in the pyruvate kinase reaction, in that it adds directly to the enzyme and forms a chelate with ADP.[87] The most important effector of pyruvate kinase is free magnesium ion.[88] Pyruvate kinase activity in the liver is also enhanced by insulin, which is thought to be dependent upon magnesium acting as its second messenger.[89]

Glycolysis converts glucose to pyruvate. If oxygen is present, the next step in generating ATP from glucose is the oxidative decarboxylation of pyruvate to form acetyl coenzyme A (acetyl COA) in the matrix of mitochondria.[81] The formation of acetyl COA links anaerobic glycolysis in the cytosol with aerobic metabolism in the mitochondria and is controlled by the elaborate, multi-enzyme, pyruvate dehydrogenase complex. Pyruvate dehydrogenase contains a number of proteins and coenzymes, including thiamine pyrophosphate, which requires magnesium for its synthesis.[8] Thus, magnesium is essential for making a key catalytic cofactor of a multi-enzyme which is poised as a regulatory switch between anaerobic and aerobic metabolism.

The citric acid cycle (also called the tricarboxylic acid or Krebs cycle) occurs within the mitochondrial matrix and is the final common pathway for the oxidation of fuel molecules, glucose, fatty acids, and amino acids.[81] During this cycle, the two-carbon acetyl unit of acetyl coenzyme A is completely oxidized to form carbon dioxide. The first of four oxidation-reduction reactions within the citric acid cycle, producing α-ketoglutarate from isocitrate, is catalyzed by the enzyme isocitrate dehydrogenase. Isocitrate dehydrogenase requires magnesium for its activity and is important in determining the overall rate of the citric acid cycle.[81,90]

Magnesium not only influences key regulatory glycolytic and oxidative enzymes, but has also been associated with ultrastructural changes in mitochondria. A deficiency of magnesium in animals has been identified with mitochondrial disruption and swelling.[44,91,92] Mitochondrial membrane changes may affect the bioenergetics of oxidative metabolism.[93]

Erythrocyte membrane disruption noted in magnesium deficiency alters transmembrane ionic flux and membrane fluidity.[94,95,96] These changes are mediated indirectly via disturbances in lipid metabolism.[93,96] Altered membrane fluidity has implications for energy production, and is proposed as an underlying mechanism to abated physical performance.

Magnesium also influences ATP production by functioning in lipid metabolism. Beta-adrenergic stimulation increases the second messenger, cyclic adenosine monophosphate (cAMP), which induces lipolysis while simultaneously decreasing extracellular magnesium. Magnesium is sequestered by adipocytes and chelated by free fatty acids. Fasting, cold exposure, and exercise, particularly endurance-type activities, stimulate lipid mobilization.[74,77,97,98] Sodium nicotinate, a derivative of the reduced coenzyme, NADH, which has an anti-lipolytic action, inhibits the production of non-esterified fatty acids and ketone bodies and prevents hypomagnesemia.[98] Hypomagnesemia has been detected in subjects who engage in continuous exercise for longer than 1 h.[26,62,99] Adrenergic outflow, which stimulates lipolysis and induces an influx of magnesium into adipocytes, may account for the reduction in serum magnesium associated with exercise. However, in a 120 min exercise session, exogenous glucose supplementation suppressed FFA increases with no effect on plasma magnesium decrements compared to placebo.[37] Other mechanisms that contribute to magnesium metabolism during exercise need to be elucidated.

Adequate magnesium may ameliorate tetany in patients with latent disease. This may be mediated by the desaturase enzyme which is highly dependent upon magnesium for its activity. Hypomagnesemia may impair the functioning of desaturase, which plays a crucial role in fatty acid metabolism and maintenance of cell membrane function and fluidity.[100] Poor dietary intake of magnesium, or an enhanced requirement of magnesium brought on by exercise training, may induce tetany and certainly would not enhance sports performance.

Since most of the studies examining the influence of magnesium on glycolysis, oxidative, and lipid metabolism have been performed using *in vitro* techniques, the generalization and application of their results to the complete, dynamic, exercising human may be limited. However, these results should not be dismissed as being insignificant, but rather point to the need for well-designed, highly controlled, *in vivo* exercise physiology research using human subjects.

All energy for muscle contraction comes from the hydrolysis of ATP, which involves the cleavage of high-energy phosphate bonds by the enzymatic addition of water.[82] An enzyme which catalyzes the hydrolysis of ATP is called an ATPase. All known ATPase reactions require magnesium for ATP hydrolysis.[81,101] In skeletal muscle, magnesium must be attached to ATP before the thick-filament myosin ATPase can hydrolyze ATP. Thus, in order for skeletal muscle contraction to proceed normally, adequate levels of magnesium are required.[102]

There is no question that the role of magnesium is pervasive in energy metabolism. Magnesium is an absolute requirement for over two-thirds of the enzymes involved in glycolysis. It is essential for phosphofructokinase (PFK), the key regulatory catalyst which controls the irreversible, committed step in glycolytic path. Magnesium is needed to synthesize a key regulatory multi-enzyme linking glycolysis with the citric acid cycle. It also helps to control a rate-limiting enzyme in the citric acid cycle. Magnesium is also necessary for the operation of hundreds of other body enzymes, including phosphate transfers involving the common energy currency ATP. Without a doubt, magnesium is essential for the efficient cytosolic and mitochondrial production of ATP, as well as the performance of all activities regardless of their anaerobic or aerobic nature. It is likely that a severe deficiency of magnesium would compromise not only the production of ATP by glycolytic and oxidative pathways, but also inhibit the steady transition between anaerobic and aerobic metabolism.

VII. MAGNESIUM AND MUSCLE

Although exercise alters the homeostatic balance in virtually all body systems, the homeostatic adaptations in skeletal muscle are likely the most conspicuous. Although far from completely understood, the direct and indirect effects of magnesium, as well as its functions which are antagonistic to calcium, have been examined primarily in skeletal muscle.

A. DISTRIBUTION IN MUSCLE

It is obvious that magnesium plays important roles in contraction and the maintenance of energy and electrochemical equilibrium given its diverse association with phosphate compounds, structural and enzymatic proteins, intracellular organelles, and cytoskeletal components in muscle. Electron-probe analyses demonstrate that approximately 20% of whole muscle magnesium is bound to ATP (Mg^{2+}-ATP), with most of the remaining amounts stored in the high-energy compound creatine phosphate, and the calcium-sensor protein parvalbumin.[103] Within the sarcoplasm, some magnesium is bound to troponin, myosin light chains, and F-actin.[104–106] Magnesium in the sarcoplasmic reticulum is bound to the calcium-pump ATPase, parvalbumin, and calmodulin.[105] Calmodulin, a multipurpose intracellular calcium sensor that bears a close structural relationship to the calcium-binding protein, troponin C, mediates most calcium-regulated processes, and is larger and more ubiquitous than parvalbumin.[81,82]

The energy requirement of exercise increases the demand for magnesium. Magnesium is required for the mechanochemical transduction of ATP hydrolysis.[101] Magnesium has an anchoring role on ADP at the myosin active site, and has a role in the interaction of nucleotides with the myosin active site.[107] In control of muscle activity, it has been postulated that magnesium acts at both troponin and the SR, as well as on ATPase directly and related fuels used in energy production.

B. DEFICIENCY AND MUSCLE

As noted previously, many of the prominent signs and symptoms of magnesium deficiency involve alterations in neuromuscular control including cramps, spasms or tremors, fasciculations, myoclonus, tetanus, seizures, and both axial and respiratory muscle weakness.[5,12,108–110] Skeletal muscle myopathy resulting from magnesium deficiency is similar to the myopathy described in alcoholism.[111–113] The underlying mechanisms contributing to hypomagnesemic-induced myopathy include magnesium's role in muscle cellular bioenergetics, excitation-contraction coupling, and functional integrity of the cell membrane.[111]

When hypomagnesemia is induced in rats, tetany and contractures are observed.[114,115] Magnesium is still heavily concentrated in the terminal cisternae despite an increased permeability of the SR membrane to magnesium during tetanus.[114] It is possible that transient contractures, spasms and cramps, during high-intensity sports performance may be induced or augmented by low levels of magnesium. A schematic paradigm for hypomagnesemic skeletal myopathy is presented in Figure 3.

C. REGULATION OF CONTRACTION

Magnesium helps to regulate muscle activity through its direct effect on the thick filament, myosin; the regulatory protein, troponin; the sarcoplasmic reticulum and other calcium storage sites; and myosin and calcium ATPases. Additionally, magnesium may exert a more subtle influence on muscle contraction by working synergistically with hormones, hexokinases, lipases, and protein kinases to alter the availability of energy nutrients.

In skeletal muscle, magnesium is needed to ensure high-energy activation of the myosin head, which contains an ATPase enzyme, as well as the subsequent interaction of the myosin head with the actin binding-site. Without magnesium attached to ATP, the myosin ATPase cannot hydrolyze the ATP,[102] and no energy would be available for cross-bridge binding, bending, and detachment. So in order for the entire sequence of cross bridge cycling in skeletal muscle to proceed normally, adequate levels of magnesium must be present. It is obvious that this absolute requirement of magnesium for cross-bridge cycling, muscle contraction, and muscle relaxation, makes it absolutely essential for the performance of all anaerobic and aerobic activities.

The interaction of calcium with the regulatory protein troponin, primarily determines whether or not a muscle fiber contracts or relaxes. Pure troponin C, the calcium-binding unit of troponin, has six divalent-cationic binding sites. Two of the

Stage of Muscle Myopathy	Biochemical Abnormalities	Acute Muscular Syndrome	Progressive Chronic Myopathy
	$\longleftrightarrow$	$\longrightarrow$	$\longrightarrow$
Serum Magnesium	normal, perhaps low normal	low normal	low normal, perhaps clinically deficient
Possible Symptoms	none muscle tenderness muscle weakness fasciculations	cramps muscle pain/tenderness muscle weakness fasciculations swelling myoglobinuria	myopathy with weakness cramps muscle pain/tenderness muscle weakness fasciculations swelling myoglobinuria
• **Physical Performance**	slight decrement; performance deficit may be obscured if chronic	noticeable decrement	unable to perform/compete

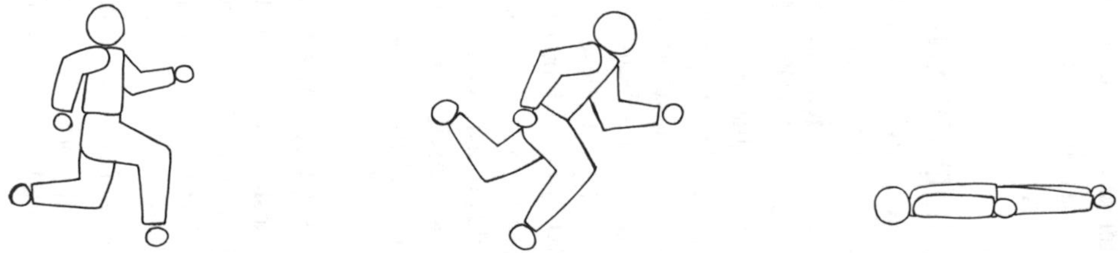

FIGURE 3. Paradigm: magnesium-deficient myopathy and effect on physical performance.

binding sites have an exclusive affinity for calcium and two bind magnesium, while the remaining two bind with either ion.[8,116,117] Magnesium alters the conformational state of troponin to inhibit the interaction of myosin and actin during contraction; this underlies the depressant effect of shortening.[104] The transitory decrease in muscle force during shortening is enhanced by increased magnesium.

In order for calcium to work as an intracellular signaling mechanism, calcium must be maintained at a low level in the cytosol. All eucaritic cells have plasma membrane calcium-ATPase enzymes that use energy from the hydrolysis of ATP to pump calcium out of the cytosol. Since magnesium and calcium are closely related, and often antagonistic, divalent cations, magnesium is involved in the regulation of calcium in all body cells.

An ATPase reaction in calcium pumps is also used to concentrate calcium in the sarcoplasmic reticulum (SR) of muscle cells. Magnesium is essential for this calcium-pump reaction sequence.

The recent discovery of calcium-sequestering compartments, similar to, but distinct from, rough endoplasmic reticulum in virtually all body cells,[82] indicates that calcium pumping, ATPase activity, and likely the regulatory role of magnesium, are even more pervasive than previously believed.

The transport of calcium by the sarcoplasmic reticulum (SR) is magnesium-dependent.[114,115,118–122] Magnesium replaces calcium on the SR calcium-ATPase,[123] while relatively fast phosphorylization of SR calcium ATPase is attributed to a magnesium-dependent accelerating effect of ATP on the enzyme's isomerization.[124] Increases in magnesium stimulate the SR active transport system for calcium,[121] but not during SR uptake of calcium as demonstrated by the low levels of calcium efflux.[120]

An adrenal medullary hormone released by sympathetic activation, epinephrine, is inactivated in the liver and kidneys by the enzyme catechol-*O*-methyltransferase. As with all methyltransferases, catechol-*O*-methyltransferase requires magnesium for its effective action.[8] When released during exercise, epinephrine activates adenylate cyclase in liver and muscle to trigger the cyclic adenosine monophosphate (cAMP) cascade. This cascade greatly amplifies the relatively weak epinephrine signal, inhibits glycogen synthesis, and stimulates its breakdown, making more glucose available for use by the active muscle. Magnesium complexed with ATP ($2Mg^{2+}$-ATP) binds to the catalytic subunit of a protein kinase enzyme, preventing its activation by cAMP, and inhibiting the release of glucose.[81] Thus, magnesium is used both extracellularly, to turn off a major hormonal signal, and intracellularly, to limit the amplification of that signal. During endurance exercise, this specific, dual, fine-tuning action of magnesium may help to preserve glucose and foster the transition from predominately sugar to fat metabolism for enhanced fat utilization in production of ATP in muscle.

D. ROLE IN MITOCHONDRIA

Mitochondria are the powerhouses of the cell, producing most of the ATP needed for energy, and are especially prevalent in cardiac and slow, oxidative skeletal muscle. Within mitochondria, a proton-motive force is used to generate ATP. ATP is synthesized by an inner-mitochondrial membrane-enzyme complex called ATP synthase, also known as F_0F_1, or H^+-ATPase.[81] ATP synthase, like all ATPase enzymes, requires magnesium for its activation. Magnesium is needed for the production of ATP by all mitochondria. This fundamental role of magnesium bears significant implications for the performance of exercises, particularly those of an aerobic nature, which rely heavily upon mitochondria abundant in highly oxidative, fatigue-resistant muscle.

Skeletal muscle mitochondria also have a highly-active, energy-dependent, magnesium transport system.[125] The mitochondrial potassium-hydrogen ion exchanger which helps to regulate mitochondrial matrix volume is inhibited by magnesium.[91] With extreme magnesium deficiency, there is severe mitochondrial swelling[44,92] together with disruption of the sarcoplasmic reticulum membrane. The alterations in membrane permeability influence the ion movement across the membrane or directly affects the membrane stability.[95,96,111]

E. ROLE IN MUSCLE SYNTHESIS AND FORCE PRODUCTION

Each of the twenty, building-block amino acids must be picked up and carried by a unique transfer ribonucleic acid (tRNA) to ribosomes, where the synthesis of all proteins, including structural and enzymatic muscle proteins, takes place. The single enzyme, aminoacyl-tRNA synthetase, which catalyzes the linkage of the tRNA with a specific amino acid, requires magnesium for its activity.[8] Thus, magnesium is required not only for the hydrolysis of ATP so that muscle contraction can proceed normally, but also is essential for the building of crucial regulatory and contractile muscle proteins. It is apparent that inadequate amounts of magnesium will compromise muscle building and subsequent contractions, and limit the performance of both anaerobic and aerobic activities. Additionally, magnesium's roles in linking amino acids to tRNA, and in ribosomal protein production, imply that it is an important limiting factor in recovery from intense exercise and in repair and healing of damaged muscle and other tissues.

Force production of muscle may be adversely affected by Mg deficiency.[30,113,126] In Mg deficient rats, marked reduction of tension was noted in both single twitch and tetanus, and half-relaxation time was significantly prolonged.[113] This was attributed to irreversible skeletal myopathy that included fiber swelling, loss of sarcomeric arrangement as indicated by loss of striations, floccular lesions, as well as swollen and vacuolated mitochondria, and reduced muscle mass. In clinical studies, maximal voluntary contraction of the quadriceps was positively correlated to serum magnesium status and muscle magnesium levels.[126,127] Lower isometric strength in hypomagnesemic patients has been reported.[112,126] In a magnesium supplementation study on strength training in humans, the supplemented group had significantly greater gains in torque production.[30] In chronic candida infection, the Mg requirement is increased and normocalcemic tetany may ensue without attention to Mg levels.[100] The effect of magnesium on force production may be related to magnesium's role on protein synthesis, one of the most sensitive functions affected by magnesium levels.[4,68,69] Magnesium depletion has resulted in conformational changes of the ribosome and muscle necrosis with rhabdomyolysis.[4,92] DNA transcription, RNA aggregation, and protein synthesis all depend on optimal Mg concentration.[68,69]

Magnesium deficiency impairs muscle potassium repletion and increases BUN.[55,65,97] This has implications for insufficiencies related to increased contractures and decreased force production. Muscle potassium levels correlate significantly ($r = 0.61$) with magnesium levels.[11] The potassium derangement may be related to the action of magnesium on the ATPase sodium-potassium pump. BUN elevations may represent high protein intake, metabolic acidosis, catabolic states possibly associated with increased muscle breakdown, dehydration, and possible renal dysfunction. As well, NH_3 is formed in muscles during exercise and may require Mg for adequate metabolism to urea and clearance, since some of the involved enzymes may require Mg salt.[40]

F. ALTERATIONS IN pH AND END-PLATE POTENTIALS

Magnesium excess increases the alkalinity of the cytosol and augments cross-bridge cycling, which could enhance buffering capacity as well as muscle contractile strength and endurance for both anaerobic and aerobic exercises.[5,104] However, too much magnesium may induce toxicity, although extremely rare,[13] and may depress muscle activity as indicated by a reduced end-plate potential amplitude.[5,104,128,129]

It is readily evident that magnesium is needed for muscle integrity including both the membranous and proteinaceous components. Magnesium influences muscle action at both the SR and troponin. The physical quality of the sarcomere requires magnesium. Protein synthesis, DNA transcription, RNA aggregation, and ribosome conformation are adversely affected and this may abate the needed muscle enhancement for sports performance. Ultimately, Mg inadequacy is manifested by decrements in force production with development of muscle hyperexcitability, including spasms, cramps, and tetany, in chronic or severe, acute Mg deficiency.

VIII. MAGNESIUM AND THE HEART, VESSELS, AND OTHER TISSUES

Adequate magnesium is needed for the normal function of the heart, vessels, and blood. Deficiencies have been associated with cardiovascular abnormalities. Patients with severe magnesium deficiency may experience cardiac arrhythmias with prolonged QRS and QT intervals and broad, flat T waves.[56,130] Loading tests have detected extreme magnesium deficiencies in patients with ischemic heart disease.[57] Communities with low concentrations of magnesium in drinking water tend to have higher rates of ischemic heart disease and acute myocardial infarction (AMI).[131,132] Patients with AMI have low serum magnesium levels, however, it appears that hypomagnesemia follows, rather than precedes, AMI.[10,57,133]

An increase in magnesium ion concentration does induce powerful local vasodilation by inhibiting smooth muscle contraction, and may help to fine-tune peripheral cardiovascular regulation during exercise.[76,134–137] Low dietary magnesium has been associated with high blood pressure, yet there are no convincing data to warrant the recommendation for increasing magnesium intake in an attempt to reduce blood pressure.[138–141]

All body cell membranes have ionic pumps, which are used to create membrane potentials. The most well-studied of these ionic pumps is the sodium-potassium pump which depends upon the sodium-potassium ATPase (Na^+-K^+ATPase) enzyme. The enzyme reaction couples the energy derived from the hydrolysis of ATP to the active movement of sodium to the outside, and potassium to the inside, of cells. As in skeletal myocytes and erythrocytes, magnesium ion is essential in cardiac myocytes for the sodium-potassium ATPase reaction.[8,142]

Although long ago magnesium was found to be concentrated highly in the ventricular myocardium of mammals, many years transpired before it was suggested that magnesium was critical in regulating tension in cardiac muscle.[85,143] Living myocardial cells accumulate magnesium in response to hypertrophic stimuli.[85,144] Ischemic heart disease is related to diminished myocardial magnesium concentration and physical inactivity.[145,146] The connection may be related to the cardiac cellular metabolism regulated by magnesium.[147]

While the function of magnesium has been established more clearly in muscular systems, it is certainly crucial for the optimal health of the nervous, endocrine, renal-excretory, skeletal, integumentary, and other body systems. Along with other ions, magnesium is thought to be conjugated to hydroxyapatite crystals as an important component of bone salts.[76,148,149]

IX. MAGNESIUM AND PHYSICAL STRESS

Physical activity is a stressor to the body, whether it is related to exercise and performance or work. Typical physiological changes ensue when an individual engages in exercise: release of neurohumoral modulators and hormones, acceleration of metabolic responses, and adaptation or collapse to chronic exposure. Magnesium has anti-stress functions and magnesium metabolism accelerates during stressful conditions, for example, hypoxia or exercise.[150] The anti-stress functions that magnesium exhibits include: anti-hypoxic, anti-allergic, anti-anaphylactic, and anti-inflammatory.

When considering exercise, it is usual to categorize the type of exercise under general headings of aerobic or anaerobic exercise, depending on the main energy source involved in the provision of energy. Typical aerobic exercise includes walking, jogging, swimming, and cycling; classic anaerobic exercise includes burst activity like throwing the discus, sprints in running, swimming, or cycling, and high-overload work like weight training. Within an exercise program, the volume or index of activity is quantitatively determined by the frequency, intensity, and duration of the physical activity.

X. MAGNESIUM AND SPORTS PERFORMANCE

The first report of the interaction of sports performance and magnesium changes was in 1970.[62] A decrement in plasma magnesium levels after a marathon was demonstrated. For the next decade, very little research was conducted on the association between magnesium and physical activity. This is readily evident in a perusal of Table 2. However, because of the roles magnesium plays in basic body functions, and especially the striking effects of magnesium on the neuromuscular system and in energy production, renewed interest in magnesium and sports physiology and performance has ensued.

For the past decade, research has shown a link between low magnesium levels and impaired endurance exercise; physical activity of a continuous nature that lasts one or more hours.[151,152] Additionally, there is some limited evidence to demonstrate that magnesium may be involved in strength exercise.[30,126] The hypothesis presented here is that marginal magnesium deficiency is widespread because of dietary practices in modern industrialized cultures, including documentation of low dietary magnesium in athletes, and a suboptimal magnesium status can interfere with sports performance.

Appraisal of magnesium's role in physical activity must be done with respect to the type of activity and whether the focus is on magnesium deficiency effects due to reduced intake, or magnesium depletion effects due to dysfunctional metabolism. Strenuous activity of long duration, or endurance activities, have received the most attention.[14,26,30,37,40,60–62,99,110,126,151,152,155–160,162–165,169–174,176–188]

More recently, anaerobic, or high-intensity, quickly exhaustive exercise and magnesium have been studied, and these studies generally demonstrate hypermagnesemia immediately post-exercise.[30,40,126,153,154,161,166–169,175] Increases in urinary magnesium, with and without magnesium loading, has been observed. Further, studies on muscle strength and magnesium have demonstrated that magnesium is required to express higher levels of strength[30,126,154] or to decrease the expression of neuromuscular hyperexcitability, such as spasms and cramps.[110,168]

A. AEROBIC EXERCISE

Unlike other major ions which are conserved in body fluids with training, magnesium is lost in sweat at about the same level in trained and untrained persons.[13,59] Compared to others, exercisers had a lower level of serum magnesium, which was still reduced even three months after they began a training program.[26] Endurance exercise may reduce plasma and bone magnesium, but is postulated to exert a protective effect in skeletal muscle in order to maintain homeostatic balance of intramuscular magnesium and ATP.[14]

Some researchers have noted that low serum magnesium has been observed in overtrained, but also in well-trained, endurance athletes.[190,191] However, there are many uncertainties regarding this distinction, since most well-trained, world-class athletes, particularly those who compete in endurance events, are consistently on the brink of over-training as demonstrated by the high rate of overuse injuries.

TABLE 2. Magnesium and Physical Activity Research Summary

Author (Year)	Sport(s)	Major Findings	Comments
Bell et al. (1988) n = 28	Weight training	Urinary Mg excretion higher in trained	≥1 year exercise; age-matched controls
Beller et al. (1975) n = 8	Walk (90 min)	↓ S-Mg[a] not explained by sweat Mg	Heat study
Beuker & Helbig (1989)	Runners; weight trained	Anabolic effect possible on strength trained	Supplement study; Ab[b]
Beuker et al. (1990) n = 23 ♂; n = 6 ♀	Weight training	N.S.[c] S-Mg with training; ↑ U-Mg with supplementation; loading saturated tissues	Supplementation study; Ab 3.5 months
Binder et al. (1990) n = 15	Fencing; ergometer	E-Mg[d]; ↓ blood glucose; ↑ glucose mobilization during exercise; ↑ glucose transfer to muscle; ↓ plasma lactate	Supplementation study; Ab 28 d
Brilla (1992)	Running	Improved economy	Supplementation study
Brilla et al. (1989) n = 32	Swimming	Slowly exchanging pools: ↓ Mg with ↓ Mg diet; exercise: ↑ skeletal muscle Mg vs. controls	Animals
Brilla and Haley (1992) n = 26	Weight training	↑ Strength gains with Mg supplement	Training study
Brilla and Lombardi (1987) n = 32	Swimming	↑ Cholesterol with ↓ diet Mg ameliorated by exercise	Animals
Caddell et al. (1986) n = 84	Shock-tetany	Massive ↑ catecholamines in ↓ diet Mg	Animals
Casoni et al. (1990) n = 11 expt. n = 30 control	25 km run	Athletes ↓ Mg with physical stress	Pre- post-race results
Chadda et al. (1985) n = 59	V̇O₂ max test	No significant change in Mg homeostasis	Patients
Conn et al. (1988) n = 22	Swimming, V̇O₂ max	P-Mg[e] correlation with $\dot{V}O_2$ max, r = +0.42	Not true in females
Cordova et al. (1988) n = 40	Swimming	Exercise and hypoxia both affect Mg homeostasis	Animals; various tissue samples
de Haan et al. (1985) n = 20 humans	Weight training	Force and local endurance not enhanced by Mg Asp.[f]	Animal and human

Reference	Exercise	Finding	Comment
Deuster et al. (1987) n = 13	Sprint intervals	Transient shift of Mg; ↑ U-Mg⁸ loss	90% $\dot{V}O_2$ max to exhaustion
Deuster and Singh (1993) n = 10	Running, 120 min	↓ P-Mg to lowest value at 120 min; glucose-electrolyte solution diminishes ↑ FFAʰ → why ↓ P-Mg?	supplementation study; replacement during run; unknown mechanism for ↓ P-Mg with smaller ↑ FFA
Fitzherbert (1982)	Running	Effect of Mg in water, food on competition	Synopsis
Flink (1983)	Prolonged	↓ Mg → aminoaciduria, ↓ S-albinin lipolysis (from cold, adrenergic administration, and exercise) → ↓ Mg	Synopsis; Ab
Franck et al. (1991) n = 56	Physical training	PE class for 8 weeks, 2 to 3 sessions per week; ↓ S-Mg after 4 weeks, S-Mg returned to normal after 8 weeks; reactive ↑ PTH	Bone and physical activity
Franz et al. (1985) n = 1	Marathon	↓ Mg post-race; related to ↑ plasma FFA	Case study
Golf et al. (1985) n = 20	1 h ergometer	14 d supplement; ↓ baseline hemoglobin and hematocrit	9 ♂, 11 ♀; supplement study; Ab
Golf et al. (1984) n = 9	1 h ergometer	Mg supplement → lowers aldosterone, and cortisol ↑ with exercise; E-Mg ↓ with exercise; NS: U-Mg	Measured serum, urine and sweat
Golf et al. (1989a)	Occlusion test	Simulate physical stress → Mg shifts → activation of fibrinolysis by local	Indirect exercise application; Ab
Golf et al. (1989) n = 14	Rowing	Improved lactate elimination following two bouts of 6 min of rowing in 5 h period	Supplement study
Helbig et al. (1989) n = 27	Body building	Prophylactic use of Mg to ameliorate spasms and cramps	Supplement study
Joborn et al. (1985) n = 10 (erg.) n = 5 (strength)	Ergometer to max; 1 h ergometer; strength	Short term → ↑ P-Mg; long term → ↓ P-Mg; adrenergic infusion → ↓ Mg	5-part comprehensive study
Laires and Alves (1991) n = 8 expt. n = 10 control	Swimming	After exercise → ↓ P-Mg; more pronounced in swimming than control	Blood and urine samples; swimmers at higher intensity than controls
Laires et al. (1989) n = 17	Swimming	↓ endurance capacity	Animal study

TABLE 2 (continued). Magnesium and Physical Activity Research Summary

Author (Year)	Sport(s)	Major Findings	Comments
Lijnen et al. (1988) n = 23	Marathon	↓ E-Mg and S-Mg after marathon; propose mechanism for Mg to enter adipocyte	Compartmental shifts
Liu et al. (1983) n = 1	Tennis	Frank hypomagnesemia with carpopedal spasms following 6 h exercise	Case study
Ljunghall et al. (1987) n = 10	Ergometer to max	Altered acid-base balance, adrenergic stimulation, and compartmental shifts of K; follows Mg change	Only K measured directly
Ljunghall et al. (1988) n = 17	Field exercise	NS: S-Mg; ↑ parathyroid hormone	Military exercise; winter
Lowney et al. (1990) n = 24	Walking/running	Reduced endurance capacity in ↓ diet Mg; no change in 2,3 DPG; Mg via water alleviates negative response	Animals
Lowney et al. (1988)	Running	↓ Endurance capacity; ↓ plasma insulin with ↓ D-Mg; ↑ tissue calcium	Animal study; 4 levels of D-Mg V̇O₂ max
Lukaski et al. (1983) n = 44 trained n = 20 control	V̇O₂ max test	P-Mg correlated to V̇O₂ max in trained only	
Mader et al. (1990)	Rowing	Intensive training produced negative Mg balance; ↑ U-Mg with Mg supplement	Supplementation study; Ab
Manore et al. (1989) n = 10	Running, 30 min	↓ S-Mg, ↑ E-Mg, ↓ haptoglobin	10 km race pace, ♀
McDonald and Keen (1988)	Various	↓ Mg with intense strenuous activity; ↓ diet Mg → ↑ endurance; no data on long-term Mg supplementation	Review: iron, zinc, Mg
Munch et al. (1990)	Various	Most Mg loss from performance in urine; disturbed membrane integrity results in ↑ V̇O₂	No detailed training protocol; Ab
Olha et al. (1982) n = 5 trained n = 5 control	Ergometer to max	Both groups ↓ S-Mg after exercise; more pronounced in trained, 6.7% vs. 2.4%; may be related to greater amount of work to reach max (↑ mito Mg in rats)	Trained vs. untrained
Rayssiguier et al. (1990)	Various	Physical exercise is a factor leading to ↓ Mg	Proposed mechanism
Refsum et al. (1973) n = 16	Cross-country skiing 70 km, 90 km	Transient ↓ S-Mg, values immediately post-race	Compartmental shifts

Study	Activity	Findings	Comments
Ripari et al. (1989) n = 16	Ergometer	Max and 70% max test; improved HR, V_e, SBP, $\dot{V}O_2$, $\dot{V}CO_2$ with supplement vs. placebo	Improved economy; Ab
Rose et al. (1970) n = 8	Marathon	↓ S-Mg post-race	First study on sport and Mg
Ruddell et al. (1985)	Running	Variations in S-Mg post-race related to supplementation	Compartmental shifts; Ab
Smith et al. (1985)	Walking	↓ Bone-Mg in trabecular bone compared to sedentary in hens	Animals; Ab
Steinacker et al. (1987) n = 29	Ergometer, treadmill	Significant ↑ physical working capacity in serum group	Supplement study; Ab
Stendig-Lindberg et al. (1987) n = 20	120 km hike	↓ S-Mg post-hike; persisted for 3 mos; ↑ S-Mg past 24 hrs may be due to exertional rhabdomyolysis on loss of membrane integrity	Recovery follow-up
Stendig-Lindberg and Rudy (1983)	Weight training	MVC[m] in quadriceps related to S-Mg	↓ S-Mg by alcoholism
Tate et al. (1978)	Running	Mitochondria accumulate Mg during acute exercise; maintain membrane integrity and offset effects of exercise Ca[n] uptake	Animal study
Tate et al. (1982) n = 8 (each group)	Swimming	Matched pairs; Mg inhibit Ca uptake in mitochondria is greater in control than exercise group	Animal study
Tibes et al. (1973) n = 15	Ergometer	During control and work, S-Mg was lower in trained than untrained; pattern similar to acidosis without exercise	Not corrected for hemoconcentration
Tiedt and Grimm (1992)	Various	No typical changes in S-Mg	Longitudinal (1 year); Ab
Verde et al. (1982) n = 8	Running	Mg concentration decreased as sweat flow increased	Heat study
Yeh et al. (1991) n = 10 (each group)	Not described	Mg absorption and retention is higher in exercise groups than sedentary or immobilization	Absorption study

[a] S-Mg = serum magnesium; [b] Ab = abstract only available; [c] N.S. = no significant difference; [d] E-Mg = erythrocyte magnesium; [e] P-Mg = plasma magnesium; [f] Mg Asp. = magnesium aspartate; [g] U-Mg = urinary magnesium; [h] FFA = free fatty acids; [i] K = potassium; [j] 2,3 DPG = 2,3-diphosphoglycerate; [k] D-Mg = dietary magnesium; [l] mito = mitochondria; [m] MVC = maximal voluntary contraction; [n] Ca = calcium.

Although inconsistencies in experimental protocol, work intensity and duration, dietary magnesium, and environmental conditions exist across the research studies, consistency is demonstrated in the expression of hypomagnesemia in response to strenuous endurance exercise. This is clearly evident despite few training studies or inclusion of females. Occasionally, environmental conditions were reported which may affect magnesium status, more so for the laboratory work than field studies. Intensity of exercise was not monitored in many studies; however, duration was consistently reported. Regardless of the mode of exercise, endurance activities result in hypomagnesemia. The effect of magnesium deficiency was to decrease endurance time when animals were run to exhaustion. Increases in physical working capacity result from magnesium supplementation, however, baseline magnesium status was not well defined.

As noted previously, plasma magnesium is fairly well maintained and may not be the best index of overall magnesium status, except in acute conditions of a single bout of endurance exercise or a prolonged exhaustive exercise routine. In the endurance studies, magnesium was measured in erythrocytes or other tissues, bone, muscle, liver, and kidney.[14,150,152] Muscle levels of magnesium are intractable. It would be expected that magnesium would leak out of the intracellular compartment of muscle because of the muscle membrane damage associated with strenuous exercise, as indicated by elevated plasma creatine kinase and LDH levels associated with exertional rhabdomyolysis.[26,99] However, it has been demonstrated in both animal and human studies that muscle magnesium is well maintained during exercise regardless of magnesium intake.[14,150,192,193]

The putative mechanisms for exercise-induced hypomagnesemia are primarily, compartmental shifts,[14,60,70,165,166,176,180,182] with some contribution from sweat production and urinary loss.[36,41,59,161,175] It is hypothesized from data results that magnesium enters muscle and adipose tissue and is removed from bone. Magnesium's role in muscle is to maintain the integrity of muscle function through control of muscle action directly at the SR and troponin, and by contributing to the energy demands as a cofactor for enzymes and as an ion important to the resonance bonds of ATP. The magnesium action in adipose tissue is to form salt complexes with the free fatty acids released in lipolysis.[60,99] This mechanism is postulated as one of the main contributors to hypomagnesemia observed in endurance exercise. However, a glucose-electrolyte supplementation study has demonstrated that serum magnesium still decreases despite blunted mobilized fatty acid levels which infers an additional contributing mechanism is acting to reduce serum magnesium.[37] Magnesium may be critical to the glucose transfer to muscle[155] and maintenance of membrane integrity to facilitate oxidative metabolism,[167,177,185,186] thereby enhancing physical working capacity.[160,174,184] To some degree, magnesium may also enter erythrocytes to act as a cofactor in glycolysis and contribute to the production of 2,3-DPG, thereby facilitating oxygen delivery by hemoglobin.[155,174,176] Other roles for magnesium include: involvement in the hexose monophosphate shunt, production of NADPH, and facilitating glutathione-reductase coenzyme which protects hemoglobin, enzymes, and membranes against oxidative damage.[158]

The reduced exercise capacity for endurance exercise has been attributed to membrane fluidity changes, among other mechanisms.[26,93,95,151,179] The membrane changes may induce erythrocyte fragility, affect electrolyte exchange, and contribute to fatigue.[193] Aberrations in fuel production may also contribute to reduced exercise capacity. This is attributed to the partial uncoupling of oxidative phosphorylation noted in hypomagnesemia which results in reduced ADP/O_2 ratio, increased O_2 uptake for ADP phosphorylation, with an increased O_2 need without a corresponding increase in ATP production.[83,167,179] This magnesium mediated mechanism also has implications for improved running economy, which has been noted in some magnesium supplementation studies.[167,181]

In addressing the timecourse of hypomagnesemia, some researchers have expressed that the magnesium fall is transient, though it may endure for some months after especially strenuous activity, and others have inferred that the hypomagnesemia is persistent due to the chronic engagement in physical activity which elicits greater magnesium needs and increases magnesium loss.[26,158] Further magnesium losses in hypomagnesemia may occur due to accumulative effects through such mechanisms as: sweat production[59,189], decreased renal concentrating mechanism as influenced by aldosterone and ADH[150,165], increased lactic acid affecting bone resorption and subsequent hypermagnesuria[41,161], the stressor of exercise increases release of catecholamines which is associated with hypermagnesuria[150,169,172], and it has been suggested that the observed hypermagnesuria is correlated with high intensity performance and the extent of lactate production and excess post-exercise oxygen consumption (EPOC).[166,179] EPOC is affected by both intensity and duration of exercise, or the overall volume of exercise.

A few studies have compared the magnesium responses of trained individuals vs. sedentary controls to a bout of exercise[158,178,187] or to a maximal graded exercise test to measure oxygen consumption.[160,174] In the exercise bouts, the trained individuals had lower plasma magnesium at rest compared to the sedentary groups and expressed a greater reduction to exercise which may be partially related to their ability to achieve higher workloads. The implications of these studies are that they do demonstrate lower magnesium status in trained individuals at rest and that this is exacerbated by a subsequent exercise bout. With respect to maximal oxygen consumption ($\dot{V}O_2$ max), there were significant correlations of $\dot{V}O_2$ max and resting plasma magnesium in trained runners (r = 0.46) and swimmers (r = 0.42), with discrepant results in these two studies in their sedentary subjects, with correlations reported of (r = –0.32)[174] and (r = 0.41).[160] Physically active individuals demonstrate a tighter relationship with indicators of magnesium status and flux, however further study is warranted.

In response to a maximal graded exercise test, magnesium levels have not changed in cardiac patients[159]; however improvements in various cardiorespiratory parameters have been described following magnesium supplementation in athletes.[167,181,184] The improvements included increased physical working capacity,[184] and decreased heart rate, systolic blood pressure, $\dot{V}_e$, and $\dot{V}O_2$ with no significant improvement in final workload.[167,181] Magnesium supplementation reduces release of cortisol during exercise which may account for the lower heart rates at similar workloads that has been noted.[165,167] In a 90% $\dot{V}O_2$ max run to exhaustion, time increased from 11 to 12 min in the supplementation treatment compared to placebo with signs of enhanced economy, as evidenced by reductions in $\dot{V}_e$ and $\dot{V}O_2$ at the final stage.[194] In rats swum to exhaustion, increased magnesium content was reported in serum, gastrocnemius muscle, and liver; when the exercise to exhaustion was coupled with environmentally induced hypoxia, magnesium was reduced in serum, gastrocnemius, and liver.[150] The relationship between magnesium status and maximal exercise testing responses, including exercise-induced hypoxia, require further study, as does the implied enhanced economy in tests to exhaustion.

B. ANAEROBIC EXERCISE

Short term tests to exhaustion are more indicative of anaerobic energy systems contributing to energy needs during exercise rather than a large aerobic component. The interaction between exercise and magnesium metabolism, with the relative contribution of anaerobic vs. aerobic influences, remain to be discerned.[60] Intense short term exercise may result in hypermagnesemia.[161,165,167,169] The increased plasma magnesium may be related to decreased plasma volume associated with strenuous exercise and increased effluent of magnesium into the vascular pool.[169] Much more research is needed in this area to further study the body magnesium response to high intensity, exhaustive exercise.

Strength training exercise is considered to be anaerobic in nature due to the overload, therefore high intensity, and relatively short duration that the individual actually spends in performing the physical activity. A few studies have reported on the relationship between magnesium and strength.[30,36,40,126,154,168] A positive relationship exists between magnesium status and strength[30,126,154] and magnesium levels may be reduced due to strength training involvement.[36,154]

Magnesium supplementation may have anabolic effects. In magnesium supplementation vs. placebo, greater strength gains were noted in the magnesium–supplemented group after seven weeks of strength training, even when adjusting for body weight and body fat differences.[30] Another study noted no strength improvements after one week of magnesium supplementation with no training.[40] Urinary magnesium levels in response to test loads are greater in individuals who strength trained for a year than controls, and was attributed to higher vitamin D levels in exercisers.[36,153] Magnesium supplementation has been used prophylactically to ameliorate spasms and cramps in body builders.[168]

The mechanisms involved in intense exhaustive exercise, such as anaerobic activities, may be related to magnesium's role in protein synthesis and muscle physiology parameters already discussed, with again possible implications on the effect of energy production. The implications marginal dietary magnesium or magnesium loading have on anaerobic performance need to be resolved. Obviously, more studies are needed on magnesium and strength relationships.

XI. PREDICTING EFFECTS OF MAGNESIUM SUPPLEMENTATION OR DEFICIENCY ON SPORTS PERFORMANCE

Magnesium maintains an intimate association with the body's common energy currency, ATP. By way of this intrinsic link, magnesium maintains important and pervasive roles in the human body including (1) the very creation of ATP and the regulation of its metabolism; and (2) the use of ATP for (a) molecular synthesis of muscle proteins and all biological enzymes; (b) for the mechanical work of muscle contraction as well as relaxation; (c) for pumping ions and developing concentration gradients needed for controlling cell volumes and for muscle cell contraction and nerve cell transmission. Magnesium is required for cellular integrity related to energetics, ionic milieu, and membrane fluidity associated with phospholipid changes. Magnesium is also critical for growth and development and optimal functioning of the nervous, endocrine, cardiovascular, digestive, reproductive, and all other body systems.

The pathological effects of magnesium deficiencies have been fairly well-established. The research on the effects of magnesium on exercise performance while not conclusive, do provide a framework for developing a model for predicting the effects of magnesium on sports performance as presented in Figure 4.

To verify the proposed model, future studies should examine the acute and chronic effects of magnesium on the performance of anaerobic and aerobic exercises by untrained and trained animals and human subjects. In examining the influence of magnesium on exercise performance, researchers should implement double-blind, placebo-controlled, cross-over designs and provide a clear distinction between supramaximal and adequate magnesium status, and marginal and severe magnesium deficiency. Magnesium load testing should be used, since it is likely the only definitive way to determine whether or not subjects are magnesium-deficient.

Given that an estimated one-third of the magnesium ingested is absorbed by way of the small intestine, it is likely that large doses of at least two times the RDA will be necessary to induce significant treatment effects. These levels of magnesium may be obtained from the diet through wise food choices, while higher doses may be achieved through supplementation. However, since divalent cations bind competitively in the small intestine, larger supplemental doses of magnesium may induce subsequent deficiencies among antagonist cations, and therefore have disadvantages which are yet unknown. For example, pharmacological doses of magnesium may induce calcium deficiencies and may predispose endurance-trained athletes to osteoporosis and stress fractures. Additionally, magnesium supplementation may exacerbate zinc deficiencies, which are quite common among athletes and the general population.

Researchers should measure the levels of antagonistic divalent cations through load testing, similar to that used for magnesium, for ions such as calcium. This will help to establish more clearly both the advantages and disadvantages of magnesium supplementation.

Continuum

DIETARY DEFICIENCY <———————————> DIETARY SUFFICIENCY

PARAMETER	SEVERE ($\leq$ 100 mg/d)	MARGINAL ($\leq$ 200 mg/d)	ADEQUATE ($\geq$ 400 mg/d)	SUPRAMAXIMAL ($\sim$ 800-1200 mg/d)
Detected by Mg^{2+} Serum Test	Yes	Yes/No	Yes/No	Yes
Detected by Mg^{2+} Loading Test	Yes	Yes	Yes	Yes
Mg^{2+} Deficiency Symptoms	Yes	Yes/No	No	No
Mg^{2+} Toxicity Symptoms	No	No	No	Yes/No
ATP Production	Severely Depressed	Depressed	Normal	Enhanced
Growth & Development (Youth)	Severely Depressed	Depressed	Normal	Enhanced
Protein Synthesis	Severely Depressed	Depressed	Normal	Enhanced
Glucose Metabolism	Severely Depressed	Depressed	Normal	Enhanced
Fat Metabolism	Enhanced (Survival)	Depressed	Normal	Enhanced (Efficiency)
Cardiovascular Endurance	Severely Depressed	Depressed	Normal	Enhanced
Muscular Strength	Severely Depressed	Depressed	Normal	Enhanced
Training Response	Minimal	Minimal	Normal	Above Average
Recovery Between Sessions	Extended	Extended	Normal	Shortened
Healing Time	Slow	Slow	Normal	Fast
Injury Frequency	Increased	Increased	Normal	Decreased
Resting Blood Pressure	Increased	Increased	Normal	Decreased
Cardiovascular Risk	High	Moderate to High	Moderate	Low
Overall Sports Performance	Poor	Poor to Average	$\geq$ Average	Above Average

FIGURE 4. Predictive model for magnesium and sports performance.

Modified according to genetic predisposition and other factors including dietary energy nutrient composition, exercise and environmental characteristics.

XII. PUTATIVE MAGNESIUM EFFECTS ON PERFORMANCE

The physiological consequences of hypomagnesemia on physical performance have not been firmly established.[61,179] There is evidence to suggest impaired endurance exercise performance with magnesium recovery varied depending on duration and extent of exercise.[26,151,152,170,171] Additionally, low plasma magnesium is implicated in spasms and cramps.[110,126,168] Magnesium supplementation has been shown to affect performance by improved economy and increases in strength, although much more research is required to elucidate metabolic and performance implications of magnesium loading.

Some researchers have suggested that the hypomagnesemia connected with exercise involvement implies that the diet of the athlete must be supplemented with magnesium. This was first intimated by Rose et al.[62] when they identified hypomagnesemia post-marathon running, and it has been recommended more recently by those studying the phenomenon.[26,158] Absorption of magnesium is approximately 30 to 50% of intake. There is a report of exercise training adaptation on increased magnesium absorption of unknown mechanism, perhaps improvement in active and passive transport systems, and retention of magnesium.[41] Metabolic depletion that may be associated with exercise potentially aggravates marginal magnesium intake, and supplementation may be warranted.

Presently, magnesium and sports performance is a nascent area for study. With the many functions of magnesium in physiology, the possible marginal dietary magnesium in sports performers, and putative magnesium depletion in strenuous exercise or training, the roles of magnesium in sports performance and sports physiology remain to be more fully elucidated.

ACKNOWLEDGMENT

Appreciation is expressed to Shannon J. Huber for the artwork provided for Figure 3.

REFERENCES

1. Durlach, J., *Magnesium in Clinical Practice*, John Libbey & Company, London, 1988.
2. Kubena, K. S. and Durlach, J., Historical review of the effects of marginal intake of magnesium in chronic experimental magnesium deficiency, *Magnesium Res.*, 3, 219, 1990.
3. Flink, E. B., Magnesium deficiency in human subjects, *J. Am. Coll. Nutr.*, 2, 271, 1983.
4. Günther, T., Functional compartmentation of intracellular magnesium, *Magnesium*, 5, 53, 1986.
5. Rude, R. K. and Singer, F. R., Magnesium deficiency and excess, *Annu. Rev. Med.*, 32, 245, 1981.
6. Wacker, W. E. C. and Parisi, A. F., Magnesium metabolism, *N. Engl. J. Med.*, 28, 712, 1968.
7. Wester, P. O., Magnesium, *Am. J. Clin. Nutr.*, 45, 1305, 1987.
8. White, A., Handler, P., Smith, E. L., Hill, R. L., and Lehman, I. R., *Principles of Biochemistry*, 6th ed., McGraw-Hill, New York, 1978.

9. Woo, J. and Cannon, D. C., Metabolic intermediates and inorganic ions, in *Clinical Diagnosis and Management by Laboratory Methods,* 17th ed., Henry, J. B., Ed., W. B. Saunders, Philadelphia, 1984.

10. Olson, R. E., Ed., Magnesium deficiency and ischemic heart disease, *Nutr. Rev.,* 46, 311, 1988.

11. Sjögren, A., Florén, C., and Nilsson, A., Magnesium and potassium status in healthy subjects as assessed by analysis of magnesium and potassium in skeletal muscle biopsies and magnesium in mononuclear cells, *Magnesium,* 6, 91, 1987.

12. Abraham, G. E. and Lubran, M. M., Serum and red cell magnesium levels in patients with premenstrual tension, *Am. J. Clin. Nutr.,* 34, 2364, 1981.

13. Hamilton, E. M. N., Whitney, E. N., Sizer, F. S., *Nutrition: Concepts and Controversies,* 5th ed., West Publishing, St. Paul, 1991.

14. Brilla, L. R., Fredrickson, J. H., and Lombardi, V. P., Effect of hypomagnesemia and exercise on slowly exchanging pools of magnesium, *Metabolism,* 38, 797, 1989.

15. Hurley, L. S., Cosens, G., and Theriault, L. L., Tetratogenic effects of magnesium deficiency in rats, *J. Nutr.,* 106, 1254, 1976.

16. Williams, M. H., Vitamin and mineral supplements to athletes: do they help? *Clin. Sports Med.,* 3, 623, 1984.

17. Pao, E. M. and Mickle, S. J., Problem nutrients in the United States, *Fd. Technol.,* 35, 58, 1981.

18. Lowenstein, F. W. and Stanton, M. F., Serum magnesium levels in the United States, 1971–1974, *J. Am. Coll. Nutr.,* 5, 399, 1986.

19. Marier, J. R., Quantitative factors regarding magnesium status in the modern-day world, *Magnesium,* 1, 3, 1982.

20. Marier, J. R., Magnesium content of the food supply in the modern-day world, *Magnesium,* 5, 1, 1986.

21. Morgan, K. J., Stampley, G. L., Zabik, M. E., and Fischer, D. R., Magnesium and calcium dietary intakes of the U. S. population, *J. Am. Coll. Nutr.,* 4, 195, 1985.

22. Altura, B. M., Altura, B. T., Gebrewold, A., Ising, H., and Günther, T., Noise-induced hypertension and magnesium in rats: relationship to microcirculation and calcium, *J. Appl. Physiol.,* 72, 194, 1992.

23. Classen, H. G., Stress and magnesium, *Artery,* 9, 182, 1981.

24. Henrotte, J. G., Type A behavior and magnesium metabolism, *Magnesium,* 5, 201, 1986.

25. Ising, H., Interaction of noise-induced stress and Mg decrease, *Artery,* 9, 205, 1981.

26. Stendig-Lindberg, G., Shapiro, Y., Epstein, Y., Galun, E., Schonberger, E., Graff, E., and Wacker, W. E. C., Changes in serum magnesium concentration after strenuous exercise, *J. Am. Coll. Nutr.,* 6, 35, 1987.

27. Benson, J., Gillien, D. M., Bourdet, K., and Loosli, A. R., Inadequate nutrition and chronic calorie restriction in adolescent ballerinas, *Phys. Sportsmed.,* 13, 79, 1985.

28. Loosli, A. R., Benson, J., Gillien, D. M., and Bourdet, K., Nutrition habits and knowledge in competitive adolescent female gymnasts, *Phys. Sportsmed.,* 8, 118, 1986.

29. Steen, S. N. and McKinney, S., Nutrition assessment of college wrestlers, *Phys. Sportsmed.,* 14, 101, 1986.

30. Brilla, L. R. and Haley, T. F., Effect of magnesium supplementation on strength training in humans, *J. Am. Coll. Nutr.,* 11, 326, 1992.

31. Singh, A., Moses, F. M., Deuster, P. A., Vitamin and mineral status in physically active men: effects of a high-potency supplement, *Am. J. Clin. Nutr.,* 55, 1, 1992.

32. Deuster, P. A., Kyle, S. B., Moser, P. B., Vigersky, R. A., Singh, A., and Schoonmaker, E. B., Nutritional survey of highly trained women runners, *Am. J. Clin. Nutr.,* 44, 954, 1986.

33. Worme, J. D., Doubt, T. J., Singh, A., Ryan, C. J., Moses, F. M., and Deuster, P. A., Dietary patterns, gastrointestinal complaints, and nutrition knowledge of recreational triathletes, *Am. J. Clin. Nutr.,* 51, 690, 1990.

34. Bazzarre, T. L., Scarpino, A., Sigmon, R., Marquart, L. F., Wu, S. L., and Izurieta, M., Vitamin-mineral supplement use and nutritional status of athletes, *J. Am. Coll. Nutr.,* 12, 162, 1993.

35. Weight, L. M., Noakes, T. D., Labadarios, D., Graves, J., Jacobs, P., and Berman, P. A., Vitamin and mineral status of trained athletes including the effects of supplementation, *Am. J. Clin. Nutr.,* 47, 186, 1988.
36. Beuker, F., Classen, H. G., and Helbig, H. J., Biokinetics of magnesium supplementation during strength training in popular athletes, *Magnesium Res.,* 3, 308, 1990.
37. Deuster, P. A. and Singh, A., Responses of plasma magnesium and other cations to fluid replacement during exercise, *J. Am. Coll. Nutr.,* 12, 286, 1993.
38. Maughan, R. J. and Sadler, D. J. M., The effects of oral administration of salts of aspartic acid on the metabolic response to prolonged exhausting exercise in man, *Int. J. Sports Med.,* 4, 119, 1983.
39. Wesson, M., McNaughton, L., Davies, P., and Tristram, S., Effects of oral administration of aspartic acid salts on the endurance capacity of trained athletes, *Res. Quart. Exer. Sport,* 59, 234, 1988.
40. de Haan, A., van Doorn, J. E., and Wesstra, H. G., Effects of potassium + magnesium aspartate on muscle metabolism and force development during short intensive static exercise, *Int. J. Sports Med.,* 6, 44, 1985.
41. Yeh, J. K. and Aloia, J. F., Effect of physical activity on the metabolism of magnesium in the rat, *J. Am. Coll. Nutr.,* 10, 487, 1991.
42. Fogelholm, M., Tikkanen, H., Näveri, H., and Härkönen, M., High-carbohydrate diet for long distance runners: a practical view-point, *Br. J. Sp. Med.,* 23, 94, 1989.
43. Kramer, L. B., Osis, D., Coffey, J., and Spencer, H., Mineral and trace element content of vegetarian diets, *J. Am. Coll. Nutr.,* 3, 3, 1984.
44. Vitale, J. J., White, P. L., Nakamura, M., Hegsted, D. M., Zamcheck, N., and Hellerstein, E. E., Interrelationships between experimental hypercholesteremia, magnesium requirement, and experimental atherosclerosis, *J. Exp. Med.,* 106, 757, 1957.
45. Holtmeier, H. J. and Kuhn, M., Problems of nutritional intake of calcium and magnesium and their possible influence on coronary disease, *Magnesium Health Dis.,* 73, 671, 1980.
46. Kubena, K. S., Landman, W. A., and Carpenter, Z. L., Suboptimal intake of magnesium in rats: effects during growth and gestation, *Nutr. Res.,* 3, 385, 1983.
47. American Institute for Cancer Research, *Report from the Executive Director, 1992–93,* HD705BS, Washington, D.C., 1993.
48. American Heart Association, *Dietary Guidelines for Americans,* American Heart Association, Dallas, Texas, 1985.
49. United States Senate Select Committee on Nutrition and Human Needs, *Dietary Goals for the United States,* U. S. Government Printing Office, Washington, D.C., 1977.
50. National Research Council, Committee on Diet and Health of the Food and Nutrition Board. National Academy of Sciences Report. Diet and health: implications for reducing chronic disease risk, *Nutr. Rev.,* 47, 142, 1989.
51. Lombardi, V. P. and Taffe, D. R., Do all modes of exercise minimize cardiovascular disease risk? *The Physiologist,* 35, 183, 1992.
52. Bunce, G. E., Reeves, P. G., Oba, T. S., and Sauberlich, H. E., Influence of dietary protein level on the magnesium requirement, *J. Nutr.,* 79, 220, 1963.
53. Schwartz, R., Wang, F. L., and Woodcock, N. A., Effect of varying dietary protein-magnesium ratios on nitrogen utilization and magnesium retention in growing rats, *J. Nutr.,* 97, 185, 1969.
54. Kitano, T., Esashi, T., and Azami, S., Effect of protein intake on mineral (calcium, magnesium, and phosphorus) balance in Japanese males, *J. Nutr. Sci. Vitaminol.,* 34, 387, 1988.
55. Whang, R., Morosi, H. J., Rodgers, D., and Reyes, R., The influence of sustained magnesium deficiency on muscle potassium repletion, *J. Lab. and Clin. Med.,* 70, 895, 1967.
56. Cerrato, P. L., Nutrition support: don't overlook this mineral deficiency, *RN,* 55, 61, 1992.
57. Rasmussen, H. S., McNair, P., Goransson, L., Balsov, S., Larsen, O. G., and Aurup, P., Magnesium load retention in IHD patients, *Arch. Intern. Med.,* 148, 329, 1988.
58. Holifield, H., Magnesium deficiency and ventricular ectopy, *Am. J. Cardiol.,* 63, 22G, 1989.

59. Beller, G. A., Maher, J. T., Hartley, L. H., Bass, D. E., and Wacker, W. E. C., Changes in serum and sweat magnesium levels during work in the heat, *Aviat., Space and Environ. Med.,* 46, 709, 1975.

60. Lijnen, P., Hespel, P., Fagard, R., Lysens, R., Vanden Eynde, E., and Amery, A., Erythrocyte, plasma and urinary magnesium in men before and after a marathon, *Eur. J. Appl. Physiol.,* 58, 252, 1988.

61. McDonald, R. and Keen, C. L., Iron, zinc and magnesium nutrition and athletic performance, *Sports Med.,* 5, 171, 1988.

62. Rose, L. I., Carroll, D. R., Lowe, S. L., Peterson, E. W., and Cooper, K. H., Serum electrolyte changes after marathon running, *J. Appl. Physiol.,* 29, 449, 1970.

63. Whitney, E. N., Hamilton, E. M. N., and Rolfes, S. R., *Understanding Nutrition,* 5th ed., West Publishing, St. Paul, 1990.

64. Fisher, P. W. F., Giroux, A., L'Abbe, M. R., and Nera, E. A., The effects of moderate magnesium deficiency in the rat, *Nutr. Reports Int.,* 24, 993, 1981.

65. Fiaccadori, E., Del Canale, S., Coffrini, E., Melej, R., Vitali, P., Guariglia, A., and Borghetti, A., Muscle and serum magnesium in pulmonary intensive care unit patients, *Crit. Care Med.,* 16, 751, 1988.

66. Kruse, H. D., Orent, E. R., McCollum, E. V., Studies on magnesium deficiency in animals. I. Symptomatology resulting from magnesium deprivation, *J. Biol. Chem.,* 96, 519, 1932.

67. Burch, G. E. and Giles, T. D., Fundamentals of clinical cardiology, *Am. Heart J.,* 94, 649, 1977.

68. Günther, T., Averdunk, R., and Ising, H., Biochemical mechanisms in magnesium deficiency, *Magnesium Health Dis.,* 8, 57, 1980.

69. Cronin, R. E., Fluids and electrolytes, in *Magnesium Disorders,* Kokko, J. P. and Tannen, R. L., Eds., W. B. Saunders, Philadelphia, 1986, 502.

70. Flink, E. B., Magnesium deficiency in human subjects, *J. Am. Coll. Nutr.,* 2, 271, 1983.

71. Rayssiguier, Y., Hypomagnesemia resulting from adrenaline infusion in ewes: its relation to lipolysis, *Horm. Metab. Res.,* 9, 309, 1977.

72. Rayssiguier, Y. and Gueux, E., Magnesium and lipids in cardiovascular disease, *J. Am. Coll. Nutr.,* 5, 507, 1986.

73. Durlach, J. and Durlach, V., Speculations on hormonal controls of magnesium homeostasis: a hypothesis, *Magnesium,* 3, 109, 1984.

74. Heroux, O., Peter, D., and Heggtveit, A., Long-term effect of suboptimal dietary magnesium on magnesium and calcium contents of organs, on cold tolerance and on lifespan, and its pathological consequences in rats, *J. Nutr.,* 107, 1640, 1977.

75. Dunn, M. J. and Walser, M., Magnesium depletion in normal man, *Metabolism,* 15, 884, 1966.

76. Guyton, A. C., *Textbook of Medical Physiology,* 8th ed., W. B. Saunders, Philadelphia, 1991.

77. Powers, S. K. and Howley, E. T., *Exercise Physiology: Theory and Application to Fitness and Performance,* Wm. C. Brown, Dubuque, 1990.

78. Lombardi, V. P., *Beginning Weight Training: The Safe and Effective Way,* Wm. C. Brown, Dubuque, 1989.

79. Pollock, M. L. and Wilmore, J. H., *Exercise in Health and Disease: Evaluation and Prescription for Prevention and Rehabilitation,* W. B. Saunders, Philadelphia, 1990.

80. American College of Sports Medicine, The Recommended quantity and quality of exercise for developing and maintaining cardiorespiratory and muscular fitness in healthy adults, *Med. and Sci. in Sport and Exer.,* 22, 265, 1990.

81. Stryer, L., *Biochemistry,* 3rd ed., W. H. Freeman and Co., New York, 1988.

82. Alberts, B., Bray, J., Lewis, G., Raff, R., Roberts, D., and Watson, P., *Molecular Biology of the Cell,* Garland Publishing, New York, 1989.

83. Garfinkel, L. and Garfinkel, D., Magnesium regulation of the glycolytic pathway and the enzymes involved, *Magnesium,* 4, 60, 1985.

84. Saks, V. A., Chernousova, G. B., Gukovsky, D. E., Smirnov, V. N., and Chazov, E. I., Studies of energy transport in heart cells, *Eur. J. Biochem.,* 57, 273, 1975.

85. Aikawa, J. K., *Magnesium: Its Biological Significance,* CRC Press, Boca Raton, 1981.

86. Wold, F. and Ballou, C. E., Studies on the enzyme enolase, *J. Biol. Chem.,* 227, 301, 1957.

87. Baek, Y. H. and Nowak, T., Kinetic evidence for a dual cation role for muscle pyruvate kinase, *Arch. Biochem. and Biophys.*, 217, 491, 1982.
88. Gregory, R. B., Ainsworth, S., and Kinderlerer, J., The regulatory properties of rabbit muscle pyruvate kinase, *Biochem. J.*, 209, 413, 1983.
89. Probst, I. and Jungermann, K., Short-term regulation of glycolysis by insulin and dexamethasone in cultured rat hepatocytes, *Eur. J. Biochem.*, 135, 151, 1983.
90. Lehninger, A. L., *Biochemistry: the Molecular Basis of Cell Structure and Function*, 2nd ed., Worth Publishers, New York, 1975.
91. Nakashima, R. A., Dordick, R. S., and Garlid, K. D., On the relative roles of Ca^{2+} and Mg^{2+} in regulating the endogenous K^+/H^+ exchanger of rat liver mitochondria, *J. Biol. Chem.*, 257, 12540, 1982.
92. Robeson, B. L., Martin, W. G., and Friedman, M. H., A biochemical and ultrastructural study of skeletal muscle from rats fed a magnesium-deficient diet, *J. Nutr.*, 110, 2078, 1980.
93. Heaton, F. W. and Elie, J. P., Metabolic activity of liver mitochondria from magnesium-deficient rats, *Magnesium*, 3, 21, 1984.
94. Elin, R. J., Utter, A., Tan, H. K. and Corash, L., Effect of magnesium deficiency on erythrocyte aging in rats, *Am. J. Pathol.*, 100, 765, 1980.
95. Hespel, P., Lijnen, P., Fiocchi, R., Denys, B., Lissens, W., M'Buyamba-Kabangu, J.R., and Amery, A., Cationic concentrations and transmembrane fluxes in erythrocytes of humans during exercise, *J. Appl. Physiol.*, 61, 37, 1986.
96. Tongyai, S., Rayssiguier, Y., Motta, C., Gueux, E., Maurois, P., and Heaton, F. W., Mechanism of increased erythrocyte membrane fluidity during magnesium deficiency in weanling rats, *Am. J. Physiol.*, 257, C270, 1989.
97. Grace, N. D. and O'Dell, B. L., Effect of magnesium deficiency on the distribution of water and cations in the muscle of the guinea pig, *J. Nutr.*, 100, 45, 1970.
98. Rayssiguier, Y. and Larvor, P., Hypomagnesemia following stimulation of lipolysis in ewes: effects of cold exposure and fasting, *Magnesium Health Dis.*, 9, 67, 1980.
99. Franz, K. B., Rüddel, H., Todd, G. L., Dorheim, T. A., Buell, J. C., and Eliot, R. S., Physiologic changes during a marathon, with special reference to magnesium, *J. Am. Coll. Nutr.*, 4, 187, 1985.
100. Galland, L., Normocalcemic tetany and candidiasis, *Magnesium*, 4, 339, 1985.
101. Miki, M., Wahl, P., and Auchet, J., Fluorescence anisotropy of labeled F-Actin: influence of divalent cations on the interaction between F-Actin and myosin heads, *Biochem.*, 21, 3661, 1982.
102. Sherwood, L., *Human Physiology: from Cells to Systems*, 2nd ed., West Publishing, St. Paul, 1993.
103. Maughan, D., Diffusible magnesium in frog skeletal muscle cells, *Biophys. J.*, 43, 75, 1983.
104. Ekelund, M. C. and Edman, K. A. P., Shortening induced deactivation of skinned fibres of frog and mouse striated muscle, *Acta Physiol. Scand.*, 116, 189, 1982.
105. Lopez, J. R., Alamo, L., Caputo, C., Vergara, J., and DiPolo, R., Direct measurement of intracellular free magnesium in frog skeletal muscle using magnesium-selective microelectrodes, *Biochim. Biophys.*, 804, 1, 1974.
106. Kitazawa, T., Shuman, H. and Somlyo, A. P., Calcium and magnesium binding to thin and thick filaments in skinned muscle fibres: electron probe analysis, *J. Muscle Res. Cell Motility*, 3, 437, 1982.
107. Watterson, J. G., Foletta, D., Kunz, P. A., and Schaub, M. C., Interaction of ADP and magnesium with the active site of myosin subfragment-1 observed by reactivity changes of the critical thiols and by direct binding methods at low and high ionic strength, *Eur. J. Biochem.*, 131, 89, 1983.
108. Cronin, R. E., Ferguson, E. R., Shannon, W. A., and Knochel, J. P., Skeletal muscle injury after magnesium depletion in the dog, *Am. J. Physiol.*, 243, F113, 1982.
109. Lorkovic, H. and Rudd, R., Influence of divalent cations on potassium contracture duration in frog fibres, *Pflügers Arch.*, 398, 114, 1983.
110. Liu, L., Borowski, G., and Rose, L. I., Hypomagnesemia in a tennis player, *Phys. Sportsmed.*, 11, 79, 1983.
111. Brautbar, N. and Carpenter, C., Skeletal myopathy and magnesium depletion: Cellular mechanisms, *Magnesium*, 3, 57, 1984.

112. Perkoff, G. T., Dioso, M. M., Bleisch, V., and Klinkerfuss, G., A spectrum of myopathy associated with alcoholism, *Ann. Intern. Med.,* 67, 481, 1967.
113. Sarkar, K., Parry, D. J., and Heggtveit, H. A., Skeletal myopathy in chronic magnesium depletion, *Magnesium Bull.,* 2, 108, 1981.
114. Somlyo, A. V., Gonzalez-Serratos, H., Shuman, H., McClellan, G., and Somlyo, A. P., Calcium release and ionic changes in the sarcoplasmic reticulum of tetanized muscle: An electron-probe study, *J. Cell Biol.,* 90, 577, 1981.
115. Yoshioka, T. and Somlyo, A. P., Calcium and magnesium contents and volume of the terminal cisternae in caffeine-treated skeletal muscle, *J. Cell Biol.,* 99, 558, 1984.
116. Potter, J. D. and Gergely, J., The calcium and magnesium binding sites on troponin and their role in the regulation of myofibrillar adenosine triphosphatase, *J. Biol. Chem.,* 250, 4628, 1975.
117. Potter, J. D., Robertson, S. P., and Johnson, J. D., Magnesium and the regulation of muscle contraction, *Fed. Proc.,* 40, 2653, 1981.
118. Hasselbach, E., Fassold, E., Migala, A. and Rauch, B., Magnesium dependence of sarcoplasmic reticulum calcium transport, *Fed. Proc.,* 40, 2657, 1981.
119. Kovács, L., Ríos, E., and Schneider, M. F., Calcium transients and intramembrane charge movement in skeletal muscle fibres, *Nature,* 279, 391, 1979.
120. Morsy, F. A. and Shamoo, A. E., Trans-magnesium dependency of ATP-dependent calcium uptake into sarcoplasmic reticulum of skeletal muscle, *Magnesium,* 4, 182, 1985.
121. Stephenson, E. W., Magnesium effects on activation of skinned fibers from striated muscle, *Fed. Proc.,* 40, 2662, 1981.
122. Stephenson, E. W. and Podolsky, R. J., Regulation by magnesium of intracellular calcium movement in skinned muscle fibers, *J. Gen. Physiol.,* 69, 1, 1977.
123. Nakamura, J., The ADP- and Mg^{2+}-reactive calcium complex of the phosphoenzyme in skeletal sarcoplasmic reticulum Ca^{2+}-ATPase, *Biochim. Biophys.,* 723, 182, 1983.
124. Champeil, P., Gingold, M. P., and Guillain, F., Effect of magnesium on the calcium-dependent transient kinetics of sarcoplasmic reticulum ATPase, studied by stopped flow fluorescence and phosphorylation, *J. Biol. Chem.,* 258, 4453, 1983.
125. Somlyo, A. P. and Somlyo, A. V., Effects and subcellular distribution of magnesium in smooth and striated muscle, *Fed. Proc.,* 40, 2667, 1981.
126. Stendig-Lindberg, G. and Rudy, N., Predictors of maximum voluntary contraction force of quadriceps muscles in man: ridge regression analysis, *Magnesium,* 2, 93, 1983.
127. Stendig-Lindberg, G., Bergstrom, J., and Hultman, E., Hypomagnesemia and muscle electrolytes and metabolites, in *Epidemiology of Magnesium in Health and Disease,* Seeling, M. S. and Heggtveit, H. A., Eds., Spectrum Publications, New York, 1980, 83.
128. Bradley, R. J., Calcium or magnesium concentration affects the severity of organophosphate-induced neuromuscular block, *Eur. J. Pharmacol.,* 127, 275, 1986.
129. McLarnon, J. G. and Quastel, D. M. J., Postsynaptic effects of magnesium and calcium at the mouse neuromuscular junction, *J. Neurosci.,* 3, 1626, 1983.
130. Berkelhammer, C. and Bear, R. A., A clinical approach to common electrolyte problems, *Hypomagnesemia,* 132, 360, 1985.
131. Anderson, T. W., Neri, L. C., Schreiber, G. B., Talbot, F. D. F., and Zdrojewski, A., Ischemic heart disease, water hardness and myocardial magnesium, *CMA Journal,* 113, 199, 1975.
132. Crawford, T. and Crawford, M. D., Prevalence and pathological changes of ischaemic heart-disease in a hard-water and in a soft-water area, *Lancet,* 7484, 229, 1967.
133. Manthey, J., Stoeppler, M., Morgenstern, W., Nüssel, E., Opherk, D., Weintraut, A., Wesch, H., and Kübler, W., Magnesium and trace metals: risk factors for coronary heart disease? *Circulation,* 64, 722, 1981.
134. Altura, B. M., Altura, B. T., Carella, A., and Turlapaty, P. D. M. V., Hypomagnesemia and vasoconstriction: Possible relationship to etiology of sudden death ischemic heart disease and hypertensive vascular diseases, *Artery,* 9, 212, 1981.
135. Siegel, G., Walter, A., Gustavsson, H., and Lindman, B., Magnesium and membrane function in vascular smooth muscle, *Artery,* 9, 232, 1981.

136. Szabo, C., Hardebo, J., and Salford, L. G., Role of endothelium in the responses of human intracranial arteries to a slight reduction of extracellular magnesium, *Exp. Physiol.,* 77, 209, 1992.

137. Zhang, A., Cheng, T. P. O., and Altura, B. M., Magnesium regulates intracellular free ionized calcium concentration and cell geometry in vascular smooth muscle cells, *Biochim. Biophys.,* 1134, 25, 1992.

138. Joffres, M. R., Reed, D. M., and Yano, K., Relationship of magnesium intake and other dietary factors to blood pressure: the Honolulu heart study, *Am. J. Clin. Nutr.,* 45, 469, 1987.

139. Mattingly, M. T., Brzezinski, W. A., and Wells, I. C., Decreased cell membrane magnesium in some essential hypertension patients, *Clin. Exper. Hyper.-Theory and Practice,* A13, 65, 1991.

140. Staessen, J., Bulpitt, C., Fagard, R., Joossens, J. V., Lijnen, P., and Amery, A., Four urinary cations and blood pressure: a population study in two Belgian towns, *Am. J. Epidemiol.,* 117, 676, 1983.

141. Yamori, Y., Nara, Y., Mizushima, S., Mano, M., Sawamura, M., Kihara, M., and Horie, R., International cooperative study on the relationship between dietary factors and blood pressure: a report from the cardiovascular diseases and alimentary comparison (CARDIAC) study, *J. Cardiovas. Pharmacol.,* 16, S43, 1990.

142. Seeling, M., Cardiovascular consequences of magnesium deficiency and loss: Pathogenesis, prevalence and manifestations—magnesium and chloride loss in refractory potassium repletion, *Am. J. Cardiol.,* 63, 4G, 1989.

143. Kerrick, W. G. L. and Donaldson, S. K. B., Effects of Mg^{++} on submaximum Ca^{++}-activated tension in skinned fibers of frog skeletal muscle, *Biochim. Biophys.,* 272, 117, 1972.

144. Pate, E., Polimeni, P.I., Zak, R., Earley, J., and Johnson, M., Myofibrillar mass in rat and rabbit heart muscle: correlation of microchemical and stereological measurements in normal and hypertrophic hearts, *Circulation Res.,* 30, 430, 1972.

145. Elwood, P. C. and Beasley, W. H., Myocardial magnesium and ischaemic heart disease, *Artery,* 9, 200, 1981.

146. Shine, K. I., Myocardial effects of magnesium, *Am. J. Physiol.,* 237, H413, 1979.

147. Garfinkel, L., Altschuld, R. A., Garfinkel, D., Magnesium in cardiac energy metabolism, *J. Mol. Cell Cardiol,* 18, 1003, 1986.

148. Cohen, L., Bitterman, H., Froom, P. and Aghai, E., Decreased bone magnesium in β Thalassemia with spinal osteoporosis, *Magnesium,* 5, 43, 1986.

149. Cohen, L., Laor, A., and Kitzes, R., Lymphocyte and bone magnesium in alcohol-associated osteoporosis, *Magnesium,* 4, 148, 1985.

150. Córdova, A., Escanero, J. F., and Gimenez, M., Magnesium distribution in rats after maximal exercise in air and under hypoxic conditions, *Magnesium Res.,* 5, 23, 1992.

151. Lowney, P., Gershwin, M. E., Hurley, L. S., Stern, J. S., and Keen, C. L., The effect of variable magnesium intake on potential factors influencing endurance capacity, *Biol. Trace Element Res.,* 16, 1, 1988.

152. Lowney, P., Stern, J. S., Gershwin, M. E., and Keen, C. L., Magnesium deficiency and blood 2,3 diphosphoglycerate concentrations in sedentary and exercised male Osborne-Mendel rats, *Metabolism,* 39, 788, 1990.

153. Bell, N. H., Godsen, R. N., Henry, D. P., Shary, J., and Epstein, S., The effects of muscle-building exercise on vitamin D and mineral metabolism, *J. Bone Mineral Res.,* 3, 369, 1988.

154. Beuker, F. and Helbig, H., Comparative study of the effect of magnesium replacement in runners and in sports involving strength (double-blind trial), *Magnesium Res.,* 2, 69, 1989.

155. Binder, F., Huntzelmann, A., and Golf, S., Biochemical effects of magnesium on glucose metabolism during a sporting event in fencers, *Magnesium Res.,* 5, 160, 1992.

156. Brilla, L. R. and Lombardi, V.P., Variable response of serum magnesium and total cholesterol to different magnesium intakes and exercise levels in rats, *Magnesium,* 6, 205, 1987.

157. Caddell, J., Kupiecki, R., Proxmire, D. L., Satoh, P., and Hutchinson, B., Plasma catecholamines in acute magnesium deficiency in weanling rats, *J. Nutr.,* 116, 1896, 1986.

158. Casoni, I., Guglielmini, C., Graziano, L., Reali, M. G., Mazzotta, D., and Abbasciano, V., Changes of magnesium concentrations in endurance athletes, *Int. J. Sports Med.,* 11, 234, 1990.

159. Chadda, K. D., Cohen, J., Werner, B. M., and Gorfien, P., Observations on serum and red blood cell magnesium changes in treadmill exercise-induced cardiac ischemia, *J. Am. Coll. Nutr.,* 4, 157, 1985.
160. Conn, C. A., Schemmel, R. A., Smith, B. W., Ryder, E., Heusner, W. W., and Ku, P., Plasma and erythrocyte magnesium concentrations and correlations with maximum oxygen consumption in nine- to twelve-year-old competitive swimmers, *Magnesium,* 7, 27, 1988.
161. Deuster, P. A., Dolev, E., Kyle, S. B., Anderson, R. A., and Schoomaker, E. B., Magnesium homeostasis during high-intensity anaerobic exercise in men, *J. Appl. Physiol.,* 62, 545, 1987.
162. Fitzherbert, J., Magnesium: the vital ingredient? *Aust. Runner,* pp. 20–21, Feb. 20, 1982.
163. Franck, H., Beuker, F., and Gurk, S., The effect of physical activity on bone turnover in young adults, *Exp. Clin. Endocrinol.,* 98, 42, 1991.
164. Golf, S., Graef, V., Happel, O., and Seim, K. E., Blood hemoglobin, erythrocytes, leukocytes, and hematocrit in physical exercise after magnesium supplementation, *J. Am. Coll. Nutr.,* 4, 393, 1985.
165. Golf, S., Happel, O., and Graef, V., Plasma aldosterone, cortisol and electrolyte concentrations in physical exercise after magnesium supplementation, *J. Clin. Chem. Clin. Biochem.,* 22, 717, 1984.
166. Golf, S., Kuhn, D., Zeblin, A., Graef, V., Temme, H., Róka, L., and Czeke, J., The role of magnesium in endogenous activation of fibrinolysis by local acidosis in dependence of predictive parameters of blood, *Magnesium Res.,* 2, 72, 1989.
167. Golf, S., Münch, J., Graef, V., Temme, H., Brüstle, A., Róka, L., Beuther, G., Heinz, N., Buhl, C., and Nowacki, P.E., Effect of a 4-week magnesium supplementation on lactate elimination in competitive rowers during exhaustive simulated rowing, *Magnesium Res.,* 2, 71, 1989.
168. Helbig, J., Beuker, F., and Munz, T., Magnesium levels in body builders during the precompetition period, *Magnesium Res.,* 2, 69, 1989.
169. Joborn, H., Åkerström, G., and Ljunghall, S., Effects of exogenous catecholamines and exercise on plasma magnesium concentrations, *Clin. Endocrinol.,* 23, 219, 1985.
170. Laires, M. J. and Alves, F., Changes in plasma, erythrocyte, and urinary magnesium with prolonged swimming exercise, *Magnesium Res.,* 4, 119, 1991.
171. Laires, M. J., Rayssiguier, Y., Guezennec, C. Y., and Alves, F., Effect of magnesium deficiency on exercise capacity in rats, *Magnesium Res.,* 2, 136, 1989.
172. Ljunghall, S., Joborn, H., Rastad, J., and Åkerström, G., Plasma potassium and phosphate concentrations: influence by adrenaline infusion, ß-blockade and physical exercise, *Acta Med. Scand.,* 221, 83, 1987.
173. Ljunghall, S., Joborn, H., Roxin, L., Skarfors, E. T., Wide, L. E., and Lithell, H. O., Increase in serum parathyroid hormone levels after prolonged physical exercise, *Med. Sci. Sports Exer.,* 20, 122, 1988.
174. Lukaski, H. C., Bolonchuk, W. W., Klevay, L. M., Milne, D. B., and Sandstead, H. H., Maximal oxygen consumption as related to magnesium, copper, and zinc nutriture, *Am. J. Clin. Nutr.,* 37, 407, 1983.
175. Mader, A., Hartmann, U., Fischer, H. G., Reinhards, G., Böhnerti, K. J., and Hollmann, W., Magnesium supplementation, magnesium excretion and general relation to training intensity and volume in elite rowers during high altitude training, *Magnesium Res.,* 3, 58, 1990.
176. Manore, M. M., Wells, C. L., and Lehman, W. R., Blood magnesium and red blood cell hemolysis following exercise in female runners consuming adequate dietary magnesium, *Nutr. Reports Int.,* 39, 787, 1989.
177. Münch, J., Golf, S. W., Graef, V., and Nowacki, P. E., Magnesium in the metabolism of high performance sportsmen, *Magnesium Res.,* 3, 307, 1990.
178. Olha, A. E., Klissouras, V., Sullivan, J. D., and Skoryna, S. C., Effect of exercise on concentration of elements in the serum, *J. Sports Med.,* 22, 414, 1982.
179. Rayssiguier, Y., Guezennec, C. Y., and Durlach, J., New experimental and clinical data on the relationship between magnesium and sport, *Magnesium Res.,* 3, 93, 1990.

180. Refsum, H. E., Meen, H. D., and Strömme, S. B., Whole blood, serum and erythrocyte magnesium concentrations after repeated heavy exercise of long duration, *Scand. J. Clin. Lab. Invest.,* 32, 123, 1973.
181. Ripari, P., Pieralisi, G., Giamberardino, M. A., Resina, A., and Vecchiet, L., Effects of magnesium pidolate on some cardiorespiratory submaximal effort parameters, *Magnesium Res.,* 2, 70, 1989.
182. Rüddel, P., Pratt, K., and Franz, K. B., Magnesium metabolism in subjects during aerobic endurance exercise, *J. Am. Coll. Nutr.,* 4, 347, 1985.
183. Smith, R. T., Miller-Ihli, N. J., Sunde, M. L., and Smith, E. L., Changes in bone magnesium content with exercise at two levels of dietary calcium intake, *J. Am. Coll. Nutr.,* 4, 392, 1985.
184. Steinacker, J. M., Grünert-Fuchs, M., Steininger, K., and Wodick, R. E., Effects of long-time-administration of magnesium on physical capacity, *Int. J. Sports Med.,* 8, 151, 1987.
185. Tate, C. A., Bonner, H. W., and Leslie, S. W., Calcium uptake in skeletal muscle mitochondria: the effects of long-term chronic and acute exercise, *Eur. J. Appl. Physiol.,* 39, 117, 1978.
186. Tate, C. A., Wolkowicz, P. E., and McMillin-Wood, J., Exercise-induced alternations of hepatic mitochondrial function, *Biochem. J.,* 208, 695, 1982.
187. Tibes, U., Hemmer, B., Schweigart, U., Böning, D., and Fotescu, D., Exercise acidosis as cause of electrolyte changes in femoral venous blood of trained and untrained man, *Pflügers Arch.,* 347, 145, 1974.
188. Tiedt, H. J. and Grimm, M., Changes in serum magnesium over a prolonged period in young competitive athletes, *Magnesium Res.,* 5, 159, 1992.
189. Verde, T., Shephard, R. J., Corey, P., and Moore, R., Sweat composition in exercise and in heat, *J. Appl. Physiol.,* 53, 1540, 1982.
190. Lehmann, M., Schnee, W., Scheu, R., Stockhausen, W., and Bachl, N., Decreased nocturnal catecholamine excretion: parameter for an overtraining syndrome in athletes? *Int. J. Sports Med.,* 13, 236, 1992.
191. Lehmann, M., Foster, C., and Keul, J., Overtraining in endurance athletes: A brief review, *Med. Sci. Sports Exer.,* 25, 854, 1993.
192. Costill, D. L., Coté, R., and Fink, W., Muscle water and electrolytes following varied levels of dehydration in man, *J. Appl. Physiol.,* 40, 6, 1976.
193. Sjøgaard, G., Electrolytes in slow and fast muscle fibers of humans at rest and with dynamic exercise, *Am. J. Physiol.,* 245, R25, 1983.
194. Brilla, L. R., Economy during endurance exercise following magnesium supplementation, *The Physiologist,* 35, 234, 1992.

Chapter **14**

LONGITUDINAL CHANGES IN MAGNESIUM STATUS IN UNTRAINED MALES: EFFECT OF TWO DIFFERENT 12-WEEK EXERCISE TRAINING PROGRAMS AND MAGNESIUM SUPPLEMENTATION

Melinda M. Manore
Jean Merkel
Julie M. Helleksen
James S. Skinner
Steven S. Carroll

CONTENTS

0-8493-7916-4/95/$0.00+$.50
© 1995 by CRC Press, Inc.

I. ABSTRACT

Magnesium (Mg) is necessary for energy metabolism during exercise, thus individuals who exercise may have increased Mg needs. The purpose of this study was to measure plasma, red cell, and urine Mg levels over two 12-week training periods to determine if type of exercise training and/or Mg supplementation alter Mg status. Untrained males were recruited for one of two consecutive exercise training programs. The first group ($n = 19$; mean age = 23 ± 3y) performed aerobic exercise, while the second group ($n = 18$; mean age = 24 ± 2y) performed both aerobic and anaerobic exercise. Within each group, subjects were randomly assigned (double-blind) to either a Mg supplement (250 mg/d) or a placebo. Blood samples and 3-d diet records were collected at baseline, midpoint, and end; 24-h urine samples were also collected at baseline and end. Both training programs increased $\dot{V}O_2$ max ($p < .01$). Mean dietary Mg intake for both groups combined was 331 mg/d ($n = 37$). Training increased plasma Mg ($p < 0.0001$) in the aerobic/anaerobic group, but had no effect on plasma Mg in the aerobic group. Training decreased ($p < .005$) red cell Mg over time; there was no effect of group or supplementation. Urine Mg did not change with training or supplementation. These data suggest that changes in plasma Mg with training may depend on the metabolic pathways stressed. Decreases in red cell Mg with training may result from an exercise induced tissue redistribution of Mg.

II. INTRODUCTION

Magnesium (Mg) is essential to the metabolic pathways stressed during physical activity[1,2] and, thus may increase the requirement for Mg.[3] It has been suggested that strenuous exercise can contribute to the development of Mg deficiency in athletes, or worsen a state of deficiency if it already exists.[3-5] This hypothesis is based on research in men showing decreased plasma Mg concentrations[4-10] and increased urine Mg[7] and sweat[8] losses during acute strenuous exercise. In addition, some endurance athletes,[4] but not all,[11-13] have been reported to have lower resting plasma Mg concentrations as compared to sedentary controls. Thus, some athletes may have suboptimal Mg status which could adversely affect their exercise performance.

No data are available on the effect of training on plasma, red cell, and urine Mg levels in untrained individuals who become trained, or whether supplementation will influence these changes. In addition, no data are available on whether modes of physical training (e.g., aerobic vs. anaerobic) alter Mg biochemical indices. The purpose of this research was to determine the effect of physical training and Mg supplementation on plasma, red cell and urinary Mg concentrations in untrained males engaged in either a 12-week aerobic or aerobic/anaerobic training program. Dietary Mg intake was also measured to determine normal dietary intakes and to determine the need for Mg supplementation.

III. METHODS

A. SUBJECTS

Healthy, untrained males were recruited for one of two consecutive training programs. The first group ($n = 19$; mean age = 23 ± 3y, mean body mass index (BMI) = 24.4 ± 2.8 kg/m^2) participated in a 12-week aerobic training program (aerobic group). The second group ($n = 18$; mean age = 24 ± 2y, mean BMI = 23.3 ± 2.5 kg/m^2) participated in a 12-week training program which emphasized both aerobic and anaerobic exercise (aerobic/anaerobic group). Untrained was defined as not presently involved in a regular exercise program and having a $\dot{V}O_2$ max ≤ 55 ml·kg^{-1}·min^{-1} using a cycle ergometer maximal test. The study was approved by the Human Subjects Institutional Review Board and informed consent was obtained prior to testing and participation in the study. Approximately 20 subjects per group started the study, data presented here are only for those who completed the 12-week training program and complied with the study protocol. Thus due to subject attrition, supplement and placebo groups have unequal sample sizes.

B. TRAINING PROTOCOL

The aerobic group trained for 35 to 40 min, three times a week, for 12 weeks at a heart rate (HR) corresponding to the onset of blood lactate accumulation (OBLA), defined as 4 mmol/L. The aerobic/anaerobic group used the same training protocol as the aerobic group, except they alternated between days of continuous (aerobic) and interval (anaerobic) training. The intensity of the interval training corresponded to the power output (Watts) at OBLA plus or minus 25 Watts for 2 min at each level, repeated continuously over the 35 to 40 min session. All training sessions included a 6-min warm-up to the desired intensity and a 3-min cool down. Every four weeks all subjects were retested for $\dot{V}O_2$ max and HR at OBLA, and training workloads were adjusted. Subjects trained on cycle ergometers equipped with HR monitors, under the supervision of an exercise physiologist in the Exercise and Sport Research Institute. A comparison of baseline and endpoint $\dot{V}O_2$ max was used to evaluate training effects. Body composition was determined before and after training using underwater weighing.

C. DIET AND Mg SUPPLEMENTS

Subjects were randomly assigned, in a double-blind procedure, to either a supplement containing 250 mg Mg or a placebo (both consumed daily). Compliance was monitored by pill counts and inquiry. No other nutritional supplements were being used besides those provided by the researchers. For both groups, 3-d diet records were collected at weeks 1, 6, and 12, three days prior to each blood draw. Subjects were trained by a researcher on how to accurately record food intake. In addition, the subjects were instructed to eat normally during the diet record period, encouraged to measure and/or weigh all foods consumed, or to save food package labels where appropriate. Upon completion of the diet record, a researcher reviewed the record in the presence of the subject to insure completeness and accuracy. The diets were then analyzed for mean energy and nutrient intakes using a computerized nutrient analysis program[14] specifically updated for Mg from the research literature. Over 90% of the foods consumed by the subjects had Mg values.

D. PLASMA AND URINE Mg

Two consecutive 24-h urine collections were done at weeks 1 and 12. Subjects were given complete instruction on how to accurately collect 24-h urine samples. Completeness of the urine collection was determined by subject questioning and measurement of urinary creatinine. All urine was collected in mineral-free containers, mixed thoroughly, volume measured, and samples were frozen at –20°C for further analyses. Fasting blood was drawn at weeks 1, 6, and 12. No exercise was allowed the day before the blood draw or the urine collection. Week 1 data (baseline) was collected before training and supplements began. Necessary precautions were taken to avoid trace mineral contamination of the blood samples. Both plasma and whole blood samples were saved in mineral-free containers and stored at –20°C until analysis. Samples (plasma, red cells, urine) were analyzed in duplicate for Mg content using atomic absorption spectrophotometry.[15-16] Mg content per liter of red cells was calculated using the method described by Archer et al.[17] All samples were done in duplicate; when agreement between samples was not <5%, samples were rerun. In addition, standards and pool samples were used to verify accuracy of analysis. All necessary precautions were made to avoid mineral contamination of containers and instruments. Only ten subjects in the aerobic/anaerobic group completed urine collections.

E. STATISTICAL ANALYSIS

A split-plot factorial ANOVA was used to analyze blood data with exercise mode (aerobic group vs. aerobic/anaerobic group) and treatment (Mg supplement vs. placebo) as the whole plot factors and time (baseline, midpoint, end blood draws) as the split-plot factor.[18] Differences between means at each time period were tested using Bonferroni contrasts. Pearson correlation coefficients were used to examine correlations between plasma Mg levels and dietary Mg (diet only) and total Mg (diet plus supplement). Pairwise t-test was used to examine changes in urinary Mg. The SAS statistical program (SAS Institute Inc., Cary, NC) was used for all data analysis. Results were determined to be significant if the p value was less than the critical value of $\alpha = 0.05$. All data are presented as mean ± standard deviation.

IV. RESULTS

Changes in weight, body fat, $\dot{V}O_2$ max, and HR at OBLA over each of the 12-week training programs are presented in Table 1. As anticipated, training significantly increased $\dot{V}O_2$ max and, thus, fitness level. However, there were no changes

TABLE 1   **Physical Characteristics of Untrained Males Participating in Either a 12-Week Aerobic or Aerobic/Anaerobic Exercise Training Program**

	Baseline	End
Aerobic Group (*n* = 19)		
Weight (kg)	79 ± 13	79 ± 13
Body fat (%)	18 ± 7	17 ± 7
V̇O$_2$ max (ml·kg^{-1}·min^{-1})	44 ± 6	50 ± 6[a]
HR at OBLA[b] (bpm)	160 ± 10	164 ± 8
Aerobic/Anaerobic Group (*n* = 18)		
Weight (kg)	76 ± 10	76 ± 9
Body fat (%)	14 ± 3	14 ± 3
V̇O$_2$ max (ml·kg^{-1}·min^{-1})	43 ± 4	49 ± 3[a]
HR at OBLA[b] (bpm)	160 ± 17	166 ± 13

[a]   Values are significantly different from baseline, $p < 0.01$.
[b]   HR at OBLA = Heart Rate at Onset of Blood Lactate Accumulation.

in body weight or percent body fat as a result of the training program. Table 2 gives the mean energy and nutrient intakes for each group over the 12-week training program. There were no significant changes in energy or nutrient intakes over time for either group. The mean dietary Mg intake for all subjects (*n* = 37; mean of three 3-d diet records) was 331 ± 128 mg/d. Group mean Mg intakes were 104% of the Recommended Dietary Allowance (RDA)[19] for the aerobic group (366 ± 143 mg/d) and 84% of the RDA for the aerobic/anaerobic group (295 ± 99 mg/d). Based on their 9-d diet records, 54% of the subjects (*n* = 20) did not meet the RDA for dietary Mg. Four subjects consumed <66% (<231 mg/d) of the RDA for Mg, but no one consumed less than 50% of the RDA for Mg.

Because high dietary calcium can interfere with intestinal absorption of Mg and increase renal Mg excretion,[20] we also examined dietary Ca intakes. As indicated in Table 2, mean dietary Ca intakes were well above the RDA at each time period. The mean Ca:Mg ratio for all subjects was 3.7. Consumption of Ca and Mg at the level of the RDA reflects a Ca:Mg ratio of 2.3. Thus, dietary Ca intake was higher in proportion to dietary Mg intake; however, for those individuals supplementing with Mg, the Ca:Mg ratio was 2.2, a ratio similar to that reflected by the RDA. The primary sources of dietary Mg were from whole-wheat breads and cereals, peanut butter, beans, and meat products. As expected, the primary sources of calcium were milk and cheese.

For each group, plasma, red cell, and urine Mg levels at each time period are given in Table 3. The normal range for plasma Mg is 0.65 to 1.05 mmol/L (1.3 to 2.1 meq/l).[15] In this study, no individual had plasma Mg concentrations below normal. ANOVA indicated a significant group by time and a significant group by treatment interaction for plasma Mg. Therefore, in the aerobic/ anaerobic group, training significantly increased plasma Mg levels from baseline to end ($p < 0.0001$); however, in the aerobic group training had no effect on plasma Mg levels over time. Thus, by the end of the 12-week training period both groups had similar plasma Mg

TABLE 2   Mean (± SD) Dietary Data From 3-d Diet Records of
Untrained Males Participating in Either a 12-Week
Aerobic or Aerobic/Anaerobic Exercise Training Program

	Baseline	Midpoint	End
Aerobic Group (n = 19)			
Energy (kcal/d)	2707 ± 653	2594 ± 723	2608 ± 673
Protein (g/d)	111 ± 29	105 ± 40	104 ± 30
Carbohydrate (g/d)	316 ± 84	328 ± 102	332 ± 98
Fat (g/d)	113 ± 35	100 ± 36	101 ± 37
Dietary fiber (g/d)	10 ± 8	15 ± 14	11 ± 11
Magnesium (mg/d)	380 ± 145	373 ± 169	344 ± 114
Calcium (mg/d)	1504 ± 423	1390 ± 658	1224 ± 373
Aerobic/Anaerobic Group (n = 18)			
Energy (kcal/d)	2675 ± 702	2549 ± 953	2581 ± 753
Protein (g/d)	103 ± 35	93 ± 40	99 ± 30
Carbohydrate (g/d)	301 ± 85	304 ± 123	329 ± 107
Fat (g/d)	115 ± 42	101 ± 43	96 ± 32
Dietary fiber (g/d)	8 ± 5	9 ± 6	7 ± 5
Magnesium (mg/d)	310 ± 84	291 ± 108	283 ± 107
Calcium (mg/d)	1198 ± 526	1039 ± 466	1055 ± 677

Note: Only 7 subjects in the aerobic group and 12 subjects in aerobic/anaerobic group
received a 250 mg/d Mg supplement. Subjects were randomly assigned to either
placebo or supplementation at the beginning of the study, and due to attrition,
unequal numbers were left in the supplement and placebo subgroups.

concentrations. Averaged over time, supplementation did not significantly change plasma Mg levels in the aerobic group, but did significantly increase plasma Mg in the aerobic/ anaerobic group ($p <.0003$). For red cell Mg, ANOVA indicated only a main effect of time. Thus, there were no differences in red cell Mg levels between the groups (aerobic vs. aerobic/anaerobic) or between supplemented and placebo subgroups. Red cell Mg significantly decreased over time (baseline vs. end) in both groups ($p <.005$). Thus, exercise training, regardless of modality, decreased red cell Mg concentrations. No significant change in urinary Mg excretion occurred over time in either group due to training mode or supplementation (see Table 2). However, the aerobic group had higher urinary Mg excretion levels than the aerobic/anaerobic group throughout the study. For all subjects, urine Mg levels were within normal ranges (1 to 10.5 mmol/d).[15]

V. DISCUSSION

Dietary Mg intake was adequate (>66% RDA) for all but 11% of subjects without supplementation. In addition, no subject had plasma Mg levels below normal. Our data support the findings of others[13,21] who report that Mg supplementation does not significantly alter plasma Mg levels in athletes doing only aerobic

TABLE 3 Mean (± SD) Plasma, Red Cell, and Urinary Magnesium (Mg) Levels Over a 12-Week Training Program in Untrained Males Participating in Either an Aerobic or Aerobic/Anaerobic Exercise Program

	Baseline	Midpoint	End
Aerobic Group (n = 19)			
Plasma Mg (mmol/L)	0.94 ± 0.07	0.95 ± 0.06	0.95 ± 0.07
Placebo (n = 12)	0.96 ± 0.08	0.96 ± 0.06	0.96 ± 0.07
Supplement (n = 7)	0.90 ± 0.05	0.94 ± 0.08	0.92 ± 0.06
Red cell Mg (mmol/L)	2.35 ± 0.38[a]	2.42 ± 0.33	2.22 ± 0.36[a]
Placebo (n = 12)	2.34 ± 0.37	2.43 ± 0.37	2.26 ± 0.40
Supplement (n = 7)	2.37 ± 0.43	2.42 ± 0.29	2.16 ± 0.28
Urine Mg (mmol/d)	6.40 ± 2.37	—	6.31 ± 2.27
Placebo (n = 11)	6.18 ± 2.17	—	6.06 ± 1.32
Supplement (n = 7)	6.67 ± 2.81	—	6.71 ± 3.37
Aerobic/Anaerobic Group (n = 18)			
Plasma Mg (mmol/L)	0.87 ± 0.05[a,b]	0.93 ± 0.07[b]	0.95 ± 0.07[a]
Placebo (n = 6)	0.85 ± 0.04	0.91 ± 0.07	0.91 ± 0.07
Supplement (n = 12)	0.88 ± 0.06	0.94 ± 0.07	0.97 ± 0.06
Red cell Mg (mmol/l)	2.49 ± 0.35[a]	2.50 ± 0.24	2.26 ± 0.27[a]
Placebo (n = 6)	2.61 ± 0.21	2.18 ± 0.27	2.12 ± 0.18
Supplement (n = 12)	2.43 ± 0.39	2.58 ± 0.20	2.34 ± 0.29
Urine Mg (mmol/d)	4.83 ± 1.34	—	4.79 ± 1.52
Placebo (n = 4)	4.77 ± 1.32	—	4.60 ± 0.91
Supplement (n = 6)	4.86 ± 1.48	—	4.92 ± 1.91

Note: Only 10 subjects completed urine collections in the aerobic/ anaerobic group.

[a,b] Values with similar letters are significantly different (*p* <.0001) within each group.

exercise. We did however observe a significant increase in serum Mg due to supplementation in the aerobic/anaerobic group.

Mean plasma Mg levels increased significantly during the aerobic/anaerobic training program, but no change occurred in the aerobic group. Therefore, changes in plasma Mg levels observed in individuals during training may depend on the intensity of the training program, the mode of exercise used (aerobic vs. anaerobic), and the metabolic pathways stressed. In addition, changes in plasma Mg concentrations over a training period may be different from acute changes in plasma Mg observed after an isolated exercise bout[4-10,22,23] or repeated days of strenuous exercise.[24] Baseline measures of blood Mg in athletes should occur after an adequate rest and rehydration period (at least 24 h) to avoid misinterpreting and/or categorizing of athletes based on plasma Mg levels which may result from acute exercise stresses.

Red cell Mg decreased in both groups as a result of exercise training. This may represent a redistribution of Mg into the muscle tissue and/or the blood. In acute exercise, red cell Mg has been reported to increase[4,7,25] or not change.[10] To date, no other data are available on the effect of an aerobic training program on red cell Mg concentrations in humans. In animals, however, exercise training significantly increases

Mg concentrations in skeletal muscle, while lowering Mg levels in plasma, erythrocytes, and bone as compared with sedentary animals fed an adequate Mg diet.[26]

Mg losses during exercise may depend on amount of Mg lost in the sweat and urine, and the type of activity (aerobic vs. anaerobic) done. High Mg losses due to strenuous exercise may compromise an athlete's Mg status if dietary Mg intakes are marginal (<50% RDA) for an extended period of time.

ACKNOWLEDGMENT

Research was supported by an Arizona State University Faculty Grant.

REFERENCES

1. Halpern, M. J., Magnesium physiopathology, in *Magnesium Deficiency*, Halpern, M. J. and Durlac J., Eds., Kager, Basel, Switzerland, 1985, 1.
2. Wacker, W. E. C., and Parisi, A. F., Magnesium metabolism, *N. Engl. J. Med.*, 278, 658, 1968.
3. Rayssiguier, Y., Guezennec, C. Y., and Durlack, J., New experimental and clinical data on the relationship between magnesium and sport, *Magnesium Res.*, 3, 93, 1990.
4. Casoni, I., Guglielmini, C., Graziano, L., Reali, M. G., Mazzotta, D., and Abbasciano, V., Changes of magnesium concentrations in endurance athletes, *Int. J. Sports Med.*, 11, 234, 1990.
5. Stendig-Lindberg, G., Shapiro, Y., Epstein, Y., Galun, E., Schonberger, E., Graff, E., and Wacker, W. E. C., Changes in serum magnesium concentration after strenuous exercise, *J. Am. Coll. Nutr.*, 6, 35, 1987.
6. Rose, L.I., Carroll, D. R., Lowe, S. L., Peterson, E. W., and Cooper, K. H., Serum electrolyte changes after marathon running, *J. Appl. Phys.*, 29, 449, 1970.
7. Refsum, H. E., Meen, H. D., and Stromme, S. B., Whole blood, serum and erythrocyte magnesium concentrations after repeated heavy exercise of long duration, *Scand. J. Clin. Lab. Invest.*, 32, 123, 1973.
8. Beller, G. A., Maher, J. T., Hartley, L. H., Bass, D. E., and Wacker, W. E. C., Changes in serum and sweat magnesium levels during work in the heat, *Aviat. Space Environ. Med.*, 46, 709, 1975.
9. Deuster, P. A., Dolev, E., Kyle, S. B., Anderson, R. A., and Shoomaker, E. B., Magnesium homeostasis during high-intensity aerobic exercise in man, *J. Appl. Physiol.*, 62, 545, 1987.
10. Laires, M. J., and Alves, F., Changes in plasma, erythrocyte, and urinary magnesium with prolonged swimming exercise, *Magnesium Res.*, 4, 119, 1991.
11. Fogelholm, G. M., Himberg, J., Alopaeus, K., Gref, C., Laakso, J., Lehto, J. J., and Mussalo-Rauhamaa, H., Dietary and biochemical indices of nutritional status in male athletes and controls, *J. Am. Coll. Nutr.*, 11, 181, 1992.
12. Fogelholm, M., Laakso, J., Lehto, J., and Ruokonen, I., Dietary intake and indicators of magnesium and zinc status in male athletes, *Nutr. Res.*, 11, 1111, 1991.
13. Singh, A., Moses, F. A., and Deuster, P. A., Vitamin and mineral status in physically active men: effects of a high-potency supplement, *Am. J. Clin. Nutr.*, 55, 1, 1992.
14. Manore, M. M., Vaughan, L. A., and Lehman, W., Development and testing of a statistical and graphics enhanced nutrient analysis program, *J. Am. Diet. Assoc.*, 89, 246, 1989.
15. Kaplan, L. A., and Pecse, A. J., *Clinical Chemistry*, C. V. Mosby, New York, 1984, 58.
16. Rousselet, F., Cherruau, B., and Granier, M. H., Methods for measuring magnesium in biological samples, in *Magnesium Deficiency*, Halpern, M. J., and Durlac, J., Eds., Karger, Basel, Switzerland, 1985.

17. Archer, W. H., Emerson, R. L., and Reusch, C. S., Intra and extracellular fluid magnesium by atomic absorption spectrophotometry, *Clin. Biochem.*, 5, 159, 1972.
18. Kirk, R. E., *Experimental design: Procedures for the behavioral sciences*, 2nd ed., Brooks/Cole Publishing, Belmont, CA, 1982.
19. Food and Nutrition Board, *Recommended Dietary Allowances*, 10th ed., National Academy of Sciences, Washington, D.C., 1989.
20. Seeling, M. S., The requirement of magnesium by the normal adult, *Am. J. Clin. Nutr.*, 14, 342, 1964.
21. Weight, L. M., Noakes, T. D., Labadarios, D., Graves, J., Jacobs, P., and Berman, P. A., Vitamin and mineral status of trained athletes including the effects of supplementation, *Am. J. Clin. Nutr.*, 47, 186, 1988.
22. Franz, K. B., Ruddel, H., Todd, G. L., Dorheim, T.A., Buell, J. C., and Eliot, R. S., Physiologic changes during a marathon, with special reference to magnesium, *J. Am. Coll. Nutr.*, 4, 187, 1985.
23. Lijnen, P., Hespel, P., Fagard, R., Lysens, R., Vander Eynde, E., and Amery, A., Erythrocyte, plasma and urinary magnesium in men before and after a marathon, *Eur. J. Appl. Physiol.*, 58, 252, 1988.
24. Dressendorfer, R. H., Wade, C. E., Keen, C. L., and Scaff, J. H., Plasma mineral levels in marathon runners during a 20-day road race, *Phys. Sportsmed.*, 10, 113, 1982.
25. Manore, M. M., Wells, C. L., and Lehman, W. R., Blood magnesium and red blood cell hemolysis following exercise in female runners consuming adequate dietary magnesium, *Nutr. Rep. Int.*, 39, 787, 1989.
26. Brill, L. R., Fredickson, J. H., and Lombardi, V. P., Effect of hypomagnesemia and exercise on slowly exchanging pools of magnesium, *Metabolism*, 38, 797, 1989.

Chapter 15

EFFECTS OF AEROBIC TRAINING AND EXERCISE ON PLASMA AND ERYTHROCYTE MAGNESIUM CONCENTRATION

Angelo Resina
Luca Gatteschi
Walter Castellani
Paola Galvan
Giuseppe Parise
Maria G. Rubenni

CONTENTS

0-8493-7916-4/95/$0.00+$.50
© 1995 by CRC Press, Inc.

I. INTRODUCTION

During the last years there has been an increasing interest in relationships between physical exercise and trace elements metabolism. Among trace elements, Magnesium (Mg^{2+}) plays an essential role in human metabolism, being the cofactor of several enzymatic activities, especially those involved in intermediary metabolism.[1-3] Several steps of glycolysis, oxydative phosphorylation, breakdown of creatine-phosphate, and gluconeogenesis are Mg^{2+} dependent processes.[3,4] So, Mg^{2+} acts both in the synthesis and in the use of high energy compounds.[4] Moreover Mg^{2+} mediates excitation-concentration coupling and it acts on the biochemical and functional integrity of cell membranes.[2]

The principal concerns about exercise and Mg status are whether acute exercise and training may increase Mg^{2+} requirements and/or enhance Mg^{2+} losses, and whether Mg^{2+} status may affect physical work capacity.

In the last years several studies have shown an influence of physical exercise on Mg^{2+} status but the results are sometimes conflicting.[2,5] Mg^{2+} status is usually assessed by determination of plasma and/or erythrocyte magnesium concentrations, but these parameters are likely not so closely related with tissue Mg^{2+} content.[6]

Plasma Mg^{2+} concentration has been observed to increase after short-term submaximal and maximal exercise while it has been reported to be unchanged during other types of exercises. Endurance exercise may lead to a progressive decrease of Mg^{2+} body content, probably increasing losses by sweating.[2]

Exercise also seems to lead to a shift of Mg^{2+} between plasma and erythrocytes, and from plasma towards other tissues, i.e., the adipocytes and the working muscle cells.[5,7,8] A delayed decrease of plasma Mg^{2+} after a prolonged aerobic exercise has been also reported.[9]

These different data may be due to different study protocols, especially concerning the time of sampling, the intensity and duration of exercise, and the metabolic pathways (aerobic or anaerobic) involved.[5]

Contradictory results may be due also to different nutritional status. A high incidence of marginal Mg^{2+} intake in the normal population has been reported.[1,10]

Athletes have a higher Mg^{2+} intake than that of non-active people, due to their high energy intake. However, such intake remains generally lower than the RDA, that is 6 mg $\cdot$ kg^{-1} $\cdot$ day^{-1}, or 400 mg/day,[1,2] so, athletes may be prone to develop hypomagnesemia.[2]

The aim of our study was to evaluate the effects of both a period of aerobic training (study A), and a single bout of aerobic exercise (study B), on Plasma and Erythrocyte Mg^{2+} concentrations.

II. SUBJECTS AND METHODS

A. STUDY A

Nine well-trained middle and long distance runners, aged 17 to 21, participated in this study. None of the athletes consumed nutritional supplements such as vitamins and trace elements during the study.

At the beginning of the study, the runners' dietary habits were evaluated by a self-reported, 3-d dietary record. A venous blood sample was drawn immediately before the start of their seasonal training (T_A), and after 1 month of training (T_B). Hemoglobin, hematocrit, and erythrocyte count were determined in quadruplicate by an automated instrument (Hemacomp 10, SEAC). Plasma Magnesium concentration [PlMg] and Erythrocyte Magnesium concentration [ErMg] were determined by flame atomic absorption spectrophotometry. Mean values of both [PlMg] and [ErMg] at T_A and at T_B were compared by *t*-test for matched pairs.[11] The significance level was set at *p* <0.05.

B. STUDY B

Five athletes from the previous group participated in the second study. The athletes performed two test sessions on an electro-magnetically braked cycle ergometer. The first test was an incremental exercise test until exhaustion. After 5 min of warm up, the initial workload of 50 Watt was increased by 30 Watts every 2 min, until exhaustion. During the exercise, the heart rate was measured by continuous electrocardiogram recording; standard techniques of open circuit spirometry were used to collect ventilatory and metabolic data. Respired gases were sampled through a low-resistance breathing mask in order to measure oxygen uptake ($\dot{V}O_2$), carbon-dioxide evolution ($\dot{V}CO_2$), external ventilation (VE), tidal volume, and respiratory exchange ratio. These parameters allowed calculation of the maximum oxygen consumption ($\dot{V}O_2$ max) and the anaerobic threshold (AT) by ventilatory methods[12] for each subject.

A week after the first test, the subjects performed a second test, consisting of 12 min of cycling at a workload near the 80% of the AT previously assessed. A blood sample was drawn before the second test (T_0), immediately after ending it (T_1), and after 12 min of recovery (T_2). On these samples, [PlMg] and [ErMg] were determined by flame atomic absorption spectrophotometry, and hemoglobin and hematocrit were determined by an automatic instrument (Hemacomp 10 SEAC).

[PlMg] was corrected on the basis of changes in plasma volume.[13] The measured [PlMg] values ($[PlMg]_M$) were compared with those expected ($[Mg]_E$) if there had been no fluxes of Mg^{2+} to or from the plasma.[11] The significance level was set at *p* <0.05.

III. RESULTS

A. GENERAL DATA

Subjects' characteristics and performance data for study B are summarized in Table 1. Analysis of the dietary records showed that the subjects had a mean daily caloric intake of 13,472 kJ. Carbohydrates contributed about 65% of the estimated total caloric intake. Mean daily Mg^{2+} intake was about 5 mg $\cdot$ kg^{-1}. However, we consider we had been able to perform only a rough estimation of Mg^{2+} intake due to differences in processing and cooking foods and in the Mg^{2+} content of drinking water.

TABLE 1   Subjects' Characteristics and Test Data

Subject	Height cm	Weight kg	$\dot{V}O_2$ max L min^{-1}	AT L min^{-1}	Test 2 Watt
M.P.	165	60	3.048	2.80	190
N.V.	165	61	3.623	3.40	210
M.A.	175	60	3.465	2.98	190
C.R.	170	62	4.244	3.19	205
P.L.	177	63	3.053	2.87	190

B. STUDY A

Hematological data were not significantly changed after 1 month of training (T_B). At T_B we have found a light, not significant, change of [PlMg] vs. T_A: 0.76 ± 0.09 mmol/l vs. 0.81 ± 011 mmol/l, respectively. [ErMg] also showed a non-significant change, 1.75 ± 0.17 mmol/l at T_B vs. 1.63 ± 0.19 mmol/l at T_A.

C. STUDY B

At the end of the test (T_1), we found a significant increase of mean hematocrit compared to baseline (T_0), 44.16 ± 2.57% vs. 40.4 ± 3.80% ($p < 0.001$); after the recovery (T_2), mean hematocrit was 42.74 ± 2.89%; it was not significantly lower than at T_1, but it was ever higher than at T_0 ($p < 0.05$). Calculated percentage changes in Plasma Volume at T_1 and at T_2 were −14.07 ± 2.9% and −8.8 ± 10.5%, respectively.

At T_1, [PlMg]$_M$ was significantly lower than [PlMg]$_E$, 0.75 ± 0.05 mmol/l vs. 0.87 ± 0.07, ($p < 0.05$). After the recovery (T_2), [PlMg]$_M$ was also different than [PlMg]$_E$, even if not significantly (Figure 1).

[ErMg] was 1.74 ± 0.18 mmol/l at T_0, and it was substantially unchanged both at T_1 and at T_2: 1.72 ± .17 and 1.75 ± 0.20 mmol/l, respectively.

IV. DISCUSSION

Previous studies have proposed that prolonged daily training may lead to a depletion of Mg body stores. In our athletes we found, after 1 month of training, a little, not significant, decrease of [PlMg] and an increase of [ErMg]. We did not find a significant correlation between changes in [PlMg] and [ErMg]. This result appears to confirm the different meaning of these two parameters.[6] However we also have to underscore that 3 of the athletes' groups at the start of training period (T_B), and 5 of them at T_A, showed [PlMg] lower than 0.73 mmol/l. This value has been reported to be associated with a significant lowering of intracellular Mg^{2+} content.[9] So, a substantial number of these athletes showed [PlMg] values suggestive of low intracellular Mg^{2+} content,[9] both at T_A and even more at T_B.

Several factors may affect Mg^{2+} balance in endurance athletes (Figure 2). These athletes often have a high carbohydrates intake, as did our athletes, and this leads to

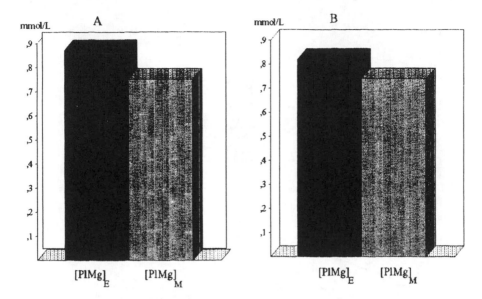

FIGURE 1. Study B: Mean [PlMg] after the test (A) and after the recovery (B); expected [PlMg]$_E$ and measured [PlMg]$_M$ values. * = p <0.05.

an increase of Mg^{2+} urinary losses.[2] Moreover, they eat a high percentage of simple carbohydrates, and such carbohydrates generally have a low Mg^{2+} content; so, in spite of a higher caloric intake than that of non-active subjects, athletes' Mg^{2+} intake generally remains less than RDA, that is 6 mg · kg^{-1} · day^{-1}.

Other factors affecting Mg balance in athletes are the hormonal status during exercise,[1] leading to an increase of urinary losses,[1,2] and increased losses due to sweating. Moreover, athletes have a greater Mg^{2+} requirement than that of non-active people due to the development of their enzymatic activities.[1] The occurrence of a marginal Mg^{2+} intake, together with an increase in Mg^{2+} requirement and/or losses, may lead to hypomagnesemia and to a depletion of body stores.[2]

In the second study, immediately after the exercise, we found [PlMg] significantly lower than expected on the basis of changes in plasma volume.[13] An acute decrease of [PlMg] may be due to high sweat and urinary losses, or to a shift toward other body compartments. If we consider the length of the exercise performed by these athletes, sweating does not seem able to explain the observed decrease of [PlMg], also taking into account the highest concentration of Mg^{2+} in athletes' sweat reported by other authors.[5] Moreover, urinary Mg^{2+} excretion has been reported to decrease during submaximal exercise.[2,5] So, the decrease of [PlMg] observed at the end of the exercise may be probably ascribed to a shift from plasma to other compartments.

We did not find significant changes in [ErMg] after the test; so, changes in [PlMg] do not seem to be related to a flux between this plasma and erythrocytes.

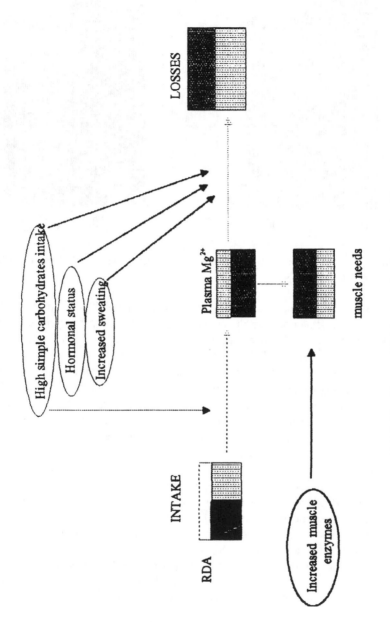

FIGURE 2. Factors affecting magnesium balance in athletes

It has been hypothesized that, during exercise, there may be an uptake of plasma Mg^{2+} from the adipocytes and/or from the working muscle cells[5] (Figure 3-A). Such a shift would be due to the increase of both enzymatic lipolytic activity,[5,7] and muscle energy production and use.[5,8]

Taking into account the submaximal intensity of exercise performed from these athletes, it seems that lipolysis might explain a great percentage of the observed [PlMg] decrease. The finding of an increase of [PlMg] after the recovery period seems to strengthen the hypothesis that the decrease, found in these athletes immediately after the exercise, may be due to the occurrence of intercompartmental shifts. In a previous study, we found a decrease of [PlMg] 24 h after a marathon run, the decrease related to the individual intensity of exercise.[14]

Several authors reported a transient lowering of [PlMg] immediately after exercise, others an increase or no changes.[5,10] Some authors have also shown a delayed fall of [PlMg] after aerobic exercise. It has been proposed that the immediate fall appears only after a strenuous effort, while the delayed fall occurs after both heavy and moderate exertion.[9]

At the end of the exercise, lipolysis decreases and then Mg^{2+} is released from adipocytes;[5] so, Mg^{2+} shift reverses to the plasma. We suggest that at the same time a shift may occur between plasma and muscle tissue. This shift might be directly from the muscles to plasma in the presence of muscle cell exertional damage.[9] Conversely, the need to restore high energy compounds and glycogen stores might lead to a decrease of this shift from muscles to plasma, or even provoke a shift from plasma to the exhausted muscles (Figure 3-B).

The shift also might be affected by the status of Mg^{2+} stores; a depletion of the stores may enhance muscle uptake, or in any case, it may decrease muscle's release to plasma.[2] In regard to magnesium muscle uptake, we have to also consider that previous studies have shown that different muscles present different contents of Mg and K; the differences may be related to the fiber composition, i.e., slow twitch and fast twitch,[15] even if not so clearly as found in species other than human.

Different types of muscle fibers also have a different enzymatic pattern, as a result of both genotype and training. This different pattern may mean a lower or higher magnesium requirement. From the results of our study, it appears that these athletes are prone to the development of hypomagnesemia. Moreover, at the end of an aerobic exercise, we have found a decrease of [PlMg] probably related to a shift between plasma and other body compartments.

We suggest that the degree and magnitude of the shifts may depend on several, also conflicting, factors, such as the energetic, metabolic pathway mainly involved (i.e., lipolysis or glycolysis), the duration of effort, the individual characteristics regarding muscle fiber composition, the kind and degree of training, and the presence or absence of adequate Mg body stores. These stores are related to dietary intake that often appears marginal in athletes.

The athletes who are involved daily in prolonged aerobic exercise may be considered as subjects with a precarious Mg^{2+}balance, due to both a marginal dietary

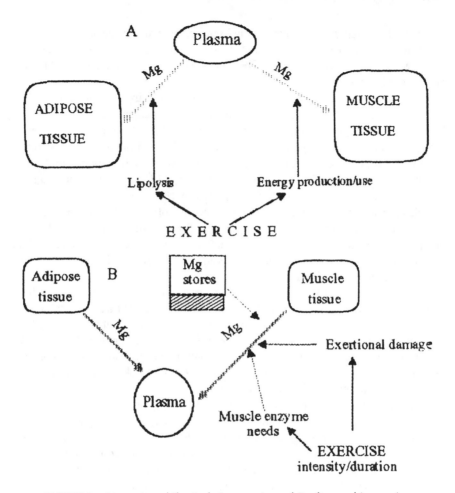

FIGURE 3. Magnesium shifts: A, during exercise and B, after aerobic exercise.

intake and a high risk of depletion. Such a precarious balance may be disrupted from acute events, like a high increase of sweat loss due to environmental conditions or exercise length; a decrease of dietary intake, an increase of magnesium-dependent enzymatic activities, and Mg^{2+} demand.

The development of a "magnesium unbalance" may lead first to an impairment of performance, and then, if not adequately corrected, to the appearance of clinical signs of Mg^{2+} deficit (Figure 4).

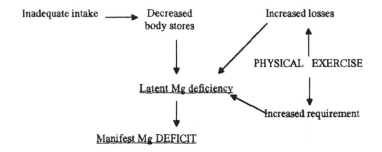

FIGURE 4. Factors inducing a magnesium deficit in athletes.

REFERENCES

1. Durlach, J., Recommended dietary amounts of magnesium: Mg RDA, *Magnesium Res.,* 2, 195, 1989.
2. Rayssiguier, Y., Guezennec, C.Y., Durlach, J., New experimental and clinical data on the relationship between magnesium and sport, *Magnesium Res.,* 3, 93, 1990.
3. Altura, B.M., Basic biochemistry and physiology of magnesium: a brief review, *Magnesium Trace Elem.,* 10, 167, 1991-2.
4. Stendig-Lindberg, G., Rudy, N., Predictors of maximum voluntary contraction force of quadriceps femoris muscle in man, *Magnesium,* 2, 93, 1983.
5. Lijnen, P., Hespel, P., Fagard, R., Lysens, R., Vanden Eynde, E., Amery, A., Erythrocyte, plasma and urinary magnesium in men before and after a marathon, *Eur. J. Appl. Physiol.,* 58, 252, 1988.
6. Elin, R.J., Laboratory tests for the assessment of magnesium status in humans, *Magnesium Trace Elem.,* 10, 172, 1991-2.
7. Vormann, J., Forster, R., Gunther, T., Hebel, H., Lipolysis-induced magnesium uptake into fat cells, *Magnesium Bull.,* 1, 39, 1983.
8. Golf, S.W., Happel, O., Graef, V., Seim, K.E., Plasma aldosterone, cortisol and electrolyte concentrations in physical exercise after magnesium supplementation, *J. Clin. Chem. Biochem.,* 22, 717, 1984.
9. Stendig-Lindberg, G., Shapiro, Y., Graff, E., Schoenberger, E., Wacker, W.E.C., Delayed metabolic changes after strenuous exertion in trained young men, *Magnesium Res.,* 2, 211, 1989.
10. McDonald, R., Keen, C.L., Iron, zinc and magnesium nutrition and athletic performance, *Sports Med.,* 5, 171, 1988.
11. Glantz, S.A., *Statistica Per Discipline Biomediche,* McGraw Hill, Milano, 1988.
12. Wasserman, K., Whipp, B.J., Koyal, N. S., Beaver, W. L., Anaerobic threshold and respiratory gas exchange during exercise, *J. Appl. Physiol.,* 35, 236, 1973.
13. Beaumont, van W., Strand, J. C., Petrofsky, J. S., Hipskind, S. G., Greenleaf, J. E., Changes in total plasma content of electrolytes and proteins with maximal exercise, *J. Appl. Physiol.,* 34, 102, 1973.
14. Gatteschi, L., Galvan, P., Orsi, F., Rubenni, M. G., Resina, A., Relationships between blood magnesium changes and physical performance, in *Proc. IV* [th] *Eur. Congress on Magnesium,* Giessen, September 21 to 23, 1992 (in press).
15. Siogaard, G., Electrolytes in slow and fast muscle fibers of humans at rest and with dynamic exercise, *Am. J. Physiol.,* 245, R25, 1983.

Chapter **16**

EFFECTS OF AEROBIC EXERCISE ON PLASMA CHROMIUM CONCENTRATIONS

Luca Gatteschi
Walter Castellani
Paola Galvan
Giuseppe Parise
Angelo Resina
Maria G. Rubenni

CONTENTS

I. INTRODUCTION

Chromium is a trace element involved in the regulation of carbohydrate and lipid metabolism.[1] It acts primarily by potentiating insulin activity.[2] Physical exercise seems to affect chromium turnover and chromium body stores.[1,2] Exercise appears to provoke increased acute urinary chromium losses. This increase has been shown in trained subjects, while it has not been found in a group of untrained runners.[3] The increase in chromium urinary excretion is likely due to increased plasma chromium concentrations, since there is virtually no renal reabsorption of chromium.[4,5] Exercise increases plasma chromium through mobilization from tissue stores.[1] The effect of exercise seems to depend on total workload,[2] and primarily on its duration.[1,2] Maybe a total exercise time that was adequately long would be needed to stimulate chromium mobilization.[1]

The aim of this study was to evaluate the effects of a single bout of not exhaustive, not prolonged, aerobic exercise on plasma chromium concentrations.

II. SUBJECTS AND METHODS

Five highly trained, long distance runners, aged 23 to 28, participated in the study, after having been informed of the risk involved. The athletes performed two test sessions on an electro-magnetically braked cycle ergometer (STS3 Cardioline). The first was an incremental exercise test: after 5 min warming up, the initial workload was increased by 30 Watts every 2 min, until exhaustion. During the exercise, standard techniques of open circuit spirometry were used to collect ventilatory and metabolic data. Respiratory gases were sampled through a low-resistance breathing mask in order to measure oxygen uptake ($\dot{V}O_2$), carbon-dioxide evolution ($\dot{V}CO_2$), external ventilation (VE), tidal volume, and respiratory exchange ratio. These parameters allowed calculation of the maximum oxygen consumption ($\dot{V}O_2$ max) and the anaerobic threshold (AT) by ventilatory methods[6] for each subject (Table 1).

A week later, the subjects performed a second test, consisting of 12 min of cycling at a workload near the 80% of the AT previously assessed (Table 1). A blood sample was drawn before the second test (T_0), immediately after ending it (T_1), and

TABLE 1   Subjects' Characteristics and Test Workloads

Subject	Height cm	Weight kg	VO$_2$ max 1/min	AT 1/min	Test B Workload (Watt)
M.P.	166	61	3.048	2.80	190
N.V.	165	61	3.623	3.40	210
M.A.	175	60	3.465	2.98	190
C.R.	170	62	4.244	3.19	205
P.L.	177	63	3.053	2.87	190

μg/dl

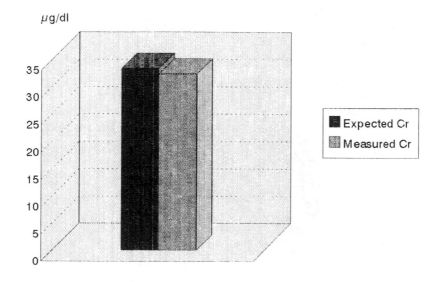

FIGURE 1.   Expected and measured chromium concentrations at the end of the test.

after 12 min of recovery (T_2). From these samples, plasma chromium concentration by flame atomic absorption spectrophotometry, and hemoglobin and hematocrit by an automatic instrument (Hemacomp 10 SEAC), were determined. The plasma chromium concentrations were corrected on the basis of changes in plasma volume.[7] The measured chromium concentrations, $[Cr]_M$, were compared with those expected $[Cr]_E$, if there were no fluxes of chromium towards or from plasma,[7] by non parametric Wilcoxon test for matched pairs.[8]

III. RESULTS

At T_1 the athletes showed a significant increase in mean hematocrit (44.16 ± 2.57 vs. 40.4 ± 3.80, $p < 0.01$); mean plasma volume was reduced to 14.07%. At T_2 mean hematocrit (42.74 ± 2.89) was not significantly different from T_1, but significantly higher than at T_0 ($p < 0.05$); the mean percentage change in plasma volume vs. baseline was -8.8%. At T_1 mean $[Cr]_E$ and mean $[Cr]_M$ were, respectively, 33.2 ± 14.2 and 32.2 ± 3.83 μg/dl, N.S. (Figure 1). At T_2 mean $[Cr]_E$ and mean $[Cr]_M$ were, respectively, 31.8 ± 14.1 and 54.8 ± 7.2 μg/dl, $p < 0.05$ (Figure 2).

IV. DISCUSSION

We found relatively high blood chromium levels with respect to those found in other studies. Blood chromium is often subject to needle-contamination at the time

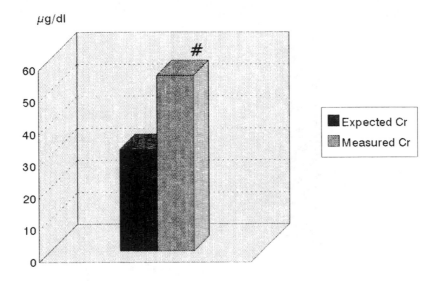

FIGURE 2. Expected and measured chromium concentrations after the recovery; $p < 0.05$.

of sampling.[2,5] So, the higher chromium levels found might be due, or partially due, to the occurrence of a contamination. However, we used the same type of needle for every sample, so the degree of contamination would not have affected time-related differences. In the absence of a shift of chromium from or towards plasma, we would have expected no differences between $[Cr]_M$ and $[Cr]_E$ values.

We did not find a significant difference between $[Cr]_M$ and $[Cr]_E$ immediately after ending the test (T_1). Considering the relative shortness of our exercise test, this data appears to strengthen the hypothesis that an appreciable amount of workload is needed to mobilize chromium from body stores.[1,2,5] However, after 12 min of recovery (T_2) we found $[Cr]_M$ values significantly higher than $[Cr]_E$ values. A suitable amount of chromium improves insulin sensitivity.[9] This increased plasma chromium might be due to a tissue mobilization to sustain an increased muscle requirement and uptake of glucose during the recovery in order to replenish glycogen stores. Chromium increase might also be due to an increase in plasma cortisol,[10] that is known to occur due to exercise.[10] However, the performed exercise was not an exhaustive one and so it would not have led to a great increase in circulating cortisol.[10]

Our data seem to confirm that exercise provokes a mobilization of chromium from tissues. Moreover, an exercise of moderate intensity and duration may also be able to mobilize chromium. Such a mobilization seems to occur with a delay from the end of this kind of exercise.

It has been reported that an increase in plasma chromium led to increased urinary losses.[1,2,3] So, taking in account the reported high incidence of suboptimal chromium dietary intake,[2] chromium balance might be affected, not only in the athletes engaged in hard daily training, but also in subjects involved in exercises only relatively prolonged and exhaustive.

REFERENCES

1. Campbell, W.W., Anderson, R.A., Effects of aerobic exercise and training on the trace minerals chromium, zinc and copper, *Sports Med.*, 4, 9,1987.
2. Anderson, R.A., New insights on the trace elements chromium, copper, and zinc and exercise, in *Advances in Nutrition and Top Sport*, Brouns, F., Karger, S., Eds, Basel, 1991, 38.
3. Anderson, R.A., Bryden, N.A., Polansky, M.M., et al., Exercise effects on chromium excretion of trained and untrained men consuming a constant diet, *J. Appl. Physiol.*, 64, 249, 1988.
4. Lefavi, G. R., Anderson, R.A., Keith, R.E., Wilson, D.G., McMillan, J.L., Stone, M.H., Efficacy of chromium supplementation in athletes: emphasis on anabolism, *Int. J. Sport Nutr.*, 2, 111, 1992.
5. Anderson, R.A., Polansky, M.M., Bryden, N.A., Bhathena, S.J., Canary, J., Effects of supplemental chromium on patients with symptoms of relative hypoglycemia, *Metabolism*, 36, 351, 1987.
6. Wasserman, K., Whipp, B.J, Koyal, N.S., Beaver, W.L., Anaerobic threshold and respiratory gas exchange during exercise, *J. Appl. Physiol.*, 35, 236, 1973.
7. Beaumont, van W., Strand, J.C., Petrofsky, J.S., Hipskind, S.G., Greenleaf, J.E., Changes in total plasma content of electrolytes and proteins with maximal exercise, *J. Appl. Physiol.*, 34, 102, 1973.
8. Glantz, S.A., *Statistica Per Discipline Biomediche,* McGraw Hill, Milano, 1988.
9. Anderson, R.A., Polansky, M.M., Bryden, N.A., Canary, J., Supplemental-chromium effects on glucose, insulin, glucagon, and urinary chromium losses in subjects consuming controlled low-chromium diets, *Am. J. Clin. Nutr.*, 54, 909, 1991.
10. Anderson, R.A., Bryden, N.A., Polansky, M.M., Thorp, J.W., Effects of carbohydrate loading and underwater exercise on circulating cortisol, insulin and urinary losses of chromium and zinc, *Eur. J. Appl. Physiol.*, 63, 146, 1991.

Chapter 17

SODIUM, POTASSIUM, AND CHLORIDE STATUS OF COLLEGE STUDENTS: COMPETITIVE ATHLETES, RECREATIONAL ATHLETES, AND NONPARTICIPANTS

Constance V. Kies

CONTENTS

0-8493-7916-4/95/$0.00+$.50
© 1995 by CRC Press, Inc.

I. INTRODUCTION

Sodium, potassium, and chloride are generally considered to be the major electrolytes found in the human body, although calcium and magnesium, among others, also have important contributory functions. In spite of their admitted importance in normal physiology and health, dietary requirements of sodium, potassium, and chloride have been, and continue to be, controversial for the athlete and non-athlete alike.[1]

II. BODY ELECTROLYTE DEPLETION

Because of sweat's obvious content of salt, heavy sweating was thought for many years to result in depletion of body reserves of sodium chloride and to necessitate the use of salt tablets. However, considerable research indicates that sweat is hypotonic and contains considerably lower amounts of electrolytes than does blood. This is coupled with controversial evidence that blood serum concentrations of both sodium and potassium may increase rather than decrease during conditions of heavy sweating has led to the conclusion that use of salt may be harmful.[1-4]

In foot races of less than 3 h in duration, electrolyte replacement during the race is unnecessary. Further evidence shows that increases in electrolyte consumption during exercise may slow the movement of water from the stomach to the intestine. This decrease in the speed of body rehydration (although disputed by other research findings) gave further strength to the argument that use of electrolyte supplements, at least during events, should be discouraged.[1] Advice given to athletes pertaining to pre-event, event, and recovery electrolyte needs may differ considerably.

Electrolyte depletion, or salt-depletion heat exhaustion, can occur in the athlete. Textbooks on sports nutrition include this as a topic of discussion but in a rather casual way. For example Williams[5] described the causes of electrolyte depletion as due to "excessive loss of electrolytes in sweat" and "inadequate electrolyte intake" and the clinical findings as being "fatigue, nausea, fainting and cramps". These rather general symptoms are, of course, difficult to differentiate from those of heat stroke. Electrolyte depletion treatment, according to Williams[5] consists of "rest in a cool environment, replace fluid and salt by mouth, and medical treatment if necessary".

In a scientific review, Noakes et al.[6] described the far more serious effects of systematic hyponatremia as being "serum sodium concentrations less than 130 mmol/l^{-1}, grand mal seizures, respiratory arrest, acute respiratory distress syndrome, coma, raised intracranial pressure, coning of cerebellar tonsils, pulmonary edema, respiratory failure, and hypotension". According to Noakes et al.[7] treatment of systematic hyponatremia consists of "hospitalization, 5% NaCl infusion, and fursemide and mannitol".

In his review, Noakes et al.[6] also summarized the reported incidences, primarily during the 1980s, of hyponatremia in athletes during prolonged ultraendurance exercise. Whether the underlying causes of hyponatremia in athletes participating in such an event is more related to over-hydration or under intake of sodium prior to or during the event is unclear.

My own interest in electrolyte status of athletes is related to an overall concern with present and future health status of these individuals rather than performance. In teaching mini-courses in nutrition, in which enrollees were primarily undergraduates from the Department of Health, Recreation and Physical Education at the University of Nebraska, I quickly found that the primary concern for the consequences of dietary practices was for future health and wellbeing.

III. ELECTROLYTE STATUS OF COLLEGE STUDENTS

A. OBJECTIVE

The objective of the study was to compare electrolyte dietary intakes, blood serum concentrations, and urinary excretions in young adult competitive athletes, recreational athletes, and nonparticipants.

B. PROCEDURES

All the subjects who participated in the study were enrolled in various sections of the Nutritional Science and Dietetics course 255, a general nutrition mini-course in which sports nutrition was stressed. Participation in the study was one of several activities by which enrollees could fulfill requirements of the course. The study was 28 d in length. During this time period, subjects kept dietary and physical activity diaries. They also completed health, dietary, and nutrition knowledge questionnaires. Fasting blood samples were drawn on days 1, 14, and 28 of the study and fasting urine samples were obtained on the same days plus days 7 and 21. Subjects signed informed consent documents prior to participation and the project, of which this study was a part, was approved by the University of Nebraska Institutional Committee for Research Involving Human Subjects.

The subjects for the study were all apparently healthy young adults. They were divided into three groups for purposes of this study: 18 competitive athletes, 28 recreational athletes, and 30 nonparticipants. Classification of the individuals was in part determined by the subjects themselves, and in part by the investigator on the basis of examination of the physical activity diaries. Individuals who did not clearly fall into one of these categories were not included in the final calculation of data. In order to equalize gender distribution within each category, some individuals were eliminated randomly in the final calculations.

Mean ages of the competitive, recreational, and nonparticipants were 21.5, 22.3, and 22.1 years, respectively. In these categories there were 18, 28, and 30 subjects, respectively, evenly divided among male and female subjects. Most of the subjects were European Americans; however, nine African Americans and one Asian American were also included.

208

Sports Nutrition: Minerals and Electrolytes

Table 1 Addition of Salt to Food

Group	Nearly Always		Sometimes		Rarely/Never	
	N	%	N	%	N	%
Competitive athletes	8	44.4	9	50.0	1	5.5
Recreational athletes	5	17.8	6	21.4	17	60.7
Nonparticipants	8	26.7	12	40.0	10	33.3

Note: No significant differences, $p < 0.05$.

Sodium, potassium, and chloride intakes of subjects were calculated using a computer program based on the U.S.D.A. bank of nutrient content of foods. Sodium and potassium content of urine and of blood serum were determined by atomic absorption spectrophotometry. Creatinine and chloride content of urine and blood serum were determined colorimetrically.

C. RESULTS AND DISCUSSION

Among the dietary practices which were investigated in this one study was the additional salting of food. Whether or not people add additional salt to food is of concern in attempting to estimate intakes of calcium and sodium from dietary diaries. As shown in Table 1, responses of the competitive athletes indicated that they nearly always added additional salt to their food 44.4% of the time, and sometimes added salt 50.0% of the time, with only 5.5% of the subjects indicating that they rarely or never added salt to food at meals. Results with the recreational athletes were quite different with 17.8% indicating that they nearly always added additional salt to foods at meals, 21.4% indicating that they sometimes did, and the majority, 60.7%, indicating that they rarely or never did. In the nonparticipant group, 26.7% indicated that they nearly always added salt to food at meals, 40.0% indicating that they sometimes did, and 33.3% indicating that they rarely or never did. Additional questions asked as part of the dietary practice questionnaire supported these findings. Other true/false questions that were asked included "athletes need more salt than do non-athletes", "I usually add salt to food before I taste it", and, if given a choice, "I usually choose regular rather than reduced-salt snack foods". A taste for salt is a learned response; hence, advice given to athletes to eat high-salt foods, or which athletes may decide upon themselves, may create a desire for highly salted food later in life. This may be undesirable relative to control/prevention of hypertension.

Some sports drinks contain appreciable amounts of electrolytes, particularly those which are designed for use during the post-exercise recovery phase. These vary considerably in proportions of sodium to potassium concentrations. Use of sports drinks was found to be somewhat higher among the recreational athletes than among the competitive athletes, with 92.8% of the recreational athletes often or sometimes using sports drinks, and 77.8% of the competitive athletes sometimes or often using them. Not surprisingly, none of the nonparticipant group subjects consumed sports drinks.

Table 2 Episodes of Diarrhea

Group	Frequent N	Frequent %	Occasionally N	Occasionally %	Rarely/never N	Rarely/never %
Competitive athletes	7	38.9	10	55.6	1	5.6
Recreational athletes	3	10.7	14	50.0	11	39.2
Nonparticipants	0	0.0	8	26.7	22	73.3

Note: No significant differences, $p < 0.05$.

Diarrhea is known to be a fairly common occurrence among competitive endurance athletes and is known to be another way in which electrolyte loss may occur. Therefore, a question on prevalence of diarrhea was included in this study. In the competitive athlete group, 38.9% indicated a frequent problem with diarrhea, 55.6% indicated occasional problems, while only 5.6% indicated that they rarely or never had problems with diarrhea. In contrast, in the recreational athlete group, 10.7, 50.0, and 39.2%, respectively indicated frequent, occasional, and rarely/never problems with diarrhea. These results are shown on Table 2.

For each group, intakes of sodium were fairly constant over time but significant differences existed among the three groups. Highest sodium intakes were found in the competitive athlete group with mean intakes during each of the 4 weeks being 231, 245, 251, and 248 meq/d, respectively. Second highest intakes were found in the nonparticipant group with mean intakes being 184, 192, 190, and 173 meq/d, respectively. The lowest intakes were calculated to be in the recreational athlete group with mean intakes being 153, 165, 148, and 156 meq/d, respectively. Based on the answers concerning attitudes toward dietary salt and dietary practices, in general, a large number of the recreational athletes also had very positive attitudes toward personal responsibilities for maintenance of personal good health.

Mean urinary fasting sodium excretion of subjects over the 4 week time span of the study were greater for the nonparticipant group than for the recreational and the competitive athlete groups. Lowest values were found among the recreational athlete group, who also had the lowest intakes of sodium. However, the competitive athlete group only had a slightly higher excretion of sodium in spite of their high intake of sodium. This was particularly surprising considering that sodium added as table salt was not included in the intake figures and the competitive exercise group indicated higher mean use of table salt. Generally, the urinary excretion of sodium is considered to be a good index of sodium intake. However, no attempt was made to estimate sodium losses in sweat in the current study and certainly these losses would have been greater in the competitive and noncompetitive exercise groups than in the nonparticipant group. It should be stressed that there were not 24-h values but were collection values per liter of urine. Another way of expressing this data would have been to calculate urinary sodium losses per gram of creatinine. When data were expressed in this fashion, highest sodium losses occurred with the nonparticipant group, in part, because of their lower creatinine excretion. This group would be expected to have a

Table 3 Electrolyte Status of College Students

	Group		
Parameter	Competitive athletes	Recreational athletes	Nonparticipants
Number	18	28	30
Sodium			
[a] Intake (mg/d)	5320	2100	2855
[a] Urinary loss (meq/l)	130	57	66
[a] Fasting blood serum (meq/l)	140	141	138
Potassium			
[a] Intake (mg/d)	1200	3940	3876
[a] Urinary loss (meq/l)	11	45	43
Fasting blood serum (meq/l)	4.12	4.24	4.51
Chloride			
Fasting blood serum (meq/l)	98.5	99.0	99.0

[a] $p < 0.05$.

lower muscle mass, and creatinine production is a function of muscle cell metabolism. In any case, these data do suggest that both the competitive and recreational athletes were meeting their sodium intake requirements.

Serum sodium concentrations were not significantly different among the three groups, nor did they differ significantly with time. This is not surprising since blood electrolytes are held in very tight check and are expected to vary only under the most extreme physiological conditions. Furthermore, these were fasting values rather than values taken following meals or during or after competitive events.

Urinary chloride excretions of subjects over the 4 weeks of the project also tended to be higher for the nonparticipant group than for the competitive or the recreational athlete groups. Intakes of chloride are difficult to estimate because of the lack of information on chloride concentration in most food products; however, they are most likely closely correlated with intakes of sodium since sodium chloride (ordinary salt) is the most important source of chloride in human diets.

Mean serum chloride concentrations were not found to differ significantly among groups, relative to time or proportional to assumed chloride intakes. As with sodium, blood serum chloride concentrations are maintained within very narrow limits in the healthy human.

Calculated intakes of potassium were found to be significantly higher in the recreational athlete group throughout the 4 weeks of the study than for the nonparticipant or the competitive athlete groups. Somewhat similar intakes for sodium and potassium were found with these latter two groups. Also, intakes of potassium tended to show more variation among these two groups than was true for the recreational athlete group. Reasons for the higher intakes of potassium among the recreational athlete group than for the other two groups might have been associated with their greater interest in health and greater knowledge of nutrition, as illustrated by scores on that part of the study. A 20 point true/false quiz developed in this department for assessing nutrition knowledge was administered the first day of the mini-course. Mean scores were 56.7% for the competitive athlete group, 68.1% for the recreational athlete group, and 61.3% for the nonparticipant group.

Mean urinary excretions of potassium for the competitive athlete, recreational athlete, and nonparticipant groups were 40.9, 63.2, and 48.3 meq/l, respectively. Unlike sodium excretions, the recreational athlete group had the highest intakes and urinary excretions of potassium. As with sodium and chloride, blood serum potassium concentrations were not found to vary among the three groups of subjects with time or with level of dietary potassium.

Ideally, intakes of sodium and potassium should be in a ratio of 1 to 1 or less. Higher ratios have been found to be associated with increased incidence of hypertension and its associated problems. In the present study, the overall sodium to potassium intake ratios for the competitive athlete, recreational athlete, and nonparticipant groups were 2.48, 0.83, and 1.80, respectively. These values were all significantly different from one another. The low mean sodium to potassium intake ratio of the recreational athlete group ties in well with this group's general interest in good health and application of this interest to self. The higher ratio found in the nonparticipant group also is not surprising considering this group's general lack of interest in activities relative to promoting good health. However, the very high intake ratios of sodium to potassium found among the competitive athlete group members are a matter of concern. It would appear that these individuals have really taken to heart the need to use diet as a means of replacing body sodium lost in sweat but either do not know, or have ignored, advice relative to potassium intake. These dietary practices certainly are not ideal for the present and may be disastrous in the future.

Urinary sodium to potassium ratios are sometimes used as predictors of sodium to potassium intake ratios. In the present study, these ratios for the competitive athlete, the recreational athlete, and the nonparticipant groups were 1.97, 0.72, and 1.80, respectively. These values are somewhat similar to those of the intake ratios but underestimate the possible problems found in the competitive athlete group.

Recently, Costill et al.[7] reported on possible effects of a low potassium diet in athletes under controlled conditions. That study involved the use of two, randomly arranged, 4-d experimental periods during which two, laboratory controlled diets were fed. Both supplied 190 meq sodium/d but one supplied 80 meq potassium/d and the other supplied 25 meq/d. Subjects exercised for 2 h/d at 50% $\dot{V}O_2$ max. Muscle biopsies, blood samples, and sweat samples were collected. Urine and feces were collected on a 24-h basis for all days.

Sodium status of these subjects on the basis of sodium balance, which included sweat losses of sodium as well as that lost in urine and feces, indicated a retention of over 100 meq/d greater when subjects were fed the low potassium diet in comparison to the control or higher potassium diet even though intakes of sodium were the same regardless of potassium intake. Nearly all of this difference was found in the urinary losses of sodium. Under these conditions, sweat losses of potassium were similar whether the lower or higher potassium diet was fed; however, urinary potassium losses were depressed. This depression in urinary potassium losses was insufficient to prevent a negative potassium balance from occurring.

In the Costill et al. study,[7] intake sodium to potassium ratios were 2.375 in the higher potassium diet and 7.600 in the low-potassium diet. Hence, even in the higher potassium diet, potassium intake figures were considerably less than used in the present study. Urinary sodium to potassium ratios in the Castill et al. study for the higher potassium diet was 1.47 and for the low potassium diet was 6.23. This suggests that even with losses of both potassium and sodium in sweat, urinary ratios of sodium to potassium may be used to predict status of these two electrolytes.

IV. FOOD SODIUM TO POTASSIUM RATIOS

Offering advice on increasing sodium intakes from diet is much easier than offering advice on increasing intakes of potassium. Part of the problem is that many foods which are ordinarily good sources of potassium may be changed through processing to have high sodium content; thus, the sodium to potassium ratio in the food which originally was thought to be low is vastly increased.

A good example of this is the potato. A raw or baked potato is a pretty good source of potassium with a sodium to potassium ratio of 0.022. However, if cheese or sour cream topping is added, the sodium to potassium ratio increases to 1.414 and 1.708, respectively. In this regard, french fries have a ratio of 0.501, still quite respectable. However, mashed potatoes from flakes, potato puffs, canned German potato salad, and canned homestyle potato salad, have sodium to potassium ratios of 2.720, 3.321, 6.702, and 4.390, respectively. Thus to tell people to eat potatoes to increase their potassium intakes may not be such good advice if the wrong type of potatoes are chosen.

Other vegetables show a similar pattern. Using data recalculated from Pennington,[8] raw tomatoes supply a good amount of potassium and have a sodium to potassium ratio of 0.066; however, canned stewed tomatoes, because of salt addition, have a sodium to potassium ratio of 3.730. Boiled beets also supply a good amount of potassium and have a sodium to potassium ratio of 0.268; however, canned pickled beets, because of salt additions, have a sodium to potassium ratio of 3.020. Plain boiled broccoli contains appreciable amounts of potassium and has a sodium to potassium ratio of 0.107; however, addition of cheddar cheese increases the ratio to 4.649. Boiled green peas have a sodium to potassium ratio of 0.036; however, canned green peas have a ratio of 2.146 and frozen peas in a butter sauce have a ratio of 6.660.

Pasta products are enjoying an increased popularity among athletes and non-athletes alike. Wheat, the principal ingredient, contains some potassium and has a very low sodium content. Hence, plain cooked macaroni and noodles have sodium to potassium ratios of 0.018 and 0.072, respectively. However, many dishes based on pasta have very high sodium to potassium ratios because of the sauces which have been used. For example, frozen parsleyed noodles, Italian pasta salad, seafood pasta salad, and macaroni and cheese were found to have sodium to potassium ratios of 45.74, 12.10, 6.17, and 11.99, respectively.

The situation is even worse with bread and bread products because considerable amounts of salt are generally added in the bread making process. Hence, white bread has a sodium to potassium ratio of 7.74 and whole wheat bread has a ratio of 5.77. One might expect that the highest ratio would be found in saltine crackers (ratio 15.35) but, of the products for which I calculated the ratios, the highest ratio was found in refrigerated butterflake rolls with a ratio of 35.37.

However, plain beef, pork, fish, and poultry contain appreciable amounts of potassium and fairly low concentrations of sodium. Thus broiled ground beef, broiled pork chops, roasted chicken, and raw sockeye salmon have sodium to potassium ratios of 0.379, 0.367, 0.545, and 0.204, respectively. However, beef frankfurters, ham, chicken roll, and canned salmon have sodium to potassium ratios of 10.463, 7.106, 4.340, and 2.340, respectively.

Whenever people think of high potassium diets, the word banana comes to mind. Bananas are an excellent source of potassium with a low sodium to potassium ratio. However, most fruits have appreciable concentrations of potassium coupled with low concentrations of sodium giving them low sodium to potassium ratios. Thus, the advice to increase intakes of raw fruits is good, relative to increasing dietary potassium intakes. Furthermore, fresh fruits taste good without the addition of salt and sauces and, if used, are more likely to be high in sucrose rather than high in salt content.

V. CONCLUSION

In conclusion, advising athletes to simply increase their intakes of high-salt foods perhaps is too simplistic an approach for maintenance of good electrolyte status for the present, and may actually be somewhat dangerous in setting food patterns for their future, noncompetitive older years. Advising athletes to increase their intakes of potassium through good food choices may offer some health advantages to the athlete and nonathlete alike. However, this is easier to say than to develop guidelines which are easy to follow.

REFERENCES

1. Pivarnik, J. M., Water and electrolytes during exercise, in *Nutrition in Exercise and Sport,* Hickson, J. F. and Wolinsky, I., Eds., CRC Press, Boca Raton, 1989, chap. 8.
2. Kaminsky, L. A. and Paul, G. L., Fluid intake during an ultramarathon running race: relationship to plasma volume and serum sodium and potassium, *J. Med. Phys. Fitness,* 31, 417, 1991.
3. Millard-Stafford, M. L., Sparling, P. B., Rosskopf, L. B., and Dicarlo, L. J., Carbohydrate-electrolyte replacement improves distance running performance in the heat, *Med. Sci. Sports Exercise,* 24, 934, 1992.
4. Fortney, S. M., Vroman, N. B., Beckett, W. S., Permutt, S., and LaFrance, N. D., Effect of hemoconcentration and hyperosmolality on exercise performance, *J. Appl. Physiol.,* 65, 519, 1988.

5. Williams, M. H., *Nutrition for Fitness and Sport,* Wm. C. Brown, Dubuque, 1992, 197–207.
6. Noakes, T. D., Norman, R. J., Buck, R. H., Godlonton, J., Stevenson, K., and Pittaway, D., The incidence of hyponatremia during prolonged ultraendurance exercise, *Med. Sci. Sports Exercise,* 22, 1651, 1990.
7. Costill, D. L., Cote, R., and Fink, W. J., Dietary potassium and heavy exercise: effects on muscle water and electrolytes, *Am. J. Clin. Nutr.,* 36, 266, 1982.
8. Pennington, J. A. T., *Bowes & Church's Food Values of Portions Commonly Used,* 16th ed., J. B. Lippincott, Philadelphia, 1994.

Chapter 18

THE REQUIREMENTS FOR FLUID REPLACEMENT DURING HEAVY SWEATING AND THE BENEFITS OF CARBOHYDRATES AND MINERALS*

—————————————————————————— Herman L. Johnson

CONTENTS

* Reference to a company or product name does not imply approval or recommendation of the product by the U.S. Department of Agriculture or Defense to the exclusion of others that may be suitable.

I. BACKGROUND

The reports on the requirements for adequate water intake and the detrimental effects of dehydration upon work performance and physiological functioning date back to the beginning of this century,[1-3] although most of the human studies on energy and water requirements in the desert were conducted by several groups[4-6] during the early 1940s. Much of this work was done for the military in preparation for, and treatment of, environmental casualties during and following desert warfare. Then little work was done until the late 1960s and 1970s when the military became concerned about prevention of dehydration and/or rehydration of military personnel operating in a hot, humid, jungle environment. Similar concerns were shown for workers in the hot gold mines in South Africa and for amateur athletes (especially young football players at the beginning of fall training); both of these groups are prone to heat injury and/or heat stroke. When the food industry saw the need to protect these young athletes from dehydration, several companies developed beverages containing minerals and carbohydrates. These were initially promoted with some greatly exaggerated claims about their rate of absorption and fatigue-prevention properties. The military was approached as a potential customer for their use during training and maneuvers in hot and humid environments and this is when our Army laboratory in Denver was asked to evaluate these beverages.

This review encompasses our initial study reported in 1973,[7] several excellent studies conducted by sports physiologists, and the recommendations that were developed in a symposium conducted by the American College of Sports Medicine in 1991. With this, I will review some of the background studies conducted during the past 30 years and present the most recent consensus of recommendations from sports physiologists on the needs for water, minerals, and carbohydrates during various types of exercise.

Our 1972 study[7,8] on three of the commercially available sport drinks was conducted in response to a Marine Corps request to evaluate these drinks during heavy physical work or training in a hot environment. For a thorough evaluation, we decided to include solutions of individual minerals with and without glucose at concentrations comparable to those in the sports drinks. These were compared to each other and to water.

TABLE 1   Composition of Test Solutions

Treat. No.	Solution[1]	Na	K	Ca mg/l	Mg mg/l	Vit. C	CHO g/l	Intake[2] ml/h
1.	Water I							475
2.	Product A[3]	651	97	10	1.0		50	616
3.	NaCl + Glu.	424					50	478
4.	NaCl	424						440
5.	NaCl + KCl	424	92					445
6.	5 × KCl		440					450
7.	Product B	740	563	103	18.4	120	99	606
8.	Water II							479
9.	KCl		92					488
10.	Product C	278	43	70	7.4	176	52	529
11.	KCl + Glu.		92				50	488
12.	Water + Vit. E							483

[1]   Each solution was given to 1 of the 6 men during each 2 weeks.
[2]   Voluntary intakes for the 4 h of exercise.
[3]   The 3 commercial products purchased Jan. 72 were Olympiad (A), Sportade (B), and Gatorade (C).

From Johnson, H. L., Nelson, R. A., and Consolazio, C. F., *Med. Sci. Sports Exerc.*, 20, 26, 1988.

II. SUBJECTS AND PROCEDURES

A. SUBJECTS AND EXPERIMENTAL DESIGN

Only six healthy male volunteers between 21 and 25 years old were available for this 12 week study; therefore we devised the 12-beverage treatments, which included water I as the control for odd-numbered weeks (See Table 1), and water II as the control for even-numbered weeks. These were assigned to subjects first. The remaining 10 treatments were randomly assigned to the men in such a way that every man received every treatment for 5 consecutive days during the 12 weeks of study and every treatment was assigned to a subject during each 2-week period of the study. Although these men were in relatively good physical condition initially, they underwent another 10 d of physical conditioning and acclimatization by exercising in the environmental room for 8 h/d. During this time they consumed a typical well-balanced American diet *ad libitum*. The volunteers consumed an all liquid diet (Table 2) in four equal meals during the experimental phase of the study. The calories in this diet were derived 14% from protein, 40% from fat, and 46% from carbohydrate. During the 12-week study, the men remained for 5 h daily in the environmental room, maintained at 35 ± 2°C and 30 to 40% relative humidity, and exercised for two 1-h periods on the treadmill alternated with two 1-h periods on the ergometer. Each hour consisted of 55 min of exercise and 5 min for drinking solutions, weighing, bathroom needs, and rest. The weekly experimental cycle began with 5 h of heat exposure that included 4 h of exercise with water ad libitum on Sunday. Each man drank one of the experimental solutions (Table 1) during the 5 h heat-exercise exposure for the next 5 d and Saturday was a day of rest without heat or exercise.

TABLE 2   Composition Of Liquid Diet

Ingredients g/d	3,200 kcals	3,500 kcals	4,000 kcals
Sodium caseinate	118	135	149
Sucrose	192	209	241
Dextri-maltose	190	210	238
Corn Oil	155	159	181
Mineral mixture	18	18	18
Vitamin mixture	10	10	10
Distilled water	1800	1800	1800
Tween (5 drops)			
Total	2483	2541	2637

Macronutrients g/d (% of calories)

Protein	110 (13.6)	126 (14.0)	138 (13.6)
Fat	145 (40.4)	159 (39.8)	181 (40.7)
Carbohydrate	371 (46.0)	414 (46.1)	473 (46.6)

Note: Minerals (in g/man/d): NaCl 7.14; KCl 5.21; $MgCl \cdot 6H_2O$ 3.34; $Ca3(PO4)_2$ 1.90. In mg/man/d; $FeSO_4 \cdot 7H_2O$ 50; $CuSO_4 \cdot 5H_2O$ 20; ZnCl 31; Mn $SO_4 \cdot H_2O$ 4.4; and KI 0.18.

From Johnson, H. L., Nelson, R. A., and Consolazio, C. F., *Med. Sci. Sports Exerc.*, 20, 26, 1988.

Each solution was coded and placed in white plastic bottles so that the subjects could not readily detect which solution they were drinking that week.

When the man entered the environmental room, he was weighed. One arm was washed with distilled water, dried, and fitted with an arm sweat collection bag. Sweat samples were collected after 2 and 4 h in the environmental room. During the first and third hours, he exercised on the cycle ergometer at a moderate work level (consuming abut 1.4 l O_2/min). During the second hour and first half of the fourth hour, he walked at 5.44 km (3.5 miles) per hour on a 4% grade. Then his energy expenditure was measured for 15 min at 4% and 15 min at 10% grade. On the fifth day, these measurements continued through a maximum performance on the treadmill using the modified Balke protocol[9] whereby the treadmill grade was increased 1% each min until the subject could not continue. Data collection continued for 10 min with the volunteer sitting at rest.

B. WORK AND ENERGY EXPENDITURE MEASUREMENTS

Expired respiratory gases were measured at all work levels using an open circuit continuous analyzer developed by the Army Medical Research and Nutrition Laboratory.[10] This analyzer served as a prototype of some of the commercial instruments now available in computerized models. Total expired volume, gas and environmental temperatures, carbon dioxide and oxygen concentrations, heart and respiratory rates, and barometric pressure and humidity were measured and recorded on a strip chart.

Oxygen consumption, carbon dioxide production, and pulmonary ventilation were calculated from these measurements. Sweat rates were calculated for the two 2-h intervals of sweat collection and for the 24-h period. During the acclimitization period, we attempted to have the men replace all of their sweat losses during exercise; however, this caused an unpleasant feeling of fullness so we permitted *ad libitum* consumption of all solutions. Intakes (shown on Table 1) were close to the amounts recommended for the commercial beverages.

C. MINERAL ANALYSES

Blood samples were obtained in the environmental room before and after exercise on days 1 and 5 of each experimental period. Complete 24-h urine specimens and 7-d fecal pools were collected. After homogenizing, aliquots of fecal and diet samples were wet-ashed. Sodium, potassium, calcium, and magnesium contents of these digests, urine, serum, and beverages were determined by absorption spectroscopy.

D. STATISTICS

Statistical analyses of the data were done by factorial or repeated measures ANOVA's and Newman-Keul's or Duncan's multiple comparisons tests, as appropriate.[11]

III. EXPERIMENTAL RESULTS

A. PERFORMANCE MEASUREMENTS

Physical performance data showed small differences among the fluids. The only significant differences (Table 3) were in the maximal performance Balke Index.[9] Apparently by chance, the Balke Index obtained for the first water treatment was significantly lower than for all other treatments except Product A. The Balke index was higher for Product B than it was for all other treatments, except Product C. Product B had twice as much carbohydrate (99 g/l) compared to other solutions that contained carbohydrate. This carbohydrate effect is well demonstrated on Table 4 where the respiratory exchange ratios (RER's, l of CO_2 produced/l of O_2 consumed) are significantly higher for carbohydrate-containing beverages compared to carbohydrate-free beverages at the 4 and 10% treadmill grades. RER's at maximum work were significantly higher only for products B & C compared to water. The average carbohydrate consumption with Product B was increased 240 grams or almost 1000 kcal/d and it was about 95 to 120 grams or 360 to 480 kcals/d for the other carbohydrate beverages compared to carbohydrate-free beverages. There was a trend for oxygen consumption during the 4% and 10% grade submaximal treadmill tests to be lower when Products B and C were provided.

TABLE 3   Mean and Standard Deviation of Recovery Heart Rates,
           Physical Fitness Index and Balke Index of Men in Hot Room

	Rec. Heart Rate		Phys. Fit. Ind.		Balke Index	
Treatment	Mean	SD	Mean	S.D.	Mean	S.D.
Water I	384	59	69	8	1700*	218
Product A	370	32	70	10	1780	315
NaCl + glucose	373	52	76	7	1890	138
NaCl	391	31	72	7	1888	145
NaCl + KCl	386	37	73	6	1888	151
5 × KCl	355	40	79	10	1883	176
Product B	381	11	79	3	2104*	104
Water II	373	48	69	5	1878	132
KCl	380	26	76	6	1857	202
Product C	416	34	70	7	1967	137
KCl + glucose	386	27	73	7	1884	137
Water + vit. E	394	30	71	8	1880	176

*   These values are significantly different ($p < 0.05$) from most other values.

From Johnson, H. L., Nelson, R. A., and Consolazio, C. F., *Med. Sci. Sports Exerc.*, 20, 26, 1988.

TABLE 4   Respiratory Exchange Ratios[1] at 3 Work Levels

	4% Grade		10% Grade		Maximum	
Treatment	Mean†	SD	Mean	S.D.	Mean	S.D.
Water I	0.77	0.04	0.79	0.04	0.91	0.07
Product A	0.87*	0.03	0.88*	0.02	0.96	0.06
NaCl + glucose	0.84*	0.04	0.84*	0.04	0.97	0.04
NaCl	0.80	0.03	0.80	0.03	0.94	0.03
NaCl + KCl	0.80	0.02	0.79	0.03	0.95	0.02
5 × KCl	0.79	0.03	0.81	0.02	0.93	0.05
Product B	0.88*	0.02	0.89*	0.03	1.01*	0.05
Water II	0.79	0.03	0.79	0.04	0.92	0.04
KCl	0.77	0.02	0.80	0.02	0.96	0.04
Product C	0.84*	0.04	0.84*	0.07	1.01*	0.05
KCl + glucose	0.84*	0.05	0.84*	0.03	0.95	0.08
Water + vit. E	0.78	0.03	0.80	0.03	0.94	0.04

[1]   Mean and S.D. from six men.
*   These values are significantly increased ($p < 0.05$) over values obtained with water treatment.

From Johnson, H. L., Nelson, R. A., and Consolazio, C. F., *Med. Sci. Sports Exerc.*, 20, 26, 1988.

B. BODY WEIGHTS AND MINERAL BALANCES

Some of the other measurements and changes that we reported[8] are summarized in Table 5. During the 12-week study, mean body weights decreased from 78 to 75 kg for a highly significant decrease of 3.25 kg. Changes during the various treatment weeks were less than 0.5 kg and were not related to the extra calories in the beverages. Some small but significant ($p < .05$) changes were observed in the blood biochemistries

TABLE 5   Other Measurements with Small Changes

Weights: Initial, 78.12; Final, 74.87; Change, 3.25 kgs; $p <.001$. Changes during 5 d on solutions ranged from –0.47 to +0.38 kg.

Blood Biochemistries: Hemoglobin, hematocrit, serum protein, osmolality, sodium, potassium, calcium, and magnesium. Small changes with significance ($p <.05$) for exercise and day-by-exercise iterations. Treatment effects were significant for osmolality and serum magnesium.

Sodium Balances were negative (2 to 3 g/d) for all drinks.

Potassium Balances were -0.5 to 1.0 g/d for all drinks.

Magnesium Balances were negative for water I and water + vitamin E (75 and 100 mg/d), positive for product C, NaCl, NaCl + KCl, and NaCl + Glucose (50 to 150 mg/d), and rest were near balance.

Calcium Balances were negative for products A & B, water I, water + vitamin E, 5 × KCl, and NaCl + Glucose; rest were near balance.

during exercise (pre vs. post) and in the day-by-exercise interactions (pre and post on Monday vs. pre and post on Friday). Significant treatment effects were noted for osmolalities and serum magnesiums. Negative sodium and potassium balances were probably the result of using the concentrations of these minerals in sweat collected in the hot room and the 24-h sweat volumes to calculate sweat losses — these concentrations were probably much lower during the remainder of the day when sweat rates were not as high. The greatest losses of calcium and magnesium were during the water treatments.

C. SERUM OSMOLALITY AND MAGNESIUM CHANGES

The significant treatment effects on osmolalities and treatment-by-day interactions on serum magnesium are shown in Table 6. Serum osmolalities for men while consuming Product C were significantly higher than during water I; osmolalities while consuming a combination of NaCl and KCl were significantly lower than while consuming Products A, B, and C, NaCl beverage, and water plus 800 mg of vitamin E daily. On the first day of treatment, serum magnesium levels were lower for men receiving Product A, high K, and water II than when they received NaCl + glucose, Product B, and C. After 5 d on the beverages, the men that received the NaCl + glucose had lower magnesium levels than those who received only NaCl or high K solutions.

D. CONCLUSIONS FROM INITIAL STUDY

The results from this study showed that men consuming a well-balanced diet could maintain a normal fluid balance while working in a hot environment by drinking water, various commercial sport drinks, and various salt/carbohydrate supplemented drinks (the additional minerals were excreted daily). The trend for reduced oxygen consumptions during submaximal work while consuming commercial products suggested improved efficiency and increased work capacity consistent with the increased Balke Index during the maximal test. The major benefit of the commercial beverages was the increased fluid consumptions during heavy sweating that helped reduce the negative water balances.[8]

TABLE 6   Treatment Effects on Serum Osmolality
(Mosm/l) and Magnesium (MG/DL)

Treatment	Osmolality* Mean	Serum Magnesium* Day 1	Day 5
Water I	293[a]	1.58	1.52
Product A	295[c]	1.50[a]	1.56
NaCl + Glucose	294	1.64b	1.45[a]
NaCl	295c	1.53	1.60b
NaCl + KCl	292d	1.53	1.53
5 × KCl	294	1.50a	1.58b
Product B	295c	1.63[b]	1.54
Water II	294	1.50[a]	1.55
KCl	293a	1.60	1.52
Product C	296[b,c]	1.64b	1.53
KCl + glucose	294	1.55	1.55
Water + vit. E	295c	1.54	1.51

*   Values with superscript a are significantly different from those
with superscript b. Values with superscript c are significantly
different from values with superscript d ($p <0.05$). Means from
6 men.

From Johnson, H. L., Nelson, R. A., and Consolazio, C. F., *Med. Sci.
Sports Exerc.*, 20, 26, 1988.

E. SUBSEQUENT STUDIES

Most of the early studies on the various carbohydrate and/or electrolyte solutions
during exercise are listed in Table 7. Two studies by Costill et al.[12,13] showed that
these electrolyte solutions and water were equally effective for replacing fluids lost
by heavy sweating during work in a hot environment. Francis[14] reported that both
water and electrolyte solutions prevented the plasma volume reduction and the serum
uric acid, cortisol, and dopamine-b-hydroxylase elevations during 2 h of moderate
work in a warm, humid environment and both reduced heart rates by 18% compared
to no fluid intake. Wells et al.[15] found no differences among water, electrolyte
solution, and a caffeine solution during a 20-mile run on work parameters, serum
electrolytes, free fatty acids or glucose, and blood hemoglobin or hematocrits. Owen
et al.[16] reported no differences among 10% glucose, 10% glucose polymers, or water
during a 2-h treadmill run (60% of max $\dot{V}O_2$) in a hot, dry room for skin and rectal
temperatures, sweat and heart rates, plasma volume changes, gastric emptying,
thermoregulation, plasma glucose, insulin, osmolality or sodium levels, and the RER.
Therefore all of these studies confirmed that the major beneficial effect of these
electrolyte solutions was the prevention of dehydration.

IV. DISCUSSION

A. DEHYDRATION

The adverse effects of various levels of dehydration are summarized in Table 8.
Since the normal body contains approximately 60% water, each 1% loss of body

TABLE 7   Early Reports on CHO/Electrolyte Solutions (ES) and Exercise

1973	Johnson, et al.[8]	Water and ES equivalent for maintaining performance in heat; CHO increased RER.
1973	Costill, Sparks[12]	Reported similar reductions in heart rates after rehydration (4% body weight) with water or ES.
1975	Costill, et al.[13]	After dehydration (3% loss of weight), water and ES were equivalent for water replenishment.
1979	Francis[14]	Both water and ES prevented loss of plasma volume and elevation of uric acid, cortisol, and dopamine-B-hydroxylase during 2 h of moderate work in warm, humid environment and heart rates were 18% lower than with no fluids.
1985	Wells, et al.[15]	No differences among water, ES, and caffeine solutions during 20-mile run on work parameters, serum electrolytes, or free fatty acids and glucose, and blood hemoglobin or hematocrits.
1986	Owen, et al.[16]	No differences among 10% glucose, 10% glucose polymer, and water during 2 h on treadmill at 50% max $\dot{V}O_2$ in 35°C, 15% RH room for rectal and skin temperatures, sweat and heart rates, plasma volume changes, gastric emptying, thermoregulation, and plasma glucose, insulin, osmolality, and Na⁺, and respiratory exchange rate.

weight is equal to 1 2/3% loss of total body water, 3% weight loss equals 5% water loss, and 6% weight loss is equal to 10% of the body water. Although increased thirst is experienced at only 1% weight loss, *ad libitum* water intake during work will be less than required to restore water balance. At 3% weight loss, hemoconcentration occurs with reduced urine production.[17] Decreased work capacity is found at 4% and mental functioning is detrimentally affected at 5% weight loss. When one loses 6% body weight or 10% of total body water, he is approaching serious problems (Table 8) and collapse is likely at a 7% weight loss, especially with heat and/or exercise.

1. Exercise and Water Absorption

Gisolfi's[18] review (Table 9) shows that fluid absorption occurs during exercise and is not reduced until the exercise approaches 60 to 70% of maximum. One can absorb between 1.9 and 2.3 l of water per h, with most occurring in the jejunum and ileum. This absorption is generally passive but can occur against an osmolar gradient. Glucose stimulates both water and Na absorption.

Na is required for fluid absorption, chloride is the best anion enhancer, and some amino acids may also enhance fluid absorption. Consequently, if minerals are added, then carbohydrate must be added to the sports drink; otherwise water is better than a mineral solution. More fluids are absorbed from carbohydrate-electrolyte beverages than from plain water under all conditions.

2. Dehydration Effects

Dehydration affects the body in a variety of ways, some of which are positive and protect physiological homeostasis, while others are negative consequences of the dehydrated condition.[19] Table 10 summarizes many of the responses to dehydration

TABLE 8   Adverse Effects of Weight (Water) Loss

% Weight Loss	Observed Effects
1%	Threshold for thirst and for impaired exercise thermoregulation leading to decrement in work capacity.
2%	Stronger thirst, vague discomfort and sense of oppression, loss of appetite.
3%	Dry mouth, increasing hemoconcentration, reduction in urinary output.
4%	Decrement of 20 to 30% in physical work capacity.
5%	Difficulty in concentrating, headache, impatience, sleepiness.
6%	Severe impairment in exercise temperature regulation, increased respiratory rate leading to tingling and numbness of extremities.
7%	Likely collapse if combined with heat and exercise.

From Greenleaf, J. E., *Med. Sci. Sports Exerc.*, 24, 645, 1992.

TABLE 9   Exercise, Intestinal Absorption and Rehydration

50 to 60% of fluid absorption is in small intestine and 1.9 to 2.3 l/h can be absorbed.

Fluid absorption is passive, but can be against a 40 to 50 mOsm gradient.

Glucose stimulates water and Na^+ absorption.

Na^+ is required for, and Cl^- enhances, fluid absorption. Amino acids, also, may enhance fluid absorption.

If minerals are added to sports drink, carbohydrate should be added, also. Water alone is better than water with minerals.

Significantly more fluid is absorbed from a carbohydrate-electrolyte beverage than from plain water, both at rest and during exercise.

Based on Gisolfi, C. V., *Sports Physiology/Biochemistry*, 4; Gatorade Sports Science Institute, Chicago, May 1991.

during exercise. Early in dehydration, gastric emptying is slowed and the rate of rehydration is reduced.[20]

The reduction in gastric emptying rate leads to sensations of bloatedness, nausea, and general gastric distress in athletes and workers in a hot environment.[21] Then, the plasma concentrations of angiotensin and vasopressin will normally rise with exercise and dehydration to help conserve body sodium and reduce urine production.[22] Both hormones promote vaso-constriction in inactive tissues, which causes the movement of fluid from these inactive tissues into plasma, helping to defend central blood volume. These circulatory changes[22] cause blood redistribution from inactive tissues (e.g., digestive organs, liver, kidneys) to the central blood volume. The decrease in urine production helps conserve body fluids.

The fluid in sweat[24] initially comes from the extracellular fluid compartment (i.e., plasma and interstitial fluid). Eventually, as the blood osmolality increases due to water losses in the sweat, intracellular water will flow into the extracellular compartment[25] and the intracellular volume will be reduced. However, even with substantial sweat losses, the body can reduce excessive plasma volume decreases by the redistribution of water from the interstitial and intracellular spaces into the

TABLE 10 Physiological Responses to Dehydration

1. Reduced rate of gastric emptying
2. Increased incidence of gastric distress
3. Increased plasma angiotensin and vasopressin
4. Decreased splanchnic and renal blood flow
5. Decreased plasma volume
6. Decreased plasma osmolality
7. Increased blood viscosity
8. Decreased central blood volume
9. Decreased central venous pressure
10. Decreased cardiac filling pressure
11. Decreased cardiac stroke volume
12. Increased heart rate
13. Decreased cardiac output
14. Decreased sweat rate and skin blood flow
15. Decreased maximal skin blood flow
16. Increased body temperature before sweating and skin blood flow increase
17. Increased core temperature

From Murray, M., *Med. Sci. Sports Exerc.*, 24, 5321–2, 1992. With permission.

plasma. The breakdown of glycogen may also contribute water to the plasma.[25] Muscle and skin apparently contribute about 70% of the total water loss[26] and this may be a protective mechanism for brain, liver, and other vital organs.[25] When plasma water is lost as sweat, the concentration of particles remaining in the blood increases. An increase in plasma osmolality is a signal that influences cardiovascular and thermoregulatory responses.[23] The loss of plasma water causes an increase in blood viscosity and a reduction in venous return; thereby reducing cardiac output.[27] The continued loss of body fluid progressively reduces the blood volume in the large vessels of the thorax and abdomen.[25] The reduction in central blood volume eventually results in an inability to maintain central venous pressure.[28]

A drop in central venous pressure reduces cardiac filling pressure.[25] This loss of venous return to the heart causes a reduction in the stroke volume.[29] To compensate for the reduced stroke volume, the heart rate is increased in an attempt to maintain cardiac output.[29] When the heart rate can no longer increase enough to make up for the drop in stroke volume, cardiac output is decreased.[29,30] Dehydration causes the body to reduce skin blood flow and sweat rate to conserve, as much as possible, body fluids and maintain central blood volume and cardiac output.[29,31] As a result, the blood flow to the skin is reduced during severe dehydration.[29]

When a person is dehydrated prior to exercise, both the increase in skin blood flow[29] and the onset of sweating[24] is delayed until the body reaches a higher body temperature; these delays represent a thermoregulatory disadvantage. The impact of dehydration on exercise performance has been recently covered in Sawka and Pandolf's excellent review.[32] Briefly, dehydration causes reductions in anaerobic capacity, muscular endurance, physical work capacity, and maximal aerobic power. As the amount of dehydration increases, the capacity to perform prolonged physical exercise decreases. Mental functioning, as shown by the ability to complete mental tasks, is compromised as the degree of dehydration is increased.[32] The inevitable result of the reductions in sweat rate and skin blood flow is an increase in core temperature.[29]

B. ACSM GUIDELINES

To develop the best means to prevent or ameliorate these consequences of dehydration, the American College of Sports Medicine conducted a symposium[33,34] on dehydration and fluid replacement to establish recommendations. The recommendations vary as the duration of exercise increases and include pre-exercise, during exercise, and post-exercise needs for fluid, carbohydrate, and electrolytes.

1. Events of Less Than 1 Hour

The exercise intensity will range from 75% to greater than 100% $\dot{V}O_2$ max for events that last less than 1 h such as most team sports (football, basketball, etc.), racket sports, many cycling events, and essentially all track events. During these events, there are few opportunities to ingest fluids, and most athletes would not sacrifice the time to do so. Also, gastric emptying is reduced at exercise intensities exceeding 75% $\dot{V}O_2$ max,[36] and drinking could produce a sensation of bloatedness, which could be detrimental to a maximal effort. The main concern in these short-term events, and especially for those conducted in a hot environment (Table 11), is to slow the rise in body temperature.[37] The sweat rate for most athletes should not exceed 2 to 3 l/h; therefore salt losses would not exceed 60 to 120 meq. Even if all of the sweat came from the plasma and interstitial fluids, and were replaced with 3 l of water, plasma sodium concentration would still be 136 meq/l (if the extracellular volume was 14 l or more). In addition, it is not likely that anyone would drink that much fluid so rapidly. Most athletes replace only half their fluid loss during, and immediately after, an event. Under these circumstances of such high-intensity exercise, they probably would drink and replace less. Therefore, the replacement of sodium under these circumstances is unnecessary. The only reason to include sodium in the drinks ingested during these short-term events would be to enhance palatability and to facilitate absorption. The addition of carbohydrate to any solution consumed will only serve to exacerbate the reduced gastric emptying that occurs during high-intensity exercise. However, glycogen depletion can occur during high-intensity exercise of less than 1 h, so the addition of carbohydrate to the pre-event drink may be beneficial.[38] In summary, 300 to 500 ml of a 6 to 10% carbohydrate beverage should be ingested before the event, and cool (5 to 15°C) water equal to about one-half of the subject's sweat rate should be ingested during exercise for events lasting less than 1 h.[35] The latter volume is about 500 to 1000 ml for athletes.

2. Events Lasting 1 to 3 Hours

The exercise intensity ranges from about 65% to 90% $\dot{V}O_2$ max for events such as soccer and most marathon contests which last for 1 to 3 h. The primary concern

TABLE 11   Fluid Requirements for Exercise of Less Than 1 Hour Duration

Exercise intensity: 80 to 130% $\dot{V}O_2$

Primary concern: Fluid replacement to attenuate rise in core temperature in heat.

Proposed formulation and intake:
  Pre-event: 6 to 10% Carbohydrate; 300 to 500 ml
  During exercise: H_2O; 500 to 1000 ml

Rational:
  Pre-event: Carbohydrate to enhance performance if glycogen depletion occurs.
             Fluid to attenuate dehydration effects.
  During exercise   Replace fluids lost in sweat and attenuate rise in core temperature.

From Gisolfi, C. V. and Duchman, S. M., *Med. Sci. Sports Exerc.*, 24, 679, 1992. With permission.

during these events is to replace body water loss and to provide a source of energy (Table 12). Events lasting this long can result in hypoglycemia, hypovolemia, hyperthermia, dehydration, and glycogen depletion.[39-41] Thus, an oral replacement solution is needed to provide both water and energy, to protect circulatory functioning, and to prevent thermal injury.[40,42] In addition, it has been shown that providing an exogenous source of energy during events of this duration can enhance performance.[43-45]

The amount of fluid to be ingested is dependent upon the sweat rate and, thus, is variable. The volume of fluid necessary to provide the amount of carbohydrate needed is 500 to 1000 ml/h;[46] while the volume required to replace the fluid lost in sweat will range from 800 to 1600 ml/hour for most athletes. The ACSM guideline is 100 to 200 ml every 2 to 3 km of the run. During a marathon (42 km), this would amount to 2.1 to 4.2 l or approximately 600 to 1400 ml/h. Mitchell and Voss[47] concluded that there was no advantage in consuming fluids in excess of 65% of the sweat loss. They found that ingesting a 7% carbohydrate solution at 65%, 83%, or 94% of sweat and respiratory water loss did not significantly affect plasma volume nor blood glucose concentration. However, the two higher rates of fluid ingestion did increase the sensations of stomach fullness.

For events lasting from 1 to 3 h, the pre-event beverage should be plain water. Fat metabolism should be promoted early in these events, so the inclusion of carbohydrate in this drink is not recommended.[34] The addition of carbohydrate would initiate carbohydrate metabolism and promote glycogen utilization and this would cause premature fatigue.[48,49]

Therefore, for events lasting from 1 to 3 h, 300 to 500 ml of water should be ingested before the event, and 800 to 1600 ml/h of a cool (5 to 15°C) 6 to 8% carbohydrate solution containing 10 to 20 meq of sodium/l are recommended during exercise. If sodium is not included in the beverage, it must be provided by intestinal secretions. The rationale for including 6 to 8% carbohydrate has been reviewed by

TABLE 12   Fluid Requirements for Exercise of 1 to 3 H Duration

Exercise intensity:	60 to 90% of $\dot{V}O_2$ max.
Primary concern:	Fluid and carbohydrate needs.
Formulation:	
Pre-event:	H_2O 300 to 500 mL
During exercise:	10 to 20 meq Na^+ and Cl^-; 6 to 8% CHO; 500 to 1000 ml/h for CHO needs up to 800 to 1600 ml 1 h for athlete's fluid needs.
Rationale:	
Pre-event:	Water is needed to attenuate dehydration during exercise.
During exercise:	CHO: to prevent depletion of muscle glycogen stores.
	Fluid: to prevent dehydration due to sweating — highly variable and depends on ambient temperature, exercise intensity, training, and heat acclimatization
	Na^+: to promote CHO and fluid absorption, enchange palatability, and help maintain ECF volume.
	Cl^-: most effective anion for fluid absorption.

From Gisolfi, C. V. and Duchman, S. M., *Med. Sci. Sports Exerc.*, 24, 679, 1992. With permission.

Lamb and Brodowicz[43] and satisfies the guidelines proposed by Coyle.[46] The form of carbohydrate does not appear to affect gastric emptying,[43] and the best form to promote intestinal absorption remains to be determined. Sodium is recommended to enhance the palatability,[13,50] and the intestinal absorption, of the fluid.[51]

3. Events Lasting More Than 3 Hours

Exercise intensity will range from 30 to 70% $\dot{V}O_2$ max for events lasting over 3 h, such as the triathlon and all ultra marathons. The concern in formulating an oral replacement solution for these events is to provide fluids, energy, and electrolytes (Table 13). This form of competition causes hypoglycemia, hypovolemia, glycogen depletion, dehydration, and possibly hyponatremia.[52] Therefore, the oral solution for these events should contain 20 to 30 meq of sodium/l. Although higher salt concentrations might be more beneficial, the drink would be unacceptable. The carbohydrate concentration is again 6 to 8% and the pre-event beverage should be water for the reasons previously mentioned.

Should potassium be added to this sport drink? Sweat concentrations of potassium are only 1 to 15 meq/l[53] and do not increase with sweat rate.[54] Some studies have reported larger losses,[55,56] but these have not been confirmed.[57] However, rehydration of the intracellular fluid compartment appears to be facilitated by potassium, and glucose ingestion causes potassium secretion into the intestine. Therefore, to replace the small sweat losses of potassium and to stimulate the rehydration of the intracellular space, the addition of 3 to 5 meq/l of K^+ to the sport drink may be beneficial.

In summary, for endurance events of more than 3 h, one should drink 300 to 500 ml of H_2O before the event, and 500 to 1000 ml/h of cool (5 to 15°C) 6 to 8% carbohydrate solution with 20 to 30 meq of sodium during exercise; the inclusion of 3 to 5 meq of potassium may provide a further benefit.

TABLE 13   Fluid, Energy, and Electrolyte Requirements for Exercise of Over 3 H Duration

Exercise intensity:	30 to 70% of $\dot{V}O_2$ max.
Concerns:	Provide adequate water, carbohydrate and sodium.

Formulation:

Pre-event:	H_2O, 300 to 500 ml
During exercise:	20 to 30 meq Na+ and Cl–; 6 to 8%
	CHO: 500 to 1000 ml/h to meet needs of most athletes

Rationale:

Pre-event:	Drink only water to attenuate dehydration during exercise.
During exercise:	CHO: to retard depletion of muscle glycogen stores.
	Fluid: to prevent dehydration–exercise intensity and sweat rates will be lower than for 1 to 3 h category.
	Na+: to promote CHO and fluid absorption, enhance palatability, and prevent hyponatremia.
	Cl–: most effective anion for promotion fluid absorption.

From Gisolfi, C.V. and Duchman, S.M., *Med. Sci. Sports Exerc.*, 24, 679–687, 1992. With permission.

4. Post Exercise Fluid Needs

Although many subjects learn to replace up to two thirds of their sweat water losses during exercise,[58] others "voluntarily" dehydrate by as much as 10% of their body weight.[53] Water and nutrients consumed during the first 2 h of recovery will markedly affect the rate of recovery and performance in a subsequent athletic event. The formulation of the recovery beverage (Table 14) should promote glycogen resynthesis, and fluid and electrolyte replacement.

Muscle glycogen resynthesis is greatest when about 25 g of carbohydrate are ingested each hour.[59,60] This amount of carbohydrate can be readily ingested in a beverage. Hyponatremia can result from water intoxication[61,62] and/or excessive sweat losses.[63] Nose et al.,[64] found that during recovery, fluid replacement was significantly enhanced when 75 meq of sodium was ingested; however, the sodium was encapsulated and this amount of sodium in solution would render a beverage unpalatable for most people. Thus, the recommendation is that the recovery drink should contain 40 meq of sodium and chloride.[35] This concentration of salt is about the maximum that is acceptable. This beverage composition appears optimal for all exercise intensities and durations that cause glycogen depletion.

V. CONCLUSION

In conclusion (Table 15), the research on fluid, carbohydrate, and mineral needs during exercise have provided these recommendations.

The first priority is to prevent large negative water balances; consequently, the exerciser should drink about 300 to 500 ml of water beginning 30 to 60 min before exercise. If the exercise is high intensity and less than 1 h long, this pre-event solution

TABLE 14　Fluid and Nutrient Requirements During Recovery

Concerns:　　　Replace glycogen, fluids, and sodium.

Formulation:　　30 to 40 meq of sodium and chloride; 6 to 8% carbohydrate so that the person receives about 25 g of carbohydrate/h

Intake:　　　　Drink to replace sweat losses of fluids.

Rationale:　　　Most fluids are replaced in first 10 to 20 min of recovery. Thus, a palatable beverage to encourage drinking, containing carbohydrate to replace glycogen stores and sodium to help restore extracellular fluid volumes, is needed. Avoid carbonated beverages that produce sensation of fullness.

From Gisolfi, C.V. and Duchman, S.M., *Med. Sci. Sports Exerc.*, 24, 679, 1992. With permission.

TABLE 15　The Recommendations for Fluids and Nutrients for Physical Exercise

First Priority: Fluid replacement — begin 30 to 60 min pre-exercise with 300 to 500 ml, may contain 6 to 10% carbohydrate preceeding exercise of less than 1 h. During exercise, drink 500 to 1000 mL/hour; for less than 1 h of exercise, use water only. Continue during recovery to replace sweat losses.

Second Priority: Add 6 to 8% carbohydrate for energy for exercise of greater than 1 h and during recovery for muscle glycogen replenishment.

Third Priority: Add 20 to 30 meq sodium and chloride to promote carbohydrate and fluid absorption, to maintain extracellular fluid volumes, and to replace sweat losses.

may contain 6 to 10% carbohydrate; otherwise, only water if the event exceeds 1 h. This volume should be increased to 500 to 1000 ml/h during the exercise session and continued during recovery until all the sweat losses are replaced. Only water is needed for exercise of less than 1 h.

The second priority is to provide the energy for exercise, maintaining blood glucose levels, and reducing glycogen depletion. Water is adequate for short exercise periods; but for events longer than 1 h, the oral solution should contain 6 to 8% carbohydrate during both exercise and recovery.

The third priority is to promote the absorption of water and carbohydrate from the intestines, to maintain extracellular fluid volumes and to replace salt losses in the sweat. This can best be accomplished by the addition of 20 to 30 meq of both sodium and chloride to the drinks. Until modified by further research, these recommendations appear to provide our best advice for the optimal maintenance of health and performance during exercise.

REFERENCES

1. Mayer, A., Essai sur la soif: ses causes et son mecanisme, Paris: Felix alcan, 1901.
2. Wettendorf, H., Modifications due sang sous l'influence de la privation d'eau: contribution a l'etude de la soif, *Travaux Lab Physiol. Inst. Solvag*, 4, 353, 1901.
3. Hunt, E. H., The regulations of body temperature in extremes of dry heat, *J. Hyg.*, 12, 479, 1912.
4. Adolph, E. F., *Physiological Regulations*, Jacques Cattell Press, Lancaster, PA, 1943, 502.
5. Pitts, G. C., Johnson, R. E., and Consolazio, F. C., Work in the heat as affected by intake of water, salt and glucose, *Am. J. Physiol.*, 142, 253, 1944.
6. Rothstein, A., Adolph, A. E., and Wills, J. H., Voluntary dehydration, in *Physiology of Man in the Desert*, Adolph, E. F. and Associates, Eds., Interscience Publishers, New York, 1947, 254.
7. Johnson, H. L., Consolazio, C. F., Daws, T. A., and Burk, R. F., The effects of various liquid supplements upon mineral balances during profuse sweating, *Fed. Proc.*, 32 (Abstr.), 913, 1973.
8. Johnson, H. L., Nelson, R. A., and Consolazio, C. F., Effects of electrolyte and nutrient solutions on performance and metabolic balance, *Med. Sci. Sports Exerc.*, 20, 26, 1988.
9. Balke, B., and Ware, R., An experimental study of physical fitness of air force personnel, *U.S. Armed Forces Med. J.*, 10, 675, 1959.
10. Nelson, R. A., Matoush, L. O., and Consolazio, C. F., *Development and Application of a Continuous Oxygen Uptake Measurement System (USAMRNL Report No. 318)*, Fitzsimmons General Hospital, Denver, CO, 1968.
11. Snedecor, G. W., and Cochran, W. G., *Statistical Methods*, 6th ed., The Iowa State University Press, Ames, IA, 1967, 271.
12. Costill, D. L., and Sparks, K. E., Rapid fluid replacement following thermal dehydration, *J. Appl. Physiol.*, 34, 299, 1973.
13. Costill, D. L., Cote, R., Miller, E., Miller, T., and Wynder S., Water and electrolyte replacement during repeated days of work in the heat, *Aviat. Space Environ. Med.*, 46, 795, 1975.
14. Francis, K. T., Effect of water and electrolyte replacement during exercise in the heat on biochemical indices of stress and performance, *Aviat. Space Environ. Med.*, 50, 115, 1979.
15. Wells, C. L., Schradeo, T. A., Stern, J. R., and Krahenbul, G. S., Physiological responses to a 20-mile rule under three fluid replacement treatments, *Med. Sci. Sports Exerc.*, 17, 364, 1985.
16. Owen, M. D., Kregel, K. C., Wall, P. T., and Gisolfi, C. V., Effects of ingesting carbohydrate beverages during exericse in the heat, *Med. Sci. Sports Exerc.*, 18, 568, 1986.
17. Greenleaf, J. E., Problem: thirst, drinking behavior, and involuntary dehydration, *Med. Sci. Sports Exerc.*, 24, 645, 1992.
18. Gisolfi, C. V., Sports Science Exchange: exercise, intestinal absorption, and rehydration, *Sports Physiology/Biochemistry*, 4(32). Gatorade Sports Science Institute, Chicago, May, 1991.
19. Murray, M., Nutrition for the marathon and other endurance sports: environmental stress and dehydration, *Med. Sci. Sports Exerc.*, 24, S319, 1992.
20. Neufer, P. D, Young, A. J., and Sawka, M. N., Gastric emptying during exercise: effects of heat stress and hypohydration, *Eur. J. Appl. Physiol.*, 58, 433, 1989.
21. Rehrer, N. J., Beckers, E. J., Brouns, F., Ten Hoor, F., and Saris, W. H. M., Effects of dehydration on gastric emptying and gastrointestinal distress while running, *Med. Sci. Sports Exerc.*, 22, 790, 1990.
22. Brandenberger, G., Candas, V., Follenius, M., Libert, J. P., and Kahn, J. M., Vascular fluids shifts and endocrine responses to exercise in the heat, *Eur. J. Appl. Physiol.*, 55, 123, 1986.
23. Rowell, L. B., Human cardiovascular adjustments to exercise and thermal stress, *Physiol. Rev.*, 54, 75, 1974.
24 Fortney, S. M., Wenger, C. B., Bove, J.R., and Nadel, E. R., Effect of hyperosmolality on control of blood flow and sweating, *J. Appl. Physiol.*, 57, 1688, 1984.
25 Sawka, M. N., and Pandolf, K. B., Effects of body water loss on physiological function and exercise performance, in *Perspectives in Exerc. Science and Sports Medicine, Vol. 3: Fluid Homeostasis During Exerc.*, Gisolfi, C. V., and Lamb, D.R., Eds., Benchmark Press, Indianapolis, 1990, 1.

26. Nose, H., Morimoto, T., and Ogura, K., Distribution of water losses among fluid compartments of tissues under thermal dehydration in the rat, *Jpn. J. Physiol.*, 33, 1019, 1983.

27. Vanderwalle, H., Lacombe, C., Lelievre, J. C., and Poirot, C., Blood viscosity after a 1-h submaximal exercise with and without drinking, *Int. J. Sports Med.*, 9, 104, 1988.

28. Kirsch, K. A., Ameln, von H., and Wicke, H. J., Fluid control mechanisms after exercise dehydration, *Eur. J. Appl. Physiol.*, 47, 191, 1981.

29. Nadel, E. R., Fortney, S. M., and Wenger, C. B., Effect of hydration on circulatory and thermal regulation, *J. Appl. Physiol.*, 49, 715, 1980.

30. Sawka, M. N., Knowlton, R. G., and Critz, J. B., Thermal and circulatory responses to repeated bouts of prolonged running, *Med. Sci. Sports Exerc.*, 11, 177, 1979.

31. Fortney, S. M., Nadel, E. R., Wenger, C. B., and Bove, J. R., Effect of blood volume on sweating rate and body fluids in exercising humans, *J. Appl. Physiol.*, 51, 1594, 1981.

32. Sawka, M. N., and Pandolf, K. B., Effects of body water loss on physiological function and exercise performance, in *Perspective in Exerc. Science and Sports Medicine, Vol. 3: Fluid Homeostasis During Exerc.*, Gisolfi, C. V., and Lamb, D. R, Eds., Benchmark Press, Indianapolis, 1990, 1.

33. Gopinathan, P. M., Pichan, G., and Sharma, V. M., Role of dehydration in heat-stress induced variations in mental performance, *Arch. Environ. Health*, 43, 15, 1988.

34. Sawka, M. N., and Greenleaf, J. E., Current concepts concerning thirst, dehydration, and fluid replacement, *Med. Sci. Sports Exerc.*, 24, 643, 1992.

35. Gisolfi, C. V., and Duchman, S. M., Guidelines for optimal replacement beverages for different athletic events, *Med. Sci. Sports Exerc.*, 24, 679, 1992.

36. Costill, D. L., and Saltin, B., Factors limiting gastric emptying during rest and exercise, *J. Appl. Physiol.*, 37, 679, 1974.

37. Robinson, S., Temperature regulation in exercise, *Pediatrics*, 32, 691, 1963.

38. Sagaki, H., Maeda, J., Usul, S., and Ishiko, T., Effect of sucrose and caffeine ingestion on performance of prolonged strennous running, *Int. J. Sports Med.*, 8, 261, 1987.

39. Coyle, E. F., Coggan, A. R., Hemmert, M. K., and Ivy, J. L., Muscle glycogen utilization during prolonged strenuous exercise when fed carbohydrate, *J. Appl. Physiol.*, 61, 165, 1986.

40. Gisolfi, C. V., and Copping, J. R., Thermal effects of prolonged treadmill exercise in the heat, *Med. Sci. Sports Exerc.*, 6, 108, 1974.

41. Pugh, L. G. C. E, Corbett J. L., and Johnson R. H., Rectal temperatures, weight losses, and sweat rates in marathon running, *J. Appl. Physiol.*, 23, 347, 1967.

42. Costill, D. L., Kammer, W. F., and Fisher, A., Fluid ingestion during distance running, *Arch. Environ. Health*, 21, 520, 1974.

43. Lamb, D. R., and Brodowicz, G. R., Optimal use of fluids of varying formulations to minimize exercise-induced disturbances in homeostasis, *Sports Med.*, 3, 247, 1985.

44. Maughan, R., Carbohydrate-electrolyte solutions during prolonged exercise, in *Perspectives in Exerc. Science and Sports Medicine, Ergogenics: Enhancement of Performance in Exerc. and Sport*, Lamb, D. R., and Williams, M. H., Eds., Benchmark Press, Indianapolis, 1991, 35.

45. Murray, R., The effects of consuming carbohydrate-electrolyte beverages on gastric emptying and fluid absorption during the following exercise, *Sports Med.*, 4, 322, 1987.

46. Coyle, E. F., Timing and methods of increased carbohydrate intake to cope with heavy training, competition and recovery, *J. Sports Sci.*, 9, 29, 1991.

47. Mitchell, J. B., and Voss, K. W., The influence of volume on gastric emptying and fluid balance during prolonged exercise, *Med. Sci. Sports Exerc.*, 23, 31, 1991.

48. Foster, C., Costill, D. L., and Fink, W. J., Effects of preexercise feeding on endurance performance, *Med. Sci. Sports Exerc.*, 11, 1, 1979.

49. Koivisto, V. O., Harkonen, M., Korone, S., Groop, P., Elovainio, R., Ferrannini, E., Sacca, L., and Defronzo, R., Glycogen depletion during prolonged exercise: influence of glucose, fructose, or placebo, *J. Appl. Physiol.*, 58, 731, 1985.

50. Hubbard, R. W., Mager, M., Bowers W. D., Leav, I., Angoff, G., Matthew, W. T, and Sils, I. V., Effect of low-potassium diet on rat exercise hyperthermia and heatstroke mortality, *J. Appl. Physiol.*, 51, 8, 1981.

51. Gisolfi, C. V., Summers, R. W, Schedl, H. P., Bleiler, T. L., and Oppliger, R. A., Human intestinal water absorption: direct vs. indirect measurements, *Am. J. Physiol.*, 258, G216, 1990.
52. Noakes, T. D., Adams, B. A., Myburgh, K. H., Greef, C., Lotz, T., and Nathan, M., The danger of an inadequate water intake during prolonged exercise, *Eur. J. Appl. Physiol.*, 57, 210, 1988.
53. Robinson, S., and Robinson, A. H., Chemical compounds of sweat, *Physiol. Rev.*, 34, 202, 1954.
54. Costill, D. L., Sweating: its composition and effects on body fluids, in *The Marathon: Physiological, Medical, Epidemiological and Psychological Studies*, Milvey, P., Ed., Ann. N.Y. Acad. Sci., 1977, 301, 160.
55. Armstrong, L. E., Hubbard, R. W., Szlyk, P. C., Matthew, W. T., and Sils, I. V., Voluntary dehydration and electrolyte losses during prolonged exercise in the heat, *Aviat. Space Environ. Med.*, 56, 765, 1985.
56. Knochel, J. P., Dotin, L. N., and Hamburger, R. J., Pathophysiology of intense physical conditioning in a hot climate, *J. Clin. Invest.*, 51, 242, 1972.
57. Costill, D. L., Muscle metabolism and electrolyte balance during heat acclimation, *Acta Physiol. Scand.*, 128, 111, 1986.
58. Pitts, G. C., Johnson, R. E., and Consolazio, F. C., Work in heat as affected by intake of water, salt and glucose, *Am. J. Physiol.*, 142, 253, 1944.
59. Blom, P. C., Hostmark, A. T., Vaage, O., Vardal, K. R., and Maehlum, S., Effect of different post-exercise sugar diets on the rate of muscle glycogen synthesis, *Med. Sci. Sports Exerc.*, 19, 491, 1987.
60. Ivy, J. L., Katz, A. L., Cutler, C. L., Sherman, W. M., and Coyle, E. F., Muscle glycogen synthesis after exercise: effect of time of carbohydrate ingestion, *J. Appl. Physiol.*, 65, 1480, 1988.
61. Frizzell, R. T., Lang, G. H., Lawrence, D. C., et al., Hyponatremia and ultramarathon running, *J.A.M.A.*, 255, 722, 1986.
62. Noakes, T. D., Goodwin, N., Rayner, B. L., Branken, T., and Taylor, R. K. N., Water intoxication: a possible complication during endurance exercise. *Med. Sci. Sports Exerc.*, 17, 370, 1985.
63. Hiller, W. D. B, O'Toole, M. L., Fortess, E. E., Laird, R. H., Imbert, P. C., and Sisk, T. D., Medical and physiological considerations in triathlons, *Am. J. Sports Med.*, 15, 164, 1987.
64. Nose, H., Mack, G. W., Shi, X., and Nadel, E. R., Role of osmolality and plasma volume during rehydration in humans, *J. Appl. Physiol.*, 65, 325, 1988.

Chapter **19**

CARBOHYDRATE, FLUID, AND ELECTROLYTE REQUIREMENTS DURING PROLONGED EXERCISE

John A. Hawley
Steven C. Dennis
Timothy D. Noakes

CONTENTS

0-8493-7916-4/95/$0.00+$.50
© 1995 by CRC Press, Inc.

I. HISTORICAL BACKGROUND

A. THE PIONEERING STUDIES OF CARBOHYDRATE METABOLISM

The pioneering studies of carbohydrate (CHO) metabolism during prolonged (i.e., >90 min) exercise began in the mid 1920s when Levine and colleagues[1] studied 12 runners in the 1923 Boston Marathon and observed a marked decline in post-race plasma glucose concentrations (<2.8 mmol/l) in three of the runners. In the race the following year they fed a number of athletes CHO in the form of candy, after 24 km of the marathon, in order to determine the possible relationship between hypoglycemia and fatigue. This practice, in combination with a high pre-race CHO diet, enhanced running performance and prevented hypoglycemia.[2]

The possibility that hypoglycemia might explain exhaustion at the end of long-distance races was next raised by Best and Partridge,[3] who studied ten athletes in the 1928 Amsterdam, Olympic Marathon. Three of the ten runners were found to be hypoglycemic at the end of the race. Best and Partridge[3] observed that "the carbohydrate reserves of the body at the start of the race" and "the ingestion of food during the race" were important factors in the prevention of hypoglycemia.

The efficacy of CHO supplementation for improving work capacity was further demonstrated by Dill and his colleagues during studies conducted at the Harvard Fatigue Laboratory in Boston in 1932.[4] They showed that when their dogs, Joe and Sally, were fed CHO (20 g/h), their running endurance increased from 4 to 6 h to 17 to 23 h. Dill et al.[4] concluded that the factor limiting the performance of prolonged moderate intensity exercise "seems to be merely the quantity of easily available fuel...in the form of blood-borne glucose" for oxidation by the working muscles.

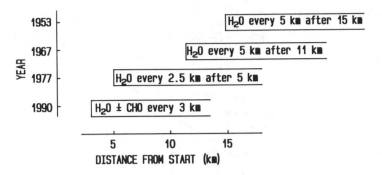

FIGURE 1. The evolution of the International Amateur Athletic Federation rules governing the intake of fluids during long-distance running.

In 1936 Boje[5] showed that feeding CHO solutions to individuals at exhaustion could restore exercise capacity. These early studies prompted Grace Eggleton[6] to surmise that "when long distance runners have run to exhaustion, the levels of blood sugar are found to be abnormally low. If the eating of sugar candy during a race was encouraged by Athletic Organisations, it seems possible that new records might be achieved in very long-distance running".

In the classic studies of Christensen and Hansen[7-9] the essential role of CHO for the performance of prolonged exercise was confirmed. Using different dietary manipulations, they found that endurance time was decreased after a high-fat diet, but markedly increased after a high-CHO diet. The premature fatigue experienced by subjects after the high-fat, low-CHO diet was accompanied by ketosis, a decreased rate of CHO oxidation, and hypoglycemia. These findings,[7-9] along with the results of the pioneering studies of CHO metabolism[1-5] were, however, largely ignored by the athletic community. Athletes were also unaware of the early industrial and military investigations showing the importance of adequate fluid replacement for exercise in the heat.[10-18]

The first official reference to fluid replacement during long-distance running can be found in the 1953 Handbook of the International Amateur Athletic Federation (IAAF). The 1953 IAAF rules controlling marathon races (Figure 1) stated that "refreshments shall (only) be provided by the organisers of a race after 15 km or 10 miles, and thereafter every 5 km or 3 miles. No refreshment may be carried or taken by a competitor other than that provided by the organisers." As water was the *only* drink made available to runners at the official refreshment stations, it was clear that the IAAF had little knowledge of the original studies which had shown the benefits of ingesting CHO during prolonged exercise.

It was not until the 1960s, with the reintroduction of the percutaneous needle muscle biopsy technique by Scandinavian physiologists, that studies of CHO utilization during exercise again became popular.[19-25] These studies demonstrated the crucial role of starting muscle glycogen stores for performance during prolonged exercise and focused attention on pre-exercise nutritional strategies aimed at maximizing working muscle glycogen content prior to exercise.

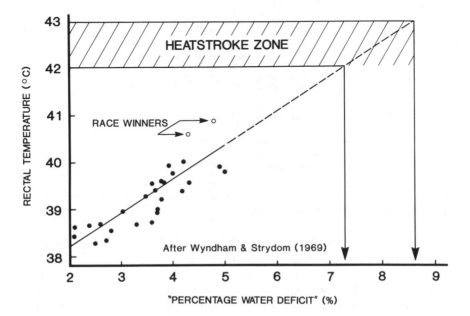

FIGURE 2.   The linear relationship between rectal temperature and water deficit after two 32 km road-running races. The highest post-race rectal temperatures were found in the fastest runners. Redrawn from Reference 26.

By this time the IAAF had *slightly* modified their rules governing the provision of refreshments during marathon races (Figure 1). Whereas in 1953 "refreshments could only be provided by the organisers of a race after 15 km or 10 miles," in 1967 the IAAF handbook stated that "refreshments could be provided after (*only*) 11 km or 7 miles" (IAAF Handbook, Rule 155, page 103, 1967). Presumably the term "refreshments" referred to water.

B.   THE CARBOHYDRATE VS. WATER DEBATE

For the next decade, the idea that water rather than CHO replacement was more important during exercise gained the ascendancy. Wyndham and Strydom[26] studied two groups of athletes competing in a 20 mile (32 km) road-race and found that those runners who became dehydrated during the race had elevated post-race rectal temperatures (Figure 2). Further, those runners who were the most dehydrated had the highest post-race temperatures. This finding led Wyndham and Strydom[26] to speculate that the athletes' level of dehydration and their elevated post-race temperatures were *causally* related, and that dehydration alone was the most important factor determining rectal temperature during prolonged exercise.[26,27] Largely, as a result of Wyndham and Strydom's[26] study, and a failure to note that rectal temperatures are more a function of metabolic rate than of dehydration,[28] the concept that fluid replacement alone was of primary importance for optimizing performance during prolonged exercise was promoted. These notions were later reinforced by the study of Costill and Saltin,[29] which showed that drinks with a high (6.25 to 37.5 g/100 ml) CHO content emptied more slowly from the stomach than water during exercise. These workers concluded that "the replacement of water was important during prolonged exercise in the heat and that only when competing in the cold could carbohydrate safely be included in solutions to be ingested during exercise". Accordingly, the CHO studies of the 1920s and 1930s were largely ignored,[30] and water, in large volumes, was considered to be the optimum fluid replacement for ingestion during prolonged exercise.

At this time the IAAF, obviously aware of the "dangers" of dehydration during long-distance events, changed their rules (Figure 1) so that competitors during a marathon could now have "refreshments provided by the organisers of the race after approximately 5 km or 3 miles." In addition, rule number 165, clause 4, stated that "the organisers shall provide sponging points where water only shall be supplied, midway between (two) refreshment stations" (IAAF Handbook, page 98, 1977). Thus, during the 1970s it was universally accepted that CHO ingestion during prolonged exercise was of little benefit. Indeed, in the "start-of-the-art" proceedings of the 1976 New York Academy of Sciences conference "The Marathon: Physiological, Medical, Epidemiological, and Psychological Studies", there was not a *single* reference to CHO ingestion during prolonged exercise.[31]

C. THE RE-EMERGENCE OF STUDIES SUPPORTING THE VALUE OF CARBOHYDRATE INGESTION DURING EXERCISE

Several studies at this time, however, did *suggest* that CHO feedings during exercise could potentially delay fatigue.[32-34] These investigations showed that when cyclists or canoeists were fed various CHO preparations during prolonged, strenuous exercise, blood glucose concentrations were elevated above pre-exercise levels, high rates of CHO were sustained during exercise, and endurance capacity was improved.

In contrast to the studies of Brooke et al.,[32-34] however, Felig et al.[35] reported that there was no difference in the time-to-fatigue during cycling at 60 to 65% of maximal oxygen uptake ($\dot{V}O_2$ max) when *untrained* subjects ingested either 5 g/100 ml (40 g/h) or 10 g/100 ml (80 g/h) glucose solutions every 15 min throughout exhausting exercise. They observed that prolonged exercise of moderate intensity precipitated hypoglycemia (<2.5 mmol/l) in 37% of subjects but, despite preventing this hypoglycemia, glucose ingestion failed to cause a consistent increase in exercise time-to-exhaustion. These results prompted Felig et al.[35] to state that "exercise can be continued in the presence of hypoglycemia, which does not support a role for glucose ingestion in improving performance during prolonged exercise."

Despite suggestions that these studies did not necessarily prove that the performance of *trained* athletes would not also be improved by the ingestion of CHO during prolonged exercise,[36] the question of whether water or CHO replacement should be emphasized during prolonged exercise was not fully resolved until the mid-to-late 1980s. At that time, commercial interests in America revived research into the value of CHO ingestion during exercise: whereas water has no marketable value, CHO added to water can be marketed and sold to millions of athletes worldwide. The studies of Coyle et al.[37,38] and Coggan and Coyle[39-41] marked the re-emergence of investigations of CHO metabolism during prolonged exercise and, in particular, the role of CHO ingestion.

In 1983, Coyle et al.[37] showed that cycling time-to-fatigue at 74% of $\dot{V}O_2$ max was significantly greater (157 ± 5 min) with CHO feedings (1 g of maltodextrin/kg bodymass in a 50 g/100 ml solution after 20 min of exercise, followed by 0.25 g of maltodextrin/kg bodymass in a 6 g/100 ml solution after 60, 90, and 120 min) than with placebo (135 ± 6 min). This was the first well-controlled experiment to *conclusively* demonstrate that CHO ingestion during prolonged, moderate-intensity exercise can delay fatigue. At the time, Coyle et al.[37] concluded that "carbohydrate administration during exercise may result in increased utilization of blood glucose with a proportional slowing of muscle glycogen depletion". However, muscle glycogen concentrations were not measured in that study and this interpretation was later shown to be incorrect.[38,42-44]

Subsequent studies by Coggan and Coyle further proved the efficacy of CHO feedings during exercise and, in particular, the important role of plasma glucose as an oxidizable substrate late in exercise.[39-41] They showed that (1) during prolonged exercise in fasted subjects not consuming CHO, blood glucose concentrations fell after 2 to 3 h when muscle glycogen levels were low; and (2) CHO ingestion maintained blood glucose at euglycemic levels (4 to 5 mmol/l) during the latter stages of exercise, preserved high rates of CHO oxidation, and improved performance. This latter finding supported the proposal of Dill et al.,[4] made some 50 years earlier.

Although the relevance for performance in actual competition of some of these conclusions has recently been questioned,[45] several other laboratories using a variety of CHO solutions and exercise performance tests have independently confirmed the efficacy of CHO feedings during prolonged running and cycling exercise.[46-59]

Although the optimal carbohydrate-electrolyte beverage has yet to be formulated, fluid consumption is not only allowed, but presently advocated by the IAAF (Figure 1) in all races of 10 km and longer (IAAF Handbook, p. 125, 1990). Beverages are normally provided by race sponsors, race organizers, coaches, or the athletes themselves. The choice of beverage, however, is typically not based upon any scientific rationale, and there still persists much mysticism as to what, and how much (if, indeed, anything) should be consumed to provide sufficient CHO, electrolytes, and fluid to replace sweat losses during exercise.

II. FLUID CHANGES DURING PROLONGED EXERCISE

A. RATES OF FLUID AND ELECTROLYTE LOSSES

Fluid loss during exercise is determined principally by the sweat rate, which is proportional to the athlete's metabolic rate.[28,60-65] Barr and Costill[66] have predicted sweat rates for athletes of different masses running at different speeds. Their predictions are in accord with the sweat rates measured in runners during longer distance races (see Noakes et al.[67]) and suggest that sweat rates in the majority of distance runners are seldom greater than 1.2 l/h.

Higher than 1.2 l/h sweat rates are usually recorded only when the environmental temperatures are higher than 25°C, especially when the humidity is high, or when the activity is held indoors without the benefit of adequate convective cooling. For example, sweat rates during out-of-doors cycling are 38% less than those measured at the same metabolic rate in wind-still conditions indoors.[68] Thus, the much higher than 1.2 l/h sweat rates measured in the laboratory[51,69] than in the field[68] could be due to the absence of adequate convective cooling during exercise indoors.

When compared to electrolyte concentrations in cellular and extracellular fluids, sweat is hypotonic. The principal ions lost in sweat are sodium and chloride ions from the extracellular compartments,[60] and their concentrations depend on an individual's level of fitness and state of heat acclimation.[70,71] Despite a 12% increase in overall sweat rate after heat acclimation, sodium losses in the sweat decrease by almost 60%.[71] Thus, for a given sweat rate, the heat acclimated individual loses less solute from the plasma.

Even the large sweat losses incurred during daily endurance training are adequately tolerated by the distance athlete. The large daily caloric intake and renal conservation of sodium in endurance athletes is normally sufficient to prevent the potential chronic dehydration and/or electrolyte deficiencies that could occur from sizeable ion losses in sweat.[60]

B. RATES OF FLUID INGESTION

Voluntary rates of fluid intake and exercise-induced weight changes in runners, cyclists, and triathletes competing over a wide range of distances have been reviewed.[67] That review suggests that the rates of fluid intake during exercise vary considerably, but are seldom more than about 0.5 l/h and are invariably less than sweat rates. During exercise lasting less than 6 h, athletes typically experience a weight loss of 2 to 3 kg and this loss of weight appears to be independent of either the type or duration of the activity.[67]

One explanation for the failure of both runners[72] and cyclists[73] to meet their fluid requirements is that they develop symptoms of "fullness" when they attempt to drink fluid at rates equal to or greater than 0.80 l/h. The discomfort of drinking large volumes of fluid repetitively is especially marked during running.[74,75] Brouns et al.[74] showed that the rate of fluid ingestion of subjects encouraged to drink as much as possible during a simulated triathlon was 2 to 3 times higher during the cycling leg (0.6 to 0.8 l/h) than during the running leg (0.1 to 0.3 l/h), suggesting that running reduces the desire to drink more than does cycling. Feelings of abdominal fullness with high rates of fluid ingestion may also be due to limited rates of small bowel fluid absorption.

Glucose absorption from ingested non-hyperosmotic CHO solutions has been shown to stimulate water absorption.[76-80] However, rates of water absorption may be less than rates of ingestion (Figure 3). Gisolfi et al.[79] have calculated that only 37%

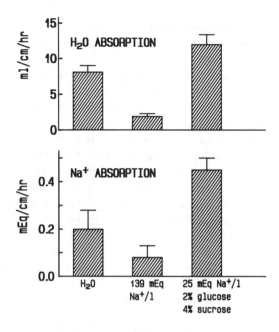

FIGURE 3.   Water and sodium flux during perfusions of the small intestine with isotonic elec-trolyte and carbohydrate-electrolyte solutions. Increases in the rate of fluid and sodium uptake in the presence of carbohydrate are significant. Redrawn from.[79] Subsequent studies by this group have shown that the type of CHO presented to the intestine is unimportant provided that the solution is not hyperosmotic.[78]

of fluid infused into the duodenum and jejunum at rates of 0.9 l/h was absorbed, while others have reported that the maximum rate of water absorption from a 100 mmol/l isotonic sodium chloride solution was only 0.8 l/h.[81] Similarly, in studies in which fluid replacement either during[66] or after[82] exercise equalled fluid losses, it was found that not all the ingested fluid could be accounted for by its appearance in the extracellular or intracellular fluid pools, suggesting that not all the fluid was rapidly absorbed.[83] Indeed Costill and Sparks[82] suggest that "a large fraction of (the) ingested water remained in the gastrointestinal tract or was shifted to the extravascular compartment". Thus, the maximum rates of fluid absorption by the small bowel during exercise are not known, but they could be less than the high rates of fluid loss incurred by some athletes during more intensive exercise.

Alternatively, unlike other mammals,[84-87] humans may dehydrate during exer-cise because only they lose sodium chloride in sweat.[13] As a result of sodium losses, serum osmolality rises less during exercise-induced dehydration in humans than in other mammals that drink sufficiently to maintain a constant serum osmolality. Nose et al.[88-90] have shown that the drinking behavior of dehydrated humans is regulated by changes in both serum osmolality and plasma volume. Hence dipsogenic drive in dehydrated humans ceases prematurely when serum osmolality is returned to isotonicity by the ingestion of plain water before either fluid or sodium losses are replaced. Ingestion of solutions containing sodium chloride also terminates drinking prematurely by restoring plasma and extracellular volumes before intracellular fluid losses are replaced. The result is that whether dehydrated humans drink plain water or sodium chloride solutions, they tend to stop drinking before they are fully rehydrated.

Perhaps it is the above complex interactions which explain why humans are unable to prevent the development of voluntary dehydration during prolonged exercise. In addition, the rapid alleviation of the symptoms which initiate drinking, such as dryness of the mouth, may cause premature cessation of drinking before full rehydration has occurred.[91] Involuntary dehydration may also depend on a hereditary predisposition to be a "heavy" or "reluctant" drinker during exercise. Szlyk et al.[92] reported that 13 of 33 men were classified as "reluctant" drinkers during exercise in the heat because they did not maintain body weight loss below 2% despite the provision of water *ad libitum*. Similarly, Itoh[93] observed an average fluid intake of only 258 ml in 18 Oriental laborers after a mean exercise-induced sweat loss of 2.2 l. Thus, thirst does not appear to be a sufficient stimulus for maintaining body water.[94]

III. THE PHYSIOLOGICAL EFFECTS OF PROGRESSIVE DEHYDRATION DURING PROLONGED EXERCISE

The physiological effects of exercise-induced dehydration have been studied by comparing the physiological responses of athletes when they ingest fluids to replace either none, some, or all of their fluid lost during prolonged exercise. In more recent studies, fluids have also been infused intravenously during exercise in order to reverse any dehydration-induced fall in plasma volume. These latter studies have attempted to differentiate the physiological effects of a reduction in plasma volume from those caused by dehydration-induced changes in serum osmolality.

A. PLASMA VOLUME

Depending on the type and intensity of exercise, and the posture adopted, plasma volume falls to varying extents in the first 5 to 10 min of exercise.[95] Thereafter, further falls in plasma volume are determined by the amount of fluid ingested during exercise[66,96-99] and can be prevented if the rate of fluid ingestion equals the rate of fluid loss.[100]

In order to prevent falls in plasma volume during exercise, perhaps the optimum fluid for ingestion is an isotonic carbohydrate-electrolyte solution. At rest, the ingestion of such solutions produces the highest rates of fluid absorption.[101] Figure 2 shows that rates of water absorption are enhanced by the presence of CHO, but this is reversed when the CHO solutions are hyperosmotic. Increasing the ingested CHO osmolality above ~280 mosmol/l suppresses water absorption, and that is thought to limit further increases in glucose uptake.[78,102]

B. SERUM OSMOLALITY AND SERUM ELECTROLYTE CONCENTRATIONS

There is some evidence that the ingestion of sodium-containing solutions during exercise may help prevent the fall in plasma volume more effectively than the ingestion of pure water.[103] Serum sodium concentrations and serum osmolality can fall when large quantities of plain water are ingested during exercise.[67,103] Since the sodium content of the extracellular space largely regulates the extracellular fluid volume,[88,104] plasma volume contracts whenever a sodium deficiency develops. A reduction of sweat sodium losses with a resultant protection of the circulating volume is an important benefit of heat acclimatization and training and explains why ingesting sodium chloride during or after exercise might be of benefit. Thus, in theory, sodium chloride ingestion should help maintain the plasma volume[82,103,105,106] although this is not always found.[97,107]

An additional advantage of adding sodium chloride to ingested solutions is that it promotes greater drinking[108,109] by increasing palatability.[110,111] Arden[112] found that the ingestion of 15 to 30 g of sodium chloride or sodium bicarbonate caused similar increased drinking in men, but that the ingestion of potassium chloride was not dipsogenic. He therefore concluded that the stimulus for drinking "was the sodium ion alone". More recently, Greenleaf[94] also reported that the intake of sodium chloride causes thirst and drinking in humans.

C. SWEAT RATE AND SKIN BLOOD FLOW

If no fluid is ingested during prolonged exercise, serum sodium concentration and osmolality rise[96,97] to values that depend on the amount of fluid lost.[99] This rise in osmolality is reduced by fluid ingestion[96,97] and is least when the rate of fluid ingestion approximates the rate of fluid loss.

Rises in serum sodium concentration and serum osmolality correlate with the increase in esophageal temperature[99] and, hence may be a stimulus for the reduction in sweating that develops at high levels of dehydration.[15] An important goal of fluid ingestion during exercise, therefore, may be to prevent rises in serum osmolality or serum sodium concentrations and thereby maintain sweat rates, as originally proposed by Dill.[13] These ideas, however, remain contentious. Some studies have shown that the sweat rate falls with increasing levels of dehydration,[15,113-115] whereas others have failed to show this effect.[66,77,96,98-100] These discrepancies may be due to the considerable individual variability in the effects of dehydration on sweat rates during exercise.[116] Pre-exercise hypohydration studies indicate that sweat rate over the trunk, but not the head, may be selectively reduced by prior dehydration.[117] Conversely, hyperhydration prior to exercise is reported to increase sweat rate and reduce rises in rectal temperature during subsequent exercise.[118]

Fluid ingestion also maintains higher rates of forearm blood flow during exercise[98,99] and of forearm and calf blood flow at rest during prolonged heat exposure.[119] The reduction of forearm blood flow is proportional to the level of dehydration.[99] Hence, fluid ingestion during exercise may attenuate the development of hyperthermia by maintaining skin blood flow.[98]

An important question is whether changes in serum osmolality or in plasma volume regulate skin blood flow, sweat rate, and body temperature. In order to differentiate between these possibilities, Fortney et al.[120] infused an isotonic saline solution to maintain plasma volume without altering serum osmolality. With infusion, they found that both the core temperature and the total sweat output during exercise were reduced. The authors concluded that the maintenance of plasma volume reduced sweat output by increasing skin blood flow and thereby raising the proportion of heat loss by convection rather than by evaporation. In contrast, increased serum osmolality raised the temperature threshold at which skin blood flow increased and delayed the onset of sweating, thereby favoring heat retention.[120,121]

Montain and Coyle[98] infused a 6% dextran solution to increase plasma volume above the level maintained by fluid ingestion during exercise in the heat (33°C, 50% relative humidity [r.h.], 2.5 m/sec wind speed). Serum sodium concentrations and serum osmolality increased when subjects did not ingest fluid during exercise but were maintained at pre-exercise concentrations by saline infusion. Unlike the findings of Fortney et al.,[121] plasma volume expansion alone did not influence either the esophageal or rectal temperature response to exercise, or forearm skin blood flow. Nor did fluid infusion prevent the rise in the rating of perceived exertion as effectively as did fluid ingestion. Thus, maintaining or increasing plasma volume by fluid ingestion may not explain the temperature-lowering effect of fluid ingestion during exercise. Rather, fluid ingestion may influence thermoregulation by preventing the rise in serum osmolality or serum sodium concentrations[98] with maintenance of forearm blood flow.[122] These findings support Dill's[13] original proposal that the goal of fluid ingestion during exercise should be the maintenance of serum osmolality and serum sodium concentrations.

D. RECTAL OR ESOPHAGEAL TEMPERATURES

After a minimum of 60 to 80 min of exercise, rises in rectal or esophageal temperature are also attenuated by fluid ingestion during exercise in the heat,[10,66,72,77,98-100,114-116] and are least when the rate of fluid ingestion approximates the sweat rate.[99,114] Hence there is a linear relationship between the rise in esophageal temperature and the level of dehydration[98,99] as was also found in some of the original field studies.[10,26] Sawka et al.[123] reported that dehydration, as measured by the percent decrease in body weight, linearly increased the core temperature by 0.15°C during exercise in the heat. Similarly, Greenleaf and Castle[114] found that core temperature was elevated 0.10°C for each percent decrease in body weight during light (i.e., 49% of $\dot{V}O_2$ max) exercise. For each percent decrease in body mass of greater than 2%, at an exercise intensity of 74% of $\dot{V}O_2$ max, Gisolfi and Copping[77] reported that core temperature was elevated by 0.4°C.

Since the magnitude of the effect of fluid ingestion on rises in rectal temperature is relatively small, its physiological relevance may be questioned.[124] Most studies indicate that levels of dehydration of up to 5% (equivalent to a weight loss of 2 to 4 kg) usually increase rectal temperature by less than 1°C.[66,77,98-100,124]

E. HEART RATE AND STROKE VOLUME

Fluid deficits that develop during exercise also proportionately increase heart rates[10,96,97,99,114,116] and reduce stroke volumes. Falls in stroke volumes and cardiac output are prevented when the rates of fluid ingestion are sufficient to maintain euhydration.[100] However, heart rate is elevated even when dehydration is prevented by adequate fluid ingestion and infusion during exercise,[98] suggesting that dehydration is not the sole cause of the progressive increase in heart rate during prolonged exercise.[100] Since the rise in heart rate and in oxygen consumption were prevented only by the addition of a glucose infusion, Hamilton et al.[100] have proposed that these components of cardiovascular drift during prolonged exercise may result from a rise in serum catecholamine concentrations that is reduced by glucose infusion.

F. HORMONAL CHANGES

In response to falls in plasma volume and rises in serum osmolality, plasma concentrations of antidiuretic hormone (ADH — also arginine vasopressin — AVP), aldosterone, renin, and atrial natriuretic peptide (ANP) increase during prolonged exercise.[105,125-127] In general, ADH activities rise in response to increasing serum osmolality,[87,127] whereas plasma renin activity may follow changes in either plasma or extracellular fluid volumes. There is also a paradoxical increase in the plasma activity of the diuretic and natriuretic hormone ANP during prolonged exercise when plasma volume is reduced.[125,127] The diuretic effects of ANP, however, are probably inhibited by the increased activity of the renin-angiotensin-aldosterone axis and the increased serum ADH concentrations.[125,128]

Fluid ingestion during or prior to exercise reduces the rises in the hormonal concentrations described above.[105] Of these, the rise in plasma ADH concentration is most affected by either hyperhydration before or after fluid ingestion during exercise and appears to be relatively independent of the nature of the fluid ingested. In contrast, the increased activity of the renin-angiotensin-aldosterone axis is reduced more by the ingestion of sodium-containing solutions compared to pure water.[105] Thrasher et al.[87] reported essentially the same findings in dehydrated dogs. In dogs, water ingestion reduced plasma ADH activity whereas ingestion of an electrolyte solution with the same composition as the extracellular fluid volume reduced plasma renin activity. Possibly these differences are due to the maintenance of higher plasma volumes when electrolyte containing solutions are ingested during exercise.[103,105]

G. PERCEPTION OF EFFORT

In the early studies of the effects of prolonged exercise-induced dehydration on physical work capacity, largely conducted on military personnel,[10,12,14-16] it was generally found that fewer subjects completed an exercise task when they did not ingest fluid. Furthermore, it was observed that fluid ingestion had more obvious effects on the psyche than on the soma. Eichna et al.[14] reported that dehydrated subjects were "reduced to apathetic, listless, plodding men straining to finish the same task" that they had completed "energetically and cheerfully" when fully hydrated.

More modern studies have shown that the perception of effort during exercise is proportional to the fluid deficit.[99] Even partial fluid replacement has a significant effect on the perception of effort during exercise of high intensity.[129] Interestingly, fluid ingestion reduces the rise in the ratings of perceived exertion more than fluid infusion.[98]

IV. THE EFFECTS OF EXERCISE-INDUCED DEHYDRATION ON PHYSICAL WORK CAPACITY

Since the early studies of exercise-induced dehydration in subjects working at relatively low work rates for many hours in the dry heat, surprisingly little attention has been paid to the effects of fluid ingestion on athletic performance. Although some studies have investigated the effects of fluid loss (hypohydration) induced by either the administration of diuretics, exposure or sauna, or fluid restriction *before* exercise, the results of such studies do not necessarily apply to dehydration induced *during* exercise. The reductions in plasma volume and in physical performance for a given level of fluid loss are greater with hypohydration than with exercise-induced dehydration.[95,98,130] The adverse effects of hypohydration on exercise tolerance have been detailed elsewhere,[131] and only exercise-induced dehydration studies are considered here.

A. PERFORMANCE STUDIES IN THE HEAT

To our knowledge, only two groups have investigated the influence of dehydration on moderate-to-high intensity exercise tolerance in the heat. Montain and Coyle[99] found that when subjects did not ingest fluid, they were less likely to complete 2 h exercise at 65% of $\dot{V}O_2$ max in the heat (33°C, 50% r.h., 2.5 m/sec wind speed). Below and Coyle[132] showed that ingestion of large volumes (1.33 l) of either water or a 6% CHO solution (80 g) during 50 min of high-intensity (80% of $\dot{V}O_2$ max) cycling in the heat (31°C, 54% r.h., 3.5 mi/sec wind speed) attenuated hyperthermia and reduced heart rate, compared to when only a small volume of fluid (0.2 l) was consumed. Performance times in a subsequent high-intensity time-trial were 6.5% faster when subjects ingested 1.33 l of fluid compared with only 0.2 l, and 6.3% faster when subjects consumed CHO versus no CHO (Below and Coyle[132]). Walsh et al.[129] also showed that when subjects ingested fluid to maintain fluid balance during a 1 h exercise bout at 70% of $\dot{V}O_2$ max in the heat (30°C, 50% r.h., 3 km/h wind speed), they were able to exercise significantly longer during a subsequent exercise bout at 90% of $\dot{V}O_2$ max than when no fluid was ingested. This effect was not due to any significant differences in any measured physiological variables, including rectal temperature, and occurred despite very modest (1.1 kg; 1.8%) dehydration in the subjects not ingesting fluid.

B. PERFORMANCE STUDIES IN NEUTRAL OR COOL ENVIRONMENTS

There have also been relatively few studies which have examined the effects of fluid ingestion on athletic performance in neutral or cool (<25°C) environments. Only two studies have compared the exercise performance of subjects when they either ingested or did not ingest fluid, or were infused with fluid during exercise at room temperature. Deschamps et al.[133] reported that intravenous saline infusion did not enhance performance at 84% of $\dot{V}O_2$ max which exhausted subjects in ~21 min. Barr et al.[66] showed that subjects who did not ingest fluid during prolonged exercise at 55% of $\dot{V}O_2$ max terminated exercise approximately 90 min earlier than when they ingested fluid. Levels of dehydration at exhaustion in their subjects were >6%.

Because the addition of high concentrations of CHO to fluid-replacement beverages may impair water absorption, while inadequate CHO ingestion may slow CHO oxidation late in exercise, recent attention has been focused on optimizing the rate of CHO ingestion during prolonged exercise.[43,134-142] In particular, the factors which could potentially limit the rate at which ingested CHO can be oxidized by the working muscles have been investigated.[141,143-145]

V. FACTORS AFFECTING THE RATE OF INGESTED CARBOHYDRATE OXIDATION DURING PROLONGED EXERCISE

A. THE RATE OF GASTRIC EMPTYING, INTESTINAL DIGESTION, AND ABSORPTION

Historically, it has been assumed that the rate of gastric emptying limits the rate of CHO delivery to the muscles.[29,146-148] Thus, there has been considerable emphasis on the factors which influence gastric emptying, such as gastric volume,[29,73,149-151] solute osmolality,[152-154] beverage temperature,[155,156] and the caloric content of the ingested beverage.[29,157,158] Since solutions containing as little as 2.5 g/100 ml of CHO have been shown to reduce the rate of gastric emptying after single feedings,[29,157,159] the practical advice to athletes[160] in the late 1980s was to "ingest solutions with a low (<2.5 g/100 ml) carbohydrate content at a rate of 100-200 ml every 2-3 km during prolonged exercise". However, as recently noted by Coyle and Montain,[161] this recommendation has limited practical value because "at the extremes it could be interpreted to suggest that slow runners (i.e. 10 km/h) drink only 330 ml/h whereas the fastest runners should be drinking up to 2000 ml/h."

More recent studies have shown that gastric volume may be a more important determinant of gastric emptying during exercise than either solute energy content or osmolality, particularly when these solutions are ingested repeatedly during exercise.[141,143,150,151,162] These studies have shown that the rates of gastric emptying of solutions with vastly different CHO contents are quite similar when these are ingested in sufficient volumes repeatedly during exercise. Under these circumstances, the pattern of gastric emptying after each drink follows an exponential time course, and falls rapidly as the volume remaining in the stomach decreases.[163,164] Thus, the maximum rate at which CHO *and* water can be delivered to the intestine from an ingested solution is strongly influenced by the average volume of fluid in the stomach at any time, which, in turn, is influenced by the drinking pattern of the athlete. Although this is not a novel finding[29,149,164-167] its importance has only recently been emphasized.[150] Thus, it is now apparent that repetitive drinking patterns can produce similar rates of both CHO *and* water delivery from a variety of different CHO solutions with markedly different concentrations.

In order to investigate the rate of oxidation of ingested CHO, recent studies have used stable (^{13}C) and radioactive (^{14}C) isotope techniques (for review see Reference 168). Pirnay et al.[169,170] were the first group to show that a significant quantity of ingested glucose is oxidized during exercise. They fed seven untrained, fasted subjects 100 g of ^{13}C-labeled glucose diluted in 400 ml of water; four subjects then walked on a treadmill for 2 h and three subjects exercised for almost 4 h. The peak rates of exogenous glucose oxidation (0.65 g/min) occurred 75 to 90 min after ingestion, and by 120 and 225 min of exercise, 57 and 95 g respectively of the 100 g glucose load had been oxidized. Thus, these workers concluded that "it would be advisable to repeat glucose intake every 60-90 min for permitting long-duration muscular exercise".

Pirnay et al.'s[169,170] findings were subsequently confirmed by other groups.[171-174] These studies showed that the peak rates of exogenous glucose oxidation (0.56 to 0.65 g/min) occurred 75 to 90 min after ingestion of 100 g of glucose. Further, the time taken to attain the peak rate of exogenous glucose oxidation was found to be independent of when the glucose was ingested during exercise,[173] or whether it was ingested as a dilute (439 mosmol/l) or a concentrated (1,204 mosmol/l) solution.[172]

Rates of exogenous glucose oxidation also appear to be relatively unaffected by the use of different feeding schedules. Comparison of the single (50 to 100 g) glucose feeding studies[170-173,175,176] to the multiple (97 to 220 g) glucose feeding studies,[134,135,177] show that the amount of ingested glucose oxidized in the first hour of exercise, and the peak rates of exogenous glucose oxidation, are quite similar. With most of the feeding schedules, around 20 g of ingested glucose was oxidized in the first hour and, in all cases, the peak rates of exogenous glucose oxidation were between 0.5 and 0.9 g/min.

Only following the repetitive ingestion of very large amounts of glucose have peak rates of exogenous glucose oxidation been observed to rise to 1 g/min. Pallikarakis et al.[178] studied six physically active males who walked uphill on a treadmill at ~45% of $\dot{V}O_2$ max for 285 min. After 15 min "adaptation" to exercise, subjects received either 200 g or 400 g of a 25 g/100 ml ^{13}C-labeled glucose solution in eight equal doses every 30 min. When subjects ingested the 200 g glucose load, the rate of ingested glucose oxidation rose progressively to a plateau of 0.66 g/min during the first 120 min of exercise. In contrast, in the subjects who were fed the 400 g glucose load, exogenous glucose oxidation continued to rise during the exercise period reaching 1.16 g/min at the end of the 285 min exercise bout. Thus, under the conditions of that study, increasing the ingestion of glucose from 25 g/30 min to 50 g/30 min increased both the peak rate of exogenous glucose oxidation and the contribution of ingested glucose to the total CHO requirements of exercise from 22% to 39%.[178]

Hawley et al.[143] studied six endurance-trained subjects who ingested a concentrated (15 g/100 ml) U-^{14}C labeled glucose solution as a 400 ml "loading" bolus immediately before, and as eight 100 ml feedings at 10 min intervals during 90 min of cycling at 70% of $\dot{V}O_2$ max. During the ride, only half of the CHO emptied from the stomach into the intestine was oxidized, indicating that the rate of gastric emptying does not limit the rate of ingested glucose oxidation. Rates of ingested glucose oxidation peaked at 0.9 g/min after 60 to 75 min and accounted for 20% of the total CHO oxidized during the 90 min of exercise.

Since, as argued previously, repetitive feedings would be expected to accelerate the delivery of glucose from the stomach to the duodenum,[73,150] the similar peak rates of ingested glucose oxidation after single and multiple feedings of moderate glucose loads (50 to 200 g) suggest that ingested CHO oxidation cannot be limited by gastric emptying, as originally proposed.[29] Instead, studies of both gastric emptying and ingested CHO oxidation[139,141,143] suggest that the oxidation of ingested CHO in the early (60 to 90 min) stages of exercise is limited either by its rate of absorption from the intestine and passage via the liver into the systemic blood supply, *or* by the rate of muscle glucose oxidation.

In this regard, the investigations into the effects of glycogen depletion[179] and fasting[177] on rates of ingested CHO oxidation during prolonged exercise are of interest. In theory, these states of CHO depletion would be expected to increase the reliance on exogenous CHO during exercise. Ravussin et al.[179] studied ingested CHO oxidation during prolonged, low-intensity exercise in untrained, glycogen-depleted and control subjects. One hour after they had ingested 100 g of ^{13}C-labeled glucose in 300 ml of water, subjects cycled for 120 min at 40% of $\dot{V}O_2$ max (97 to 107 W). Under both glycogen-depleted or normal (control) states, ingested glucose oxidation peaked at 0.4 g/min after 75 min of exercise. Further, during the 120 min exercise bout, oxidation of exogenous glucose was the same for control and glycogen depleted subjects (41 g vs. 38 g, respectively), although, these amounts accounted for vastly different contributions to total CHO oxidation (37% for controls vs. 72% for glycogen-depleted subjects). Ravussin et al.[179] concluded that "depletion of the (muscle) glycogen stores does not increase the rate of ingested glucose utilization." However, it should be noted that at such low intensity workloads (40% of $\dot{V}O_2$ max), fat, and *not* CHO oxidation might be expected to account for most of the energy demands of exercise.

Massicotte et al.[177] studied the effects of fasting on ingested glucose oxidation in 10 subjects during 2 h of cycling at 52 to 56% of $\dot{V}O_2$ max. Subjects ingested ~100 g of ^{13}C labeled glucose dissolved in 230 ml of water given as six feedings every 20 min throughout the exercise bout. The amount of glucose oxidized during exercise was the same under both experimental conditions (fed state 56 g; fasted 58 g). Thus, neither glycogen depletion[179] nor fasting[177] increased ingested glucose oxidation.

As glucose ingestion prior to and during exercise has been shown to inhibit lipolysis by increasing plasma insulin concentrations,[144,180,181] there has been some interest in the use of fructose as an alternate CHO source. Compared to glucose ingestion, fructose ingestion produces a 20 to 30% lower rise in plasma insulin concentrations,[182,183] and hence does not inhibit lipolysis to the same extent.

Decombaz et al.[175] were the first workers to investigate the oxidation of ingested fructose using isotopic techniques. They compared the effects of the ingestion of 70 g of ^{13}C-labeled fructose and glucose on ingested CHO oxidation during moderate intensity exercise. Subjects ingested either fructose or glucose in 350 ml of water 1 h prior to a 60 min ride. For the first 45 min of exercise, subjects cycled at 61% of $\dot{V}O_2$ max, and were then told to "work as hard as possible" for the next 15 min. Two hours after ingestion, 30 g of the 70 g of fructose, and 26 g of the 70 g of glucose, had been oxidized. The amount of work produced during the last 15 min of the exercise bout did not differ between the two types of CHO, indicating that fructose ingested *before* exercise was oxidized *during* exercise to the same extent as was glucose ingested *before* exercise. Data from other studies, however, indicate that the rate of oxidation of fructose ingested during 2 to 3 h of moderate-intensity (52 to 55% of $\dot{V}O_2$ max) exercise is slower than that of glucose, at least in the fed state.[134,135,176]

Perhaps surprisingly, only three studies have investigated the effects of sucrose ingestion during prolonged exercise. Benade et al.[184] had four trained subjects cycle for 6 h (50 min exercise followed by 10 min rest/h) at 44 to 50% of $\dot{V}O_2$ max. After 4 h, subjects ingested 100 g of U-^{14}C-labeled sucrose in 400 to 500 ml of water in one feeding. Peak rates of exogenous sucrose oxidation were observed approximately 70 min after ingestion and accounted for 44% of total CHO oxidation at that time.

Utilizing stable isotope techniques, Gerard et al.[185] investigated the effects of sucrose ingestion (100 g in 400 ml of water given as a single feeding 15 min after the start of exercise) during 4 h of walking at ~50% of $\dot{V}O_2$ max. They reported that 93 ± 4 g of ingested sucrose was oxidized during the exercise bout, and proposed that there was a significant sparing of endogenous CHO.[185] Muscle glycogen utilization, however, was not directly determined.

Moodley et al.[139] investigated the effects of ingesting varying concentrations of U-^{14}C-labeled sucrose (7.5 g/100 ml, 10 g/100 ml, and 15 g/100 ml), consumed as nine 100 ml feedings every 10 min during 90 min of exercise at 70% of $\dot{V}O_2$ max, on the rates of gastric emptying and ingested CHO oxidation. Although gastric emptying fell as the sucrose content of the drink increased, CHO delivery to the intestine and exogenous CHO oxidation increased linearly with increasing CHO concentration. As only 15 to 20 g (26 to 34%) of the CHO delivered to the intestine was oxidized, these workers speculated that the low rates of exogenous sucrose oxidation were not due to a lack of demand by the working muscles, but rather must have resulted from low rates of absorption from the intestine.[139]

Glucose polymer ingestion during prolonged exercise has been thought to be preferable to the ingestion of equivalent concentrations of glucose, fructose, or sucrose.[50,142,159] The ~20% lower osmotic pressure of a glucose polymer solution than of an isocaloric glucose solution was presumed to (1) increase the rate of gastric emptying; (2) decrease the movement of water from the plasma into the intestinal lumen; and (3) lower rates of gastric secretion.[148,159] Recent studies, however, have raised the question of whether the ingestion of glucose polymer solutions offer any advantage over the ingestion of glucose solutions in terms of exogenous CHO oxidation or water balance.[135,141]

Massicotte et al.[135] compared the oxidation of 7 g/100 ml concentrations of ^{13}C-labeled glucose polymer with glucose and fructose ingested as repetitive feedings (six 16 g feedings in 235 ml of water every 20 min) throughout 120 min of cycling at 53% of $\dot{V}O_2$ max. They found that the oxidation rates of ingested glucose and glucose polymers were similar throughout the 2 h exercise bout (70 vs. 64 g, respectively), and both were higher than rates of exogenous fructose oxidation (53 g). Massicotte et al.[135] concluded that "despite a lower osmotic pressure, glucose ingested in the form of a glucose polymer does not appear to be delivered more quickly and to be oxidised in larger amounts than when ingested in the form of an isocaloric free glucose solution".

Rehrer et al.[141] studied both the rates of gastric emptying and ingested CHO oxidation in eight trained subjects who cycled at 70% of $\dot{V}O_2$ max for 80 min while ingesting 17 g/100 ml ^{13}C-labeled glucose or glucose polymer solutions. They found no significant differences in the rates of gastric emptying (glucose 781 ml/80 min; glucose polymer 864 ml/80 min), or the calculated intestinal CHO delivery (glucose 133 g; glucose polymer 147 g). Again, the amount of ingested CHO oxidized during the 80 min exercise bout was similar for both drinks (glucose 42 g; glucose polymer 39 g). Thus, the results of Rehrer et al.[141] and Massicotte et al.[135] show that glucose polymer solutions do not confer any advantages in terms of gastric emptying, intestinal CHO delivery, or exogenous CHO oxidation over an equicaloric free glucose solution. Further, the similar rates of ingested glucose polymer and glucose oxidation suggest that the digestion of polymers (at least with a chain-length of up to ~20 glucose units) is not rate-limiting.

The studies reviewed above, therefore, suggest that (1) the amount of CHO emptied from the stomach after the repeated ingestion of solutions containing a variety of mono-, di-, and oligosaccharides is at least double the amount that is oxidized; and (2) irrespective of the ingestion regimen, peak rates of ingested CHO oxidation rise to ~1 g/min during the latter stages of prolonged exercise. Hence, rates of ingested CHO oxidation may be limited either by the release of the CHO into the systemic circulation, *or* the rate of working muscle glucose oxidation.

B. THE RATE OF HEPATIC GLUCOSE APPEARANCE IN THE SYSTEMIC CIRCULATION

In order to determine if by-passing both intestinal absorption and hepatic glucose uptake via an intravenous glucose infusion might increase the rate of muscle glucose oxidation above 1 g/min, we recently studied ten endurance-trained subjects during 125 min of cycling at 70% of $\dot{V}O_2$ max.[144] During exercise, subjects ingested either a 15 g/100 ml U-^{14}C-labeled glucose solution or, in the case of the subjects who were infused with glucose, water labeled with traces of U-^{14}C-glucose for the determination of the rates of plasma glucose oxidation. In subjects not ingesting CHO, unlabeled glucose (25% dextrose) was infused to maintain plasma glucose concentration at 5 mmol/l. Despite similar plasma glucose concentrations (ingestion 5.3 mmol/l; infusion 5.0 mmol/l), CHO ingestion significantly increased plasma insulin concentrations, elevated overall CHO oxidation, and reduced fat oxidation compared to when subjects received an intravenous glucose infusion. However, the rates of plasma glucose oxidation eventually increased to similar values (~1 g/min) with both glucose infusion and glucose ingestion, suggesting that when sufficient CHO is ingested, the appearance of ingested glucose in the systemic blood supply does not limit the rate of ingested glucose oxidation.[144] Rather, the finding that a more or less unlimited rate of intravenous glucose infusion did not elicit higher rates of muscle glucose oxidation than CHO ingestion indicates that physiological plasma glucose concentrations regulate the rates of ingested CHO oxidation. A limit to the oxidation rate of euglycemic plasma glucose concentrations would explain why the ingestion of a variety of CHOs, all of which elicit similar (i.e., 5 mmol/l) plasma glucose concentrations, are limited to ~1 g/min.

Another interesting finding of this study was an increased reliance on CHO metabolism with CHO ingestion, which was associated with a suppression of fat oxidation. Whereas the contribution from fat oxidation to energy production rose to $51 \pm 10\%$ after 2 h of exercise with glucose infusion, it only reached $18 \pm 4\%$ with glucose ingestion. Thus, conditions which elevate plasma insulin concentrations during the first 90 to 120 min of prolonged (i.e., 3 to 4 h) exhaustive exercise *may* decrease endurance by inhibiting fat metabolism and accelerating CHO oxidation. The latter effect is the opposite to that which is believed to aid performance during prolonged exercise.[186]

C. THE RATE OF GLUCOSE OXIDATION BY MUSCLE

In order to determine whether the rate of muscle glucose oxidation can be increased when plasma glucose and insulin concentrations are raised above normal physiological values, we also studied 12 trained subjects during 2 h of cycling when blood glucose concentration was either maintained at 5 mmol/l (euglycemia) or 10 mmol/l (hyperglycemia) by continuous variable-rate intravenous infusion.[145] Hyperglycemia and the concomitant hyperinsulinemia (i.e., 25 μU/ml) increased CHO oxidation and suppressed fat oxidation throughout exercise compared to euglycemia. Hyperglycemia was also associated with an increasing glucose disposal throughout the 2 h ride, such that during the latter stages of exercise, whereas euglycemic subjects utilized plasma glucose at rates of ~1 g/min, hyperglycemic subjects oxidized plasma glucose at rates of 1.8 g/min. That the rates of plasma glucose oxidation are concentration-dependent further suggests that the physiological concentrations of glucose and insulin normally present during prolonged, moderate-intensity exercise may produce an upper limit to the rate of glucose uptake and oxidation by skeletal muscle.[145]

VI. SUMMARY AND RECOMMENDATIONS FOR THE OPTIMAL REPLACEMENT BEVERAGE DURING PROLONGED EXERCISE

A. FLUID INGESTION

The principal aims of adequate fluid ingestion during prolonged exercise are to (1) prevent any rise in serum osmolality; (2) limit any dehydration-induced decreases in plasma volume, skin blood flow, stroke volume, and cardiac output; (3) diminish progressive rises in heart rate and rectal temperature; and (4) decrease the perception of effort and hence improve athletic performance.

It has been assumed that the optimum rate of fluid ingestion is that which equals the rate of fluid loss. However, the precise composition of the fluid that will optimize electrolyte and fluid replacement of the extracellular space is not established. Neither is the precise volume of fluid to be ingested by athletes during prolonged exercise known. The rates of fluid ingestion needed to replace high (>1 l/h) sweat rates may exceed the maximum intestinal absorptive capacity for water. Furthermore, such high rates of fluid intake (>1 l/h) are achieved only with difficulty during exercise, especially when running, and are likely to lead to feelings of fullness and abdominal discomfort.

Most athletes are "reluctant" drinkers who do not ingest fluid at rates sufficient to offset their rates of fluid loss; hence they develop progressive (voluntary) dehydration during prolonged exercise. A question of practical relevance, as recently noted by Coyle and Montain,[161] is "are the physiological benefits of high rates (i.e., >1 l/h) of fluid ingestion worth the possible discomfort and time that might be lost attempting to drink such large volumes during competition?"

Fluid consumption can be maximized by attention to a number of factors, including the temperature and palatability of the drink,[10,91,92,187-193] the simultaneous consumption of food while drinking,[10,193] and the addition of electrolytes, particularly sodium, to the beverage.[88,89,190,194,195]

In events of 60 to 80 min duration, during which exercise intensity will range from 60 to 100% of $\dot{V}O_2$ max, there is usually little opportunity to ingest fluids. The prime consideration in such events is to *partially* replace the athlete's fluid losses. The addition of CHO to an oral rehydration solution for ingestion during exercise lasting <80 min is probably not warranted.[163]

B. CARBOHYDRATE INGESTION

The primary purposes of CHO ingestion during exercise are to maintain blood glucose concentration and high rates of CHO oxidation during the latter stages of prolonged exercise when muscle glycogen content is low. Under these conditions, ingested CHO may provide virtually all of total blood glucose oxidation.[186] Thus, CHO ingestion can be recommended whenever the exercise is of sufficient duration or intensity to deplete endogenous CHO stores, which will impair exercise performance.

Provided most CHOs are ingested frequently enough in appropriate volumes, the type of CHO consumed does not appear greatly to influence rates of gastric emptying.[168] Further, as only ~50% of any CHO emptied from the stomach into the intestine is oxidized during exercise, the rate of gastric emptying cannot limit the rate of ingested CHO oxidation. There does not seem to be any physiologically important differences in the rates of ingested CHO oxidation from a variety of mono-, di-, and oligosaccharides ingested repetitively during exercise; all are ultimately oxidized at ~1 g/min after the first 70 to 90 min of exercise.[168] This is because the physiological concentrations of glucose and insulin normally present during prolonged, moderate-intensity exercise may set the upper limit for the rate of glucose uptake and oxidation by skeletal muscle.[144] The ingestion of highly concentrated (i.e., >10 g/100 ml) CHO beverages in the early (i.e. <75 min) stages of prolonged, exhaustive exercise should probably be avoided. Such beverages attenuate fat oxidation and accelerate CHO utilization[144] and could lead to premature fatigue.[159,163,183]

On the basis of the most recent findings detailed in this review, the following practical guidelines are tentatively made to athletes participating in prolonged, moderate-intensity (i.e., 60 to 80% of $\dot{V}O_2$ max) exercise of up to 8 h duration.

1. Immediately prior to the beginning of exercise (i.e., during the warm-up), the athlete should attempt to fill the stomach to tolerable limits by consuming 300 to 400 ml of cool (i.e., 10°C) flavored water.

2. For the first 60 to 75 min of exercise, the athlete should consume 100 to 150 ml of a cool, dilute (i.e., 2.5 to 5.0 g/100 ml) glucose polymer solution at regular (i.e., 10 to 15 min) intervals, As only ~20 g of ingested CHO are oxidized in the first hour of moderate-intensity exercise, irrespective of the type of CHO consumed or the drinking regimen, it seems unnecessary to ingest CHO in amounts much greater than ~30 g during this period. Indeed, the inclusion of more concentrated CHOs may increase plasma insulin concentrations, thereby suppressing fat oxidation during the early stages of exercise, with a concomitant acceleration of CHO utilization. An increased reliance of carbohydrate oxidation for the provision of energy could lead to premature fatigue.

3. After 90 min of exercise, or during the last quarter of an athlete's anticipated race time, 200 to 300 ml of a cool, mildly concentrated (i.e., 10 to 12 g/100 ml) glucose polymer solution containing 20 mEq/l of sodium should be ingested. Although higher sodium concentrations may promote intestinal absorption more effectively, such solutions are probably not palatable to the majority of athletes. As potassium may facilitate rehydration of the intracellular fluid compartment, replacing the small (i.e., 7 to 10 mEq/l) amounts of potassium lost in sweat *may* be advantageous. Thus, perhaps 2 to 4 mEq/l of potassium could be included in the replacement beverage.

4. For the remainder of the race the athlete should be encouraged to consume 100 to 150 ml of the same solution at 10 to 15 min intervals. Such a drinking regimen will optimize fluid delivery by maintaining high gastric volumes, while maintaining blood glucose concentrations at euglycemic (i.e., 4 to 5 mmol/l) levels, thereby sustaining high rates of CHO oxidation in the latter stages of exercise.

**TABLE 1   Carbohydrate and Electrolyte Concentrations
and Osmolalities of Various "Sports"
Beverages, Soft Drinks and Water**

	CHO (g/l)	Na+ (mEq)	K+ (mEq)	Osmolality (mosmol/l)
Appletizer	94	2.4	16.9	710
Coca cola	107	2.0	0	650
Cranberry juice	150	2.0	7.0	890
Exceed	72	10.0	5.0	250
Gatorade	60	21.0	3.0	280
Isostar	73	24.0	4.0	296
Orange juice	118	0.5	58.0	690
Pepsi cola	81	1.7	0.1	568
Water	0	Trace	Trace	10 to 20

Note: CHO, carbohydrate; Na+, sodium; K+, potassium. Data are from
References 157, 163, 196.

Although we, and others,[161,163] currently consider there is sufficient data available from which to estimate the rates of CHO ingestion necessary to maintain euglycemia and enhance performance during prolonged, moderate-intensity exhaustive exercise lasting up to ~8 h, there is less precise information regarding the formulation of the most effective oral hydration solution to be ingested during such events.[163] None of the beverages listed in Table 1, for example, fulfill the specific needs of athletes for both CHO and electrolyte replacement *during* exercise. There are also limited data available regarding the extent to which fluid ingestion should offset exercise-induced dehydration during both prolonged exercise in cool, neutral environments, and the heat. Further experimentation will be required to answer these questions before additional scientifically based recommendations can be made.

REFERENCES

1. Levine, S. A., Gordon, B., and Derick, C. L., Some changes in the chemical constituents of the blood following a marathon race, *JAMA*, 82, 1778, 1924.
2. Gordon, B., Kohn, L. A., Levine, S. A., Matton, M., Schriver, W., and Whiting, W. B., Sugar content of the blood in runners following a marathon race, *JAMA*, 185, 508, 1925.
3. Best, C. H., and Partridge, R. C., Observations on Olympic athletes, *Proc. R. Soc. London*, Ser. B, 105, 323, 1930.
4. Dill, D. B., Edwards, H. T., and Talbott, J. H., Studies in muscular activity: VII. Factors limiting the capacity for work, *J. Physiol., (London)*, 77, 49, 1932.
5. Boje, O., Der blutzucker wahrend und nach korperlicher arbeit, *Scand. Arch. Physiol.*, 74 (Suppl. 10), 1, 1936.
6. Grace Eggleton, M., *Muscular Exercise*, Kegan Paul, Trench Trubner and Company Limited, London, 1936, 153.
7. Christensen, E. H., and Hansen, O., II. Untersuchungen uber die Verbrennungsvorgange bei langdauernder, scwherer Muskerlarbeit, *Scand. Arch. Physiol.*, 81, 152, 1939.

8. Christensen, E. H., and Hansen, O., Arbeitsfahigkeit und ernahrung, *Scand. Arch. Physiol.*, 81, 162, 1939.
9. Christensen, E. H., and Hansen, O., IV. Hypoglykamie, Arbeitafahigkeit und Eraudung, *Scand. Arch. Physiol.*, 81, 172, 1939.
10. Adolph, E. F., *Physiology Of Man In The Desert*, Interscience, New York, 1947.
11. Adolph, E. F., and Dill, D. B., Observations on water metabolism in the desert, *Am. J. Physiol.*, 123, 369, 1938.
12. Bean, W. B., and Eichna, L. W., Performance in relation to environmental temperature. Reactions of normal young men to simulated desert environment, *Fed. Proc.*, 2, 144, 1943.
13. Dill, D. B., *Life, Heat, and Altitude. Physiological Effects of Hot Climates and Great Heights*, Harvard University Press, Cambridge, 1938.
14. Eichna, L. W., Bean, W. B., Ashe, W. F., and Nelson, N., Performance in relation to environmental temperature. Reactions of normal young men to hot, humid (simulated jungle) environment, *Bull. Johns Hopkins Hosp.*, 76, 25, 1945.
15. Ladell, W. S. S., The effects of water and salt intake upon the performance of men working in hot and humid environments, *J. Physiol.*, 127, 11, 1955.
16. Pitts, G. C., Johnson, R. E., and Consolazio, F. C., Work in the heat as affected by intake of water, salt and glucose, *Am. J. Physiol.*, 142, 253, 1944.
17. Talbott, J. H., Dill, D. B., Edwards, H. T., Stumme, E. H., and Consolazio, W. V., The ill effects of heat upon workmen, *J. Hyg. Toxicol.*, 19, 258, 1937.
18. Talbott, J. H., Edwards, H. T., Dill, D. B., and Drastich, L., Physiological responses to high environment and temperature, *J. Trop. Med. Hyg.*, 13, 381, 1933.
19. Ahlborg, G., Bergstrom, J., Brohult, J., Ekelund, L. G., Hultman, E., and Maschio, G., Human muscle glycogen content and capacity for prolonged exercise after different diets, *Forvarsmedicin*, 3, 85, 1967.
20. Ahlborg, G., Bergstrom, J., Brohult, J., Ekelund, L. G., and Hultman, E., Muscle glycogen and muscle electrolytes during prolonged physical exercise, *Acta Physiol. Scand.*, 70, 129, 1967.
21. Bergstrom, J., Hermansen, L., Hultman, E., and Saltin, B., Diet, muscle glycogen and physical performance, *Acta Physiol. Scand.*, 71, 140, 1967.
22. Bergstrom, J., Hultman, E., Jordfeldt, L., Pernow, B., and Wahren, J., Effect of nicotinic acid on physical working capacity and on metabolism of muscle glycogen in man, *J. Appl. Physiol.*, 26, 170, 1969.
23. Bergstrom, J., and Hultman, E., Muscle glycogen synthesis after exercise: an enhancing factor localised to the muscle cell in man, *Nature*, 210, 309, 1966.
24. Bergstrom, J., and Hultman, E., A study of the glycogen metabolism during exercise in man, *Scand. J. Clin. Lab. Invest.*, 19, 218, 1967.
25. Hermansen, L., Hultman, E., and Saltin, B., Muscle glycogen during prolonged severe exercise, *Acta Physiol. Scand.*, 71, 129, 1967.
26. Wyndham, C. H., and Strydom, N. B., The danger of an inadequate water intake during marathon running, *S. Afr. Med. J.*, 43, 893, 1969.
27. Wyndham, C. H., Heat stroke and hyperthermia in marathon runners, in *The Marathon: Physiological, Medical Epidemiological and Psychological Studies*, Vol. 301, Milvy, P. Ed., Ann. N.Y. Acad. Sci., 1977, 160.
28. Noakes, T. D., Myburgh, K. H., Du Plessis, J., Lang, L., Lambert, M., Van Der Riet, C., and Schall, R., Metabolic rate, not percent dehydration, predicts rectal temperature in marathon runners, *Med. Sci. Sports Exercise*, 23, 443, 1991.
29. Costill, D. L., and Saltin, B., Factors limiting gastric emptying during rest and exercise, *J. Appl. Physiol.*, 37, 679, 1974.
30. Noakes, T. D., Energy utilization and repletion during endurance exercise: an historical perspective, *J. Hum. Nutr. Dietet.* 4, 45, 1991.
31. Milvy, P., Ed., *The Marathon: Physiological, Medical, Epidemiological, and Psychological Studies*, Volume 301, The New York Academy of Sciences, New York, 1977.

32. Brooke, J. D., and Green, L. F., The effect of a high carbohydrate diet on recovery following prolonged work to exhaustion, *Ergonomics*, 17, 480, 1974.
33. Brooke, J. D., Davies, G. J., and Green, L.F., The effects of normal and glucose syrup work diets on the performance of racing cyclists, *J. Sports Med.*, 15, 257, 1975.
34. Green, L. F., and Bagley, R., Ingestion of a glucose syrup drink during long distance canoeing, *Brit. J. Sports Med.*, 6, 125, 1972.
35. Felig, P., Cherif, A., Minagawa, A., and Wahren, J., Hypoglycemia during prolonged exercise in normal men, *N. Engl. J. Med.*, 306, 895, 1982.
36. Noakes, T. D., Koeslag, J. H., and McArthur, P., Hypoglycemia during exercise, *N. Engl. J. Med.*, 308, 279, 1983.
37. Coyle, E. F., Hagberg, J. M., Hurley, B. F., Martin, W. H., Ehsani, A. A., and Holloszy, J. O., Carbohydrate feeding during prolonged exercise can delay fatigue, *J. Appl. Physiol.*, 55, 230, 1983.
38. Coyle, E. F., Coggan, A. R., Hemmert, M. K., and Ivy, J. L., Muscle glycogen utilization during prolonged strenuous exercise when fed carbohydrate, *J. Appl. Physiol.*, 61, 165, 1986.
39. Coggan, A. R., and Coyle, E. F., Reversal of fatigue during prolonged exercise by carbohydrate infusion or ingestion, *J. Appl. Physiol.*, 63, 2388, 1987.
40. Coggan, A. R., and Coyle, E. F., Effect of carbohydrate feedings during high-intensity exercise, *J. Appl. Physiol.*, 65, 1703, 1988.
41. Coggan, A. R., and Coyle, E. F., Metabolism and performance following carbohydrate ingestion late in exercise, *Med. Sci. Sports Exercise*, 21, 59, 1989.
42. Bosch, A. N., Dennis, S. C., and Noakes, T. D., Influence of carbohydrate-loading on fuel substrate turnover and oxidation during prolonged exercise, *J. Appl. Physiol.*, 74, 1921, 1993.
43. Flynn, M. G., Costill, D. L., Hawley, J. A., Fink, W. J., Neufer, P. D., Fielding, R. A., and Sleeper, M. A., Influence of selected carbohydrate drinks on cycling performance and glycogen use, *Med. Sci. Sports Exercise*, 19, 37, 1987.
44. Hargreaves, M., and Briggs, C. A., Effect of carbohydrate ingestion on exercise metabolism, *J. Appl. Physiol.*, 65, 1553, 1988.
45. Valeriani, A., The need for carbohydrate intake during endurance exercise, *Sports Med.*, 12, 349, 1991.
46. Davies, J. M., Burgess, W. A., Slentz, C. A., Bartoli, W. P., and Pate, R. R., Effects of ingesting 6% and 12% glucose/electrolyte beverages during prolonged intermittent cycling in the heat, *Eur. J. Appl. Physiol.*, 57, 563, 1988.
47. Davies, J. M., Lamb, D. R., Pate, R. R., Slentz, C. A., Burgess, W. A., and Bartoli, W. P., Carbohydrate-electrolyte drinks; effects on endurance cycling in the heat, *Am. J. Clin. Nutr.*, 48, 1023, 1988.
48. Hargreaves, M., Costill, D. L., Coggan, A. R., Fink, W. J., and Nishibata. I., Effect of carbohydrate feedings on muscle glycogen utilization and exercise performance, *Med. Sci. Sports Exercise*, 16, 219, 1984.
49. Ivy, J. L., Costill, D. L., Fink, W. J., and Lower, R. W., Influence of caffeine and carbohydrate feedings on endurance performance, *Med. Sci. Sport*, 11, 6, 1979.
50. Ivy, J. L., Miller, W., Dover, V., Goodyear, L. G., Sherman, W. M., Farrell, S., and Williams, H., Endurance improved by ingestion of a glucose polymer supplement, *Med. Sci. Sports Exercise*, 15, 466, 1983.
51. Millard-Stafford, M., Sparling, P. B., Rosskopf, L. B., Hinson, B. T., and Dicarlo, L. J., Carbohydrate-electrolyte replacement during a simulated triathlon in the heat, *Med. Sci. Sports Exercise*, 22, 621, 1990.
52. Murdoch, S. D., Bazzarre, T. L., Snider, I. P., and Goldfarb, A. H., Differences in the effects of carbohydrate food form on endurance performance to exhaustion, *Int. J. Sports Nutr.*, 3, 55, 1993.
53. Murray, R., Eddy, D. E., Murray, T. W., Siefert, J. G., Gregory, L. P., and Halaby, G. A., The effect of fluid and carbohydrate feeding during intermittent cycling exercise, *Med. Sci. Sport Exercise*, 19, 597, 1987,
54. Murray, R., Paul, G. L., Siefert, J. G., Eddy, D. E., and Halaby, G. A., The effects of glucose, fructose, and sucrose ingestion during exercise, *Med. Sci. Sports Exercise*, 21, 275, 1989.

55. Murray, R., Paul, G. L., Siefert, J. G., and Eddy, D. E., Responses to varying rates of carbohydrate ingestion during exercise, *Med. Sci. Sport Exercise*, 23, 713, 1991.
56. Murray, R., Siefert, J. G., Eddy, D. E., Paul, G. L., and Halaby, G. A., Carbohydrate feeding and exercise: effect of beverage carbohydrate content, *Eur. J. Appl. Physiol.*, 59, 152, 1989.
57. Neufer, P. D., Costill, D. L., Flynn, M. G., Kirwan, J. P., Mitchell, J. B., and Houmard, J., Improvements in exercise performance: effects of carbohydrate feedings and diet, *J. Appl. Physiol.*, 62, 983, 1987.
58. Williams, C., Nute, M. G., Broadbank, L., and Vinall, S., Influence of fluid intake on endurance running performance. A comparison between water, glucose and fructose solutions, *Eur. J. Appl. Physiol.*, 60, 112, 1990.
59. Wright, D. A., Sherman, W. M., and Dernbach, A. R., Carbohydrate feedings before, during, or in combination improve cycling endurance performance, *J. Appl. Physiol.*, 71, 1082, 1991.
60. Costill, D. L., Sweating: its composition and effects on body fluids, in *The Marathon: Physiological, Medical Epidemiological and Psychological Studies*, Vol. 301, Milvy, P., Ed., Ann. N.Y. Acad. Sci., 1977, 160.
61. Davies, C. T. M., Influence of skin temperature on sweating and aerobic performance during severe work, *J. Appl. Physiol.*, 47, 770, 1979.
62. Davies, C. T. M., Brotherhood, J. R., and Zeidifard, E., Temperature regulation during severe exercise with some observations on effects of skin wetting, *J. Appl. Physiol.*, 41, 772, 1976.
63. Greenhaff, P. L., Cardiovascular fitness and thermoregulation during prolonged exercise in man, *Br. J. Sports Med.*, 23, 109, 1989.
64. Greenhaff, P. L., and Clough, P. J., Predictors of sweat loss in man during prolonged exercise, *Eur. J. Appl. Physiol.*, 58, 348, 1989.
65. Wyndham, C. H., Strydom, N. B., Van Rensburg, A. J., Benade, A. J. S., and Heyns, A. J., Relation between VO_2max and body temperature in hot humid air conditions, *J. Appl. Physiol.*, 29,45, 1970.
66. Barr, S. I., Costill, D. L., and Fink, W. J., Fluid replacement during prolonged exercise: effects of water, saline, or no fluid, *Med. Sci. Sports Exercise*, 23, 811, 1991.
67. Noakes, T. D., Fluid replacement during exercise, in *Exercise and Sports Science Reviews*, Vol. 21, Holloszy, J. O., Ed., Williams and Wilkins, Baltimore, 1993, 297.
68. Brown, S. L., and Banister, E. W., Thermoregulation during prolonged actual and laboratory-simulated bicycling, *Eur. J. Appl. Physiol.*, 54, 125, 1985.
69. Armstrong, L. E., Hubbard, R. W., Jones, B. H., and Daniels, J. T., Preparing Alberto Salazar for the heat of the 1984 Olympic Games, *Phys. Sportsmed.*, 14, 73, 1986.
70. Allan, T. E., and Wilson, C. G., Influence of acclimatization on sweat sodium concentration, *J. Appl. Physiol.*, 30, 708, 1971.
71. Kirby, C. R., and Convertino, V. A., Plasma aldosterone and sweat sodium concentrations after exercise and heat acclimation, *J. Appl. Physiol.*, 61, 967, 1986.
72. Costill, D. L., Kammer, W. H., and Fisher, A., Fluid ingestion during distance running, *Arch. Environ. Health*, 21, 520, 1970.
73. Mitchell, J. B., and Voss, K. W., The influence of volume on gastric emptying during prolonged exercise, *Med. Sci. Sports Exercise*, 23, 314, 1991.
74. Brouns, F., Beckers, E., Knopfli, B., Villiger, B., and Saris, W., Rehydration during exercise: effect of electrolyte supplementation on selective blood parameters, *Med. Sci. Sports Exercise*, 23, S84, 1991.
75. Brouns, F., Saris, W. H. M., and Rehrer, N.J., Abdominal complaints and gastrointestinal function during long-lasting exercise, *Int. J. Sports Med.*, 8, 175, 1987.
76. Fordtran, J. S., Stimulation of active and passive sodium absorption by sugars in the human jejunum, *J. Clin. Invest.*, 55, 728, 1975.
77. Gisolfi, C. V., and Copping, J. R., Thermal effects of prolonged treadmill exercise in the heat, *Med. Sci. Sports Exercise*, 6, 108, 1974.
78. Gisolfi, C. V., Summers, R. W., Schedl, H. P., and Bleiler, T. L., Intestinal water absorption from select carbohydrate solutions in humans, *J. Appl. Physiol.*, 73, 2142, 1992.

79. Gisolfi, C. V., Spranger, K. J., Summers, R. W., Schedl, H. P., and Bleiler, T. L., Effects of cycle exercise on intestinal absorption in humans, *J. Appl. Physiol.*, 71, 2518, 1991.

80. Schedl, H. P., Clifton, J. A., Solute and water absorption by the human small intestine, *Nature*, 199, 1264, 1963.

81. Davis, G. R., Santa Ana, C. A., Morawski, S. G., and Fordtran, J. S., Development of a large solution associated with minimal water and electrolyte absorption or secretion, *Gastroenterology*, 78, 991, 1980.

82. Costill, D. L., and Sparks, K. E., Rapid fluid replacement following thermal dehydration, *J. Appl. Physiol.*, 34, 299, 1973.

83. Noakes, T. D., Hyponatremia during endurance running: a physiological and clinical interpretation, *Med. Sci. Sports Exercise*, 24, 403, 1992.

84. Adolph, E. F., Measurement of water drinking in dogs, *Am. J. Physiol.*, 125, 75-86, 1939.

85. Arnauld, E., and Du Pont, J., Vasopressin release and firing of supraoptic neurosecretory neurones during drinking in the dehydrated monkey, *Pflügers. Arch.*, 394, 195, 1982.

86. Choshniak, I., Wittenberg, C., and Saham, D., Rehydrating Bedouin goats with saline: rumen and kidney function, *Physiol. Zool.*, 60, 373, 1987.

87. Thrasher, T. N., Nistal-Herrera, J. F., Keil, L. C., and Ramsay, D. J., Satiety and inhibition of vasopressin secretion after drinking in dehydrated dogs, *Am. J. Physiol.*, 240, E394, 1981.

88. Nose, H., Mack, G. W., Shi, X., and Nadel, E. R., Shift in body fluid compartments after dehydration in humans, *J. Appl. Physiol.*, 65, 318, 1988.

89. Nose, H., Mack, G. W., Shi, X., and Nadel, E. R., Role of osmolality and plasma volume during rehydration in humans, *J. Appl. Physiol.*, 65, 325, 1988.

90. Nose, H., Mack, G. W., Shi, X., and Nadel, E. R., Involvement of sodium retention hormones during rehydration in humans, *J. Appl. Physiol.*, 65, 332, 1988.

91. Hubbard, R. W., Szlyk, P. C., and Armstrong, L. E., Influence of thirst and fluid palatability on fluid ingestion during exercise, in *Perspectives in Exercise Science and Sports Medicine, Fluid Homeostasis During Exercise*, Vol. 3., Gisolfi, C. V., and Lamb, D. R., Eds., Benchmark Press, 1990, 39.

92. Szlyk, P. C., Sils, I. V., Francesconi, R. P., Hubbard R. W., and Matthew, W. T., Variability in intake and dehydration in young men during a simulated desert walk, *Aviat. Space Environ. Med.*, 60, 422, 1989.

93. Itoh, S., The water loss and blood changes by prolonged sweating without intake of food and drink, *Jap. J. Physiol.*, 3, 148, 1953.

94. Greenleaf, J. E., Problem: thirst, drinking behavior, and involuntary dehydration, *Med. Sci. Sports Exercise*, 24, 645, 1992.

95. Coyle, E. F., and Hamilton, M., Fluid replacement during exercise: effects on physiological homeostasis and performance, in *Perspectives in Exercise Science and Sports Medicine, Fluid Homeostasis During Exercise*, Vol. 3., Gisolfi, C. V., and Lamb, D. R., Eds., Benchmark Press, 1990, 281.

96. Candas, V., Libert, J. P., Brandenberger, G., Sagot, J. C., and Kahn, J. M., Thermal and circulatory responses during prolonged exercise at different levels of hydration, *J. Physiol.,(Paris)*, 83, 11, 1988.

97. Maughan, R. J., Fenn, C. E., Gleeson, M., and Leiper, J.P., Metabolic and circulatory responses to the ingestion of glucose polymer and glucose/electrolyte solutions during exercise in man, *Eur. J. Appl. Physiol.*, 56, 356, 1987.

98. Montain, S. J., and Coyle, E. F., Fluid ingestion during exercise increases skin blood flow independent of increases in blood volume, *J. Appl. Physiol.*, 73, 903, 1992.

99. Montain, S. J., and Coyle, E. F., The influence of graded dehydration on hyperthermia and cardiovascular drift during exercise, *J. Appl. Physiol.*, 73, 1340, 1992.

100. Hamilton, M. C., Gonzalez-Alonso, J., Montain, S., and Coyle, E. F., Fluid replacement and glucose infusion during exercise prevent cardiovascular drift, *J. Appl. Physiol.*, 71, 871, 1991.

101. Gisolfi, C. V., Summers, R. W., Schedl, H. P., Bleiler, T. L., and Oppliger, R. A., Human intestinal water absorption: direct vs. indirect measurements, *Am. J. Physiol.*, 258, G216, 1990.

102. Abbott, W. O., Karr, W. G., and Miller, T. G., Absorption of glucose from the human small intestine (Abstract), *Am. J. Med. Sci.*, 191: 874, 1936.

103. Candas, V., Liebert, J. P., Brandenberger, G., Sagot, J. C., Amoros, C., and Kahn, J. M., Hydration during exercise. Effects on thermal and cardiovascular adjustments, *Eur. J. Appl. Physiol.*, 55, 113, 1986.

104. Nadel, E. R., Mack, G. W., and Nose, H., Influence of fluid replacement beverages on body fluid homeostasis during exercise and recovery, in *Perspectives in Exercise Science and Sports Medicine, Fluid Homeostasis During Exercise*, Vol. 3., Gisolfi, C. V., and Lamb, D. R., Eds., Benchmark Press, 1990, 181.

105. Brandenberger, G., Candas, V. M., Follenius, M., and Kahn, K. M., The influence of the initial state of hydration on endocrine responses to exercise in the heat, *Eur. J. Appl. Physiol.*, 58, 674, 1989.

106. Nielsen, B., Sjogaard, G., Ugelvig, J., Knudsen, B., and Dohlmann, B., Fluid balance in exercise dehydration and rehydration with different glucose-electrolyte drinks, *Eur. J. Appl. Physiol.*, 55, 318, 1986.

107. Powers, S. K., Lawler, J., Dodd, S., Tulley, R., Landry, G., and Wheeler, K., Fluid replacement drinks during high intensity exercise: effects on minimizing exercise-induced disturbances in homeostasis, *Eur. J. Appl. Physiol.*, 60, 54, 1990.

108. Gamble, J. L., McKhann, C. F., Butler, A. M., and Tuthill, E., An economy of water in renal function referable to urea, *Am. J. Physiol.*, 109, 139, 1934.

109. Gamble, J. L., Putnam, M. C., and McKhann, C. F., The optimal water requirements in renal functions. I. Measurements of water drinking by rats according to increments of urea and of several salts in the food, *Am. J. Physiol.*, 88, 571, 1929.

110. Costill, D. L., Cote, R., Miller, E., Miller, T., and Wynder, S. Water and electrolyte replacement during repeated days of work in the heat, *Aviat. Space Environ. Med.*, 46, 795, 1975.

111. Hubbard, R. W., Mager, M., and Bowers, W. D., Effect of low-potassium diet on rat exercise hyperthermia and heatstroke, *J. Appl. Physiol.*, 51, 8, 1981.

112. Arden, F., Experimental observations upon thirst and potassium overdosage, *Aust. J. Exp. Biol. Med. Sci.*, 12, 111, 1934

113. Ekblom, B., Greenleaf, C. J., Greenleaf, J. E., and Hermansen, L., Temperature regulation during exercise dehydration in man, *Acta Physiol. Scand.*, 79, 475, 1970.

114. Greenleaf, J. E., and Castle, B. L., Exercise temperature regulation in man during hypohydration and hyperhydration, *J. Appl. Physiol.*, 30, 847, 1971.

115. Strydom, N. B., Benade, A. J. S., and Van Rensburg, A. J., The state of hydration and the physiological responses of men during work in heat, *Aust. J. Sports Med.*, 7, 28, 1975.

116. Strydom, N. B., and Holdsworth, L. D., The effects of different levels of water deficit on physiological responses during heat stress, *Int. Z. Angew. Physiol.* 26: 95, 1968.

117. Caputa, M., and Cabanac, M., Precedence of head homeothermia over trunk homeothermia in dehydrated men, *Eur. J. Appl. Physiol.*, 57, 611, 1988.

118. Moroff, S. V., and Bass, D. E., Effects of overhydration on man's physiological responses to work in the heat, *J. Appl. Physiol.*, 20, 267, 1965.

119. Horstman, D. H., and Horvath, S. M., Cardiovascular and temperature regulatory changes during progressive dehydration and euhydration, *J. Appl. Physiol.* 33, 446, 1972.

120. Fortney, S. M., Vroman, N. B., Beckett, W. S., Permutt, S., and LaFrance, N. D., Effect of exercise hemoconcentration and hyperosmolality on exercise responses, *J. Appl. Physiol.*, 65, 519, 1988.

121. Fortney, S. M., Wenger, C. B., Bove, J. R., and Nadel, E. R., Effect of hyperosmolality on control of blood flow and sweating, *J. Appl. Physiol.*, 57, 1688, 1984.

122. Nose, H., Mack, G. W., Shi, X., Morimoto, K., and Nadel, E. R., Effect of saline infusion during exercise on thermal and circulatory regulations, *J. Appl. Physiol.*, 69, 609, 1990.

123. Sawka, M. N., Young, A. J., Caderette, B. S., Levine, L., and Pandolf, K. B., Influence of heat stress and acclimation on maximal aerobic power, *Eur. J. Appl. Physiol.*, 53, 294, 1985.

124. Noakes, T. D., Adams, B. A., Myburgh, K. H., Greeff, C., Lotz, T., and Nathan, M., The danger of an inadequate water intake during prolonged exercise, *Eur. J. Appl. Physiol.*, 57, 210, 1988
125. Altenkirch, H. U., Gerzer, R., Kirsch, K. A., Weil, J., Heyduck, B., Schultes, I., and Rocker, L., Effect of prolonged physical exercise on fluid regulating hormones, *Eur. J. Appl. Physiol.*, 61, 209, 1990.
126. Freund, B. J., Claybaugh, J. R., Hashiro, G. M., Buono, M., and Chrisney, S., Exaggerated ANF response to exercise in middle-aged vs. young runners, *J. Appl. Physiol.*, 69, 1607, 1990.
127. Wade, C. E., and Freund, B. J., Hormonal control of blood volume during and following exercise, in *Perspectives in Exercise Science and Sports Medicine, Fluid Homeostasis During Exercise*, Vol. 3., Gisolfi, C. V., and Lamb, D. R., Eds., Benchmark Press, 1990, 207.
128. Vitali, E., DeP., Malacarne, F., Vedovato, M., Cavallini, R., Bagni, B., Nunzi, L., and Gilli, P., Atrial natriuretic peptide and urinary sodium balance during physical exercise, *Nephron* 57, 60, 1991.
129. Walsh, R. M., Noakes, T. D., Hawley, J. A., and Dennis, S. C., Impaired high-intensity cycling performance time at low levels of dehydration, *Int. J. Sports Med.*, 15, 392, 1994.
130. Caldwell, J. E., Ahonen, E. S. A., and Nousiainen, U., Differential effects of sauna-, diuretic-, and exercise-induced hypohydration, *J. Appl. Physiol.*, 57, 1018, 1984.
131. Sawka, M. N., and Pandolf, K. B., Effects of body water loss on physiological function and exercise performance, in *Perspectives in Exercise Science and Sports Medicine, Fluid Homeostasis During Exercise*, Vol. 3., Gisolfi, C. V., and Lamb, D. R., Eds., Benchmark Press, 1990, 1.
132. Below, P. R., and Coyle E. F. Fluid and carbohydrate ingestion individually benefit exercise lasting one-hour (Abstract), *Med. Sci. Sports Exercise,* 25 (Suppl.), S3, 1993.
133. Deschamps, A., Levy, R. D., Cosio, M. G., Marliss, E. B., and Magder, S., Effect of saline infusion on body temperature and endurance during heavy exercise, *J. Appl. Physiol.*, 66, 2799, 1989.
134. Massicotte, D., Peronnet, F., Allah, C., Hillaire-Marcel, C., Ledoux, M., and Brisson, G., Metabolic response to [^{13}C] glucose and [^{13}C] fructose ingestion during exercise, *J. Appl. Physiol.*, 61: 1180, 1986
135. Massicotte, D., Peronnet, F., Brisson, G., Bakkouch, K., and Marcel, C. H., Oxidation of glucose polymer during exercise: comparison with glucose or fructose, *J. Appl. Physiol.*, 66: 179, 1989
136. Mitchell, J. B., Costill, D. L., Houmard, J. A., Fink, W. J., Pascoe, D. D., and Pearson, D. R., Influence of carbohydrate dosage on exercise performance and glycogen metabolism, *J. Appl. Physiol.*, 67: 1843, 1989.
137. Mitchell, J. B., Costill, D. L., Houmard, J. A., Flynn, M. G, Fink, W. J., and Beltz, J. D., Effects of carbohydrate ingestion on gastric emptying and exercise performance, *Med. Sci. Sports Exercise*, 20, 110, 1988.
138. Mitchell, J. B., Costill, D. L., Houmard, J. A., Fink, W. J., Robergs, R. A., and Davis, J. A., Gastric emptying: influence of prolonged exercise and carbohydrate concentration, *Med. Sci. Sports Exercise*, 21, 269, 1989.
139. Moodley, D. G., Noakes, T. D., Bosch, A. N., Hawley, J. A., Schall, R., and Dennis, S. C., Exogenous carbohydrate oxidation during prolonged exercise: the effect of carbohydrate type and its concentration, *Eur. J. Appl. Physiol.*, 64, 328, 1992.
140. Neufer, P. D., Costill, D. L., Fink, W. J., Kirwan, J. P., Fielding, R. A., and Flynn, M. G., Effects of exercise and carbohydrate composition on gastric emptying, *Med. Sci. Sports Exercise*, 18, 658, 1986.
141. Rehrer, N. J., Wagenmakers, A. J. M., Beckers, E. J., Halliday, D., Leiper, J. B., Brouns, F., Maughan, R. J., Westerterp, K., and Saris, W. H, M., Gastric emptying, absorption, and carbohydrate oxidation during prolonged exercise, *J. Appl. Physiol.*, 72, 468, 1992.
142. Sole, C. C., and Noakes, T. D., Faster gastric emptying for glucose-polymer and fructose solutions than for glucose in humans, *Eur. J. Appl. Physiol.*, 58, 605, 1989.
143. Hawley, J. A., Dennis, S. C., Nowitz, A., Brouns, F., and Noakes, T. D., Exogenous carbohydrate oxidation from maltose and glucose ingested during prolonged exercise, *Eur. J. Appl. Physiol.*, 64, 523, 1992.

144. Hawley, J. A., Bosch, A. N., Weltan, S. M., Dennis, S. C., and Noakes, T. D., Effects of glucose ingestion or glucose infusion on fuel substrate kinetics during prolonged exercise, *Eur. J. Appl. Physiol.*, 68, 381, 1994.

145. Hawley, J. A., Bosch, A. N., Weltan, S. M., Dennis, S. C., and Noakes, T. D., Glucose kinetics during prolonged exercise in euglycaemic and hyperglycaemic subjects, *Pflügers Arch.*, 426, 378, 1994.

146. Houmard, J. A., Egan, P. C., Johns, A. R., Neufer, P. D., Chenier, T. C., and Israel, R. G., Gastric emptying during 1 h of cycling and running at 75% VO$_2$max, *Med. Sci. Sports Exercise*, 23, 320, 1991.

147. Maughan, R. J., Carbohydrate-electrolyte solutions during prolonged exercise, in *Perspectives in Exercise Science and Sports Medicine. Fluid Homeostasis During Exercise*, Vol. 4, Lamb, D. R., and Williams, M., Eds, 1991, 35.

148. Wheeler, K. B., and Banwell, J. G., Intestinal water and electrolyte flux of glucose-polymer electrolyte solutions, *Med. Sci. Sports Exercise*, 18, 436, 1986.

149. Marbaix, O., Le passage pylorique, *Cellule*, 14, 332, 1898.

150. Noakes, T. D., Maughan, R. J., and Rehrer, N. J., The importance of volume in regulating gastric emptying, *Med. Sci. Sports Exercise*, 23: 307, 1991.

151. Rehrer, N. J., Brouns, F., Beckers, E. J., Ten Hoor, F., and Saris, W. H. M., Gastric emptying with repeated drinking during running and bicycling, *Int. J. Sports Med.*, 11, 238, 1990.

152. Carnot, P., and Chassevant, A., Modifications subies dans l'estomac et le duodenum par les solutions salines suivant leu concentration moleculaire. Le reflex regulateur de sphincter pylorue, *Contemp. Soc. Biol.*, 58, 173, 1905.

153. Hunt, J. N., and Pathak, J. D., The osmotic effect of some simple molecules and ions on gastric emptying, *J. Physiol.*, 154, 254, 1960.

154. Rehrer, N. J., Beckers, E. J., Brouns, F., Saris, W. H. M., and Ten Hoor, F., Effects of electrolytes in carbohydrate beverages on gastric emptying and secretion, *Med. Sci. Sports Exercise*, 25, 42, 1993.

155. McArthur, K. E., and Feldman, M., Gastric acid secretion, gastrin release, and gastric temperature in humans as affected by liquid meal temperature, *Am. J. Clin. Nutr.*, 49, 51, 1989.

156. Sun, W. M., Houghton, L. A., Read, N. W., Grundy, D. G., and Johnson, A. G., Effect of meal temperature on gastric emptying of liquids in man, *Gut*, 29, 302, 1988.

157. Coyle, E. F., Costill, D. L., Fink, W. J., and Hoopes, D. G., Gastric emptying rates for selected athletic drinks, *Res. Quart.*, 49, 119, 1978.

158. Fordtran, J. S., and Saltin, B., Gastric emptying and intestinal absorption during prolonged severe exercise, *J. Appl. Physiol.*, 23, 331, 1967.

159. Foster, C., Costill, D. L., and Fink, W. J., Gastric emptying characteristics of glucose and glucose polymer solution, *Res. Quart. Exercise Sport*, 51, 299, 1980.

160. American College of Sports Medicine, Position stand on prevention of thermal injuries during distance running, *Med. Sci. Sports Exercise*, 19, 529, 1987.

161. Coyle, E. F., and Montain, S. J., Carbohydrate and fluid ingestion during exercise: are there trade-offs? *Med. Sci. Sports Exercise*, 24, 671, 1992.

162. Maughan, R. J., and Noakes, T. D., Fluid replacement and exercise stress. A brief review of the studies on fluid replacement and some guidelines for the athlete, *Sports Med.*, 12, 16, 1991

163. Gisolfi, C. V., and Duchman, S. M., Guidelines for optimal replacement beverages for different athletic events, *Med. Sci. Sports Exercise*, 24, 679, 1992.

164. Hunt, J. N., and Knox, M. T., Regulation of Gastric Emptying, in *Handbook of Physiology IV. Alimentary Canal*, American Physiological Society, Washington D.C., 1969, 1917.

165. Hunt, J. N., and MacDonald, I., The influence of volume on gastric emptying, *J. Physiol.*, 126, 459, 1954.

166. Hunt, J. N., and Spurrell, W. R., The pattern of emptying of the human stomach, *J. Physiol.*, 113, 157, 1951.

167. Minami, H., and MaCallum, R. W., The physiology and pathophysiology of gastric emptying in humans, *Gastroenterology*, 86, 1592, 1984.

168. Hawley, J. A., Dennis, S. C., and Noakes, T. D., Oxidation of carbohydrate ingested during prolonged endurance exercise, *Sports Med.,* 14, 27, 1992.

169. Pirnay, F., Lacroix, M., Morosa, F., Luyckx, A., and Lefebvre, P., Glucose oxidation during prolonged exercise evaluated with naturally labelled [¹³C] glucose, *J. Appl. Physiol.,* 43, 258, 1977.

170. Pirnay, F., Lacroix, M., Morosa, F., Luyckx, A., and Lefebvre, P., Effect of glucose ingestion on energy substrate utilization during prolonged exercise in man, *Eur. J. Appl. Physiol.,* 36, 247, 1977.

171. Jandrain, B., Krzentowski. G., Pirnay, F., Morosa, F., Lacroix, M., Luyckx, A., and Lefebvre, P., Metabolic availability of glucose ingested 3 h before prolonged exercise in humans, *J. Appl. Physiol.,* 56, 1314, 1984.

172. Jandrain, B. J., Pirnay, F., Lacroix, M., Morosa, F., Scheen, A. J., and Lefebvre, P. J., Effect of osmolality on availability of glucose ingested during prolonged exercise in humans, *J. Appl. Physiol.,* 67, 76, 1989.

173. Krzentowski, G. B., Jandrain, F., Pirnay, F., Morosa, M., Lacroix, A. S., Luyckx, A., and Lefebvre, P. J., Availability of glucose given orally during exercise, *J. Appl. Physiol.,* 56, 315, 1984.

174. Krzentowski, G. B., Pirnay, F., Luyckx, A. S., Lacroix, M., Morosa, F., and Lefebvre, P. J., Effect of physical training on utilization of a glucose load given orally during exercise, *Am. J. Physiol.,* 246, E412, 1984.

175. Decombaz, J., Sartori, D., Arnaud, M. J., Thelin, A. L., Schurch, P., and Howald, H., Oxidation and metabolic effects of fructose or glucose ingested before exercise, *Int. J. Sports Med.,* 6, 282, 1985.

176. Guezennec, C. Y., Satabin, P., Duforez, F., Merino, D., Peronnet, F., and Koziet, J., Oxidation of corn starch, glucose, and fructose ingested before exercise, *Med. Sci. Sports Exercise,* 21, 45, 1989.

177. Massicotte, D., Peronnet, F., Brisson, G., Boivin, L., and Hillaire-Marcel, C., Oxidation of exogenous carbohydrate during prolonged exercise in fed and fasted conditions, *Int. J. Sports Med.,* 11, 253, 1990.

178. Pallikarakis, N., Jandrain, B., Pirnay, F., Morosa, F., Lacroix, M., Luyckx, A. S., and Lefebvre, P. J., Remarkable metabolic availability of oral glucose during long-duration exercise in humans, *J. Appl. Physiol.,* 60, 1035, 1986.

179. Ravussin, E., Pahud, P., Dorner, A., Arnaud, M. J., and Jequier, E., Substrate utilization during prolonged exercise preceded by ingestion of ¹³C-Glucose in glycogen depleted and control subjects, *Pflügers Arch.,* 382, 197, 1979.

180. Ahlborg, G., and Felig, P., Influence of glucose ingestion on fuel-hormone response during prolonged exercise, *J. Appl. Physiol.,* 41, 683, 1976.

181. Galbo, H., Holst, J. J., and Christensen, H. J., The effect of different diets and of insulin on the hormonal response to prolonged exercise, *Acta Physiol. Scand.,* 107, 19, 1979.

182. Koivisto, V. A., Fructose as a dietary sweetener in diabetes mellitus, *Diabetes Care,* 1, 241, 1978.

183. Koivisto, V. A., Karonen, S. L., and Nikkila, E. A., Carbohydrate ingestion before exercise: comparison of glucose, fructose, and sweet placebo, *J. Appl. Physiol.,* 51, 783, 1981.

184. Benade, A. J. S., Jansen, C. R., Rogers, G. G., Wyndham, C. H., and Strydom, N. B., The significance of an increased RQ after sucrose ingestion during prolonged aerobic exercise, *Pflügers Arch.,* 342, 199, 1973.

185. Gerard, J., Jandrain, B., Pirnay, F., Krzentowski, G., Lacroix, M., Morosa, F., and Luyckx, A. S., Utilization of oral sucrose load during exercise in humans. Effect of alpha-glucosidase inhibitor arcabose, *Diabetes,* 35, 1294, 1986.

186. Coggan, A. R., and Coyle, E. F., Carbohydrate ingestion during prolonged exercise: effects on metabolism and performance, in *Exercise and Sports Science Reviews,* Vol. 19, Holloszy, J. O., Ed., Williams and Wilkins, Baltimore, 1991, 1.

187. Boulze, D., Montastruc, P., and Cabanac, M., Water intake, pleasure and water temperature, *Physiol. Behav.,* 30, 97, 1983.

188. Epstein, Y., and Sohar, E., Fluid balance in hot climates: sweating, water intake, and prevention of dehydration, *Public Health Rev.*, 13, 115, 1985.
189. Hubbard, R. W., Sandick, B. L., and Matthew, W. T., Voluntary dehydration and alliesthesia for water, *J. Appl. Physiol.*, 57, 868, 1984.
190. Sohar, E., Adar, R., Gilat, T., Tennenbaum, J., and Nir, M., Reduction of voluntary dehydration during effort in hot environments, *Harefuah*, 60, 319, 1961.
191. Sandick, B. L., Engell, D. B., and Maller, O., Perception of drinking water temperature and effects for humans after exercise, *Physiol. Behav.*, 32, 851, 1984.
192. Szlyk, P. C., Hubbard, R. W., Matthew, W. T., Armstrong, L. E., and Kerstein, M. D., Mechanisms of voluntary dehydration among troops in the field, *Mil. Med.*, 152, 405, 1987.
193. Szlyk, P. C., Sils, I. V., Francesconi, R. P., and Hubbard, R.W., Patterns of human drinking: effects of exercise, water temperature, and food consumption, *Aviat. Space Environ. Med.*, 61, 43, 1990.
194. Greenleaf, J. E., Geelen, G., and Saumet, J. L., Vascular uptake of rehydration fluids in resting hypohydrated men, *IFASEB J.*, 5, A1147, 1991.
195. Spioch, F. M., and Nowara, M., Voluntary dehydration in men working in heat. *Int. Arch. Occup. Environ. Health*, 46, 233, 1980.
196. Van der Horst, G., Wesso, I., Burger, A. P., Dietrich, D. L. L., and Grobeler, S. R., Chemical analysis of selected cooldrinks and pure fruit juices: some implications for clinicians, *S. Afr. Med. J.*, 66, 755, 1984.

Chapter 20

INTERACTIONS AMONG INDICES OF MINERAL ELEMENT NUTRITURE AND PHYSICAL PERFORMANCE OF SWIMMERS

Henry C. Lukaski

CONTENTS

I. INTRODUCTION

For more than two decades, Americans have been responding to recommendations from public action agencies and private service organizations and increasing
physical activity as a means to prevent chronic disease and enhance the quality of life.
With increased participation in a variety of types of recreational and sporting activities by children, adolescents, and adults, an important question arises regarding the
interaction among nutrition, physical activity, and performance. As shown in Figure
1, this question includes two concerns. These issues refer to the influence of physical
activity per se on nutritional status and, conversely, the effect of nutritional status on
performance.

Two experimental designs have been used to address these relevant issues. The
first approach relies on cross-sectional and longitudinal surveys of physically active
individuals, and comparisons among athletes and nontraining control subjects before,
during, and after physical training. This method, which describes differences in
nutrient intakes and blood biochemical indices of nutritional status, provides some
insight into the influence of increased energy expenditure on nutrient intake and
nutritional status.

Another experimental design employs longitudinal assessment of blood biochemical indices of nutritional status of physically active individuals, and nutritional
intervention when impaired nutritional status occurs. Changes in performance are
monitored as a function of nutritional status indicators. Findings from such

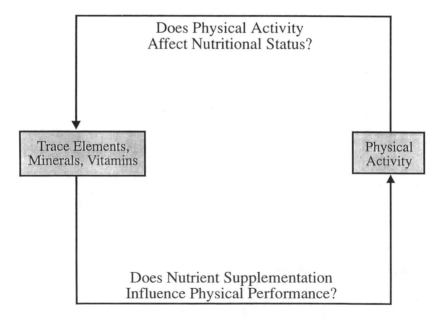

FIGURE 1.   Theoretical interactions between nutrients and physical activity.

investigations provide evidence of the prevalence of impaired nutritional status and its effect on physical performance.

Based on investigations using these experimental designs, some generalizations can be made. Among the macronutrients, it is generally accepted that carbohydrate intake and water consumption are limiting factors in endurance activities.[1] However, information about the role of micronutrients, particularly the mineral elements, on human performance is quite limited.[2-4]

This review describes the relationships among mineral element intakes, blood biochemical indices of mineral nutriture, and measurements of performance of swimmers during the competitive season. A model, based on assessments of mineral nutriture, is derived for the prediction of swimming performance.

II. MINERAL ELEMENTS AND ENERGY METABOLISM

Mineral elements play an important role in the production and utilization of energy in the body. Their function is to serve as mandatory components of enzymes needed for the generation of energy and to facilitate the performance of physical work. Some of these roles are summarized below.

A. IRON

A major role of iron is the transport of oxygen to cells and its utilization within cells. These functions are accomplished by means of hemoglobin and myoglobin, which together account for approximately 74% of body iron. In addition, about 1% of body iron is found in the many oxidative enzymes, including the mitochondrial cytochromes, iron-sulfur proteins, or non-heme enzymes, and other mitochondrial proteins.[5] Although these compounds constitute only a small fraction of iron in the body, their metabolic functions are as vital to oxidative metabolism, and thus work performance, as that of hemoglobin.

B. COPPER

In contrast to the relatively large amount of iron in the body, about 3.5 g in an adult man, the estimated copper content of the body is less than 100 mg.[6] Nevertheless, this small amount of copper serves critical roles in oxidative metabolism.

One copper-containing compound, ceruloplasmin, also known as feroxidase, indirectly affects energy utilization because of its proposed role in regulating iron utilization in the body.[7] More directly, copper in the form of the enzyme cytochrome-*C*-oxidase affects cellular oxidative metabolism.[8] Another copper-containing enzyme, superoxide dismutase, is an oxygen free-radical scavenger.[9]

C. ZINC

The total amount of zinc in the body has been estimated to be 2 to 3 g.[10] Although many biological functions have been associated with zinc, its role in energy metabolism has been linked with two specific enzymes. As a necessary component of lactate dehydrogenase and carbonic anhydrase, zinc acts to regulate energy expenditure and to facilitate carbon dioxide removal from the cells.[11-13] Zinc is required at the catalytic sites of these compounds for optimal enzyme function.

D. MAGNESIUM

In an adult human, the magnesium content of the body ranges from 21 to 28 g.[14] As such, magnesium is the most abundant cation in the body and the second most plentiful intracellular cation. Although bone has the greatest content of magnesium in the body, liver and skeletal muscle have the greatest magnesium concentrations. Many biological roles have been demonstrated for magnesium.[15] As an activator of enzymes that hydrolyze and transfer phosphate groups, and those involved with adenosine triphosphate metabolism, magnesium is required for macronutrient metabolism and muscle contraction. It is also required as a cofactor for oxidative phosphorylation.

III. MINERAL NUTRITURE AND SWIMMING PERFORMANCE

A study was designed to examine the relationships among indices of mineral element nutriture and swimming performance. Members of the University of North Dakota men's and women's swimming teams were studied at the start and conclusion of the competitive season. Women ($n = 10$) and men ($n = 6$) specializing in the 100-yard, free-style event were studied. The participants were free-living volunteers who did not consume vitamin or mineral supplements. Performance was determined during intercollegiate swim meets scheduled early in, and at the end of, the competitive season.

A. MINERAL ELEMENT INTAKES

Nutrient intakes were estimated by analysis of self-reported, 7-d dietary records. Participants consumed self-selected diets from foods available in dormitory dining facilities. Diet records were reviewed for completeness of food descriptions and amounts of food consumed. Nutrient intakes were calculated by using a computerized dietary analysis system.

Estimated mineral element intakes did not change during training. Among the female swimmers, intakes of copper (1.23 ± 0.12 and 1.11 ± 0.12 mg/d; mean $\pm$ SE), iron (12.4 ± 1.0 and 11.6 ± 0.8 mg/d), magnesium (268 ± 26 and 244 ± 26 mg/d), and zinc (10.5 ± 0.8 and 9.5 ± 0.8 mg/d) were not different over time. Similarly, daily intakes of copper (2.10 ± 0.20 and 1.98 ± 0.18 mg/d), iron (21.7 ± 1.8 and 19.2 ± 2.1 mg/d), magnesium (449 ± 46 and 394 ± 36 mg/d), and zinc (17.6 ± 1.9 and 16.4 ± 1.2 mg/d) were unchanged during the competitive season among the male swimmers.

The adequacy of the estimated mineral intakes was assessed in relation to a general guideline representing 67% of the specific mineral element intakes proposed for American adults.[16] Among the female swimmers, the average iron and magnesium intakes exceeded the guidelines for iron and magnesium (10 and 188 mg/d, respectively). Zinc intake was similar to the guideline of 10 mg/d. Similarly, estimated copper intake was not different than the guideline for safe and adequate intake. The average intakes of copper, iron, magnesium, and zinc of the male swimmers exceeded the guidelines for these minerals (1.5, 7, 235, and 10 mg/d, respectively).

Because of the differences ($p < 0.01$) in estimated energy intakes between the women and the men (2110 ± 100 vs. 3890 ± 236 kcal/d), mineral intakes were normalized for a standardized energy intake. On the average, there were no significant differences by either gender or time for mineral intakes expressed per 1000 kcal/d.

B. BLOOD INDICES OF MINERAL NUTRITURE

Mineral element nutriture, assessed by plasma and red blood cell concentrations of minerals, was unchanged by physical training (Table 1). All values of plasma and red blood cell mineral concentrations were within the range of normal values for adult residents of Grand Forks.

Iron status was unaffected by training. No differences in hematocrit or hemoglobin concentration were found. Serum ferritin and transferrin saturation were significantly less in the female, as compared to the male, swimmers.

Specific indices of copper nutriture also were not significantly affected by training. In the men, however, there was a tendency for an increase in ceruloplasmin activity and superoxide dismutase activity late in the competitive season.

C. SWIM PERFORMANCE AND MINERAL NUTRITURE

Times in the 100-yard free-style decreased ($p < 0.05$) in each group of swimmers during the competitive season. The women had a 3.3% decrease (61.1 ± 1.9 to 59.1 ± 1.5 sec) and the men had a 4.8% decrease (52.3 ± 0.9 to 49.8 ± 1.0 sec) in time.

Swim times in the 100-yard free-style event were significantly associated with some measurements of mineral element intake (Table 2). Data for early and late season nutritional and performance assessments were combined by gender. Daily zinc intake among the men was the only significant dietary mineral variable to predict swim time.

Among the blood biochemical indicators of mineral nutritional status, some significant relationships with swim time were observed (Table 3). Among the women, plasma iron concentration, serum ferritin concentration, and transferrin saturation were significant individual predictors of swim time. None of the biochemical determinations were significant predictors of performance for the men.

Step-wise multiple regression models, using mineral element intake and blood biochemical measurements of mineral nutriture as independent variables, were developed to predict swim time (Table 4). Among the women, swim time was related

TABLE 1   Blood Biochemical Indices of Copper (Cu), Iron (Fe), Magnesium (Mg), and Zinc (Zn) Status of Female and Male Swimmers Assessed During the Early and End of a Competitive Season.

	Women (n = 10)		Men (n = 6)	
	Early	End	Early	End
Plasma				
Cu, μmol/l	17.9 ± 1.9	17.8 ± 1.8	13.9 ± 0.6	13.3 ± 0.7
Fe, μmol/l	16.0 ± 1.6^A	15.1 ± 1.5^A	21.3 ± 1.8^B	18.9 ± 1.4^B
Mg, μmol/l	820 ± 36	821 ± 22	883 ± 64	870 ± 28
Zn, μmol/l	13.3 ± 0.6^A	11.8 ± 0.6^A	14.9 ± 0.9^B	12.8 ± 0.4^B
RBC[a]				
Cu, μmol/g Hgb[b]	0.31 ± 0.01	0.31 ± 0.01	0.30 ± 0.01	0.33 ± 0.02
Mg, mmol/g Hgb	63.2 ± 2.5	63.9 ± 1.2	60.8 ± 1.3	61.1 ± 1.5
Zn, μmol/g Hgb	5.4 ± 0.2	5.6 ± 0.3	5.3 ± 0.2	5.2 ± 0.2
Iron status				
Hematocrit, %	38.2 ± 0.7^A	38.2 ± 0.8^A	43.0 ± 0.8^B	42.8 ± 0.9^B
Hemoglobin, g/l	135.9 ± 2.3^A	135.7 ± 3.1^A	154.8 ± 2.3^B	153.0 ± 2.8^B
Ferritin, μg/l	30.2 ± 7.9^A	26.5 ± 6.2^A	73.2 ± 12.2^B	45.5 ± 14.0^B
Transferrin,[c] %	27.0 ± 3.2^A	26.0 ± 3.0^A	38.3 ± 3.2^B	35.7 ± 2.8^B
Copper status				
Cp-ENZ,[d] mg/l	51.4 ± 3.9	50.0 ± 4.1	45.1 ± 2.7	51.3 ± 6.9
SOD,[e] U/g Hgb	2850 ± 196	2167 ± 213	2171 ± 34	2349 ± 114

Note: Values are mean ± SEM

[A,B]   Values in a row with different superscripts are different ($p < 0.05$).
[a]   RBC = red blood cell.
[b]   Hgb = hemoglobin.
[c]   Transferrin, % = transferrin saturation.
[d]   Cp-ENZ = enzymatic activity of ceruloplasmin.
[e]   SOD = superoxide dismutase activity.

to magnesium, iron, and zinc intakes as well as blood measurements of iron, magnesium, and copper nutriture. In contrast, zinc and copper intakes, together with circulating iron variables, were the important predictors of swim time in the men.

IV. MINERAL NUTRITION AND PERFORMANCE: AN INTERPRETATION

The data presented suggest that some individual measurements of mineral element nutritional status are significant predictors of 100-yard free-style swim times of collegiate athletes. To interpret the significance and practical implication of these findings, it is necessary to examine these relationships with respect to some basic hypotheses relating nutritional status and physical activity.

As shown in Figure 2, there are two prevalent hypotheses regarding the interactions between nutrition and physical activity. It is generally assumed that nutritional status affects performance; as nutritional status improves, event time decreases and,

TABLE 2   Correlation Coefficients Relating Time in 100-Yard Free-Style and Measurements of Trace Element Intakes of Female and Male Swimmers

	Women	Men
Cu, mg/d	−0.37	0.42
Fe, mg/d	−0.08	0.28
Mg, mg/d	−0.31	0.46
Zn, mg/d	−0.23	−0.11
Cu, mg/1000 kcal/d	−0.35	0.38
Fe, mg/1000 kcal/d	0.17	0.08
Mg, mg/1000 kcal/d	−0.36	0.44
Zn, mg/1000 kcal/d	−0.08	0.57[a]

[a] $p < 0.05$

TABLE 3   Correlation Coefficients Relating 100-Yard Free-style Time and Blood Biochemical Indices of Trace Element Status in Swimmers

	Women $n = 20$	Men $n = 12$
Plasma concentrations		
Cu, μmol/l	0.10	0.02
Fe, μmol/l	0.56[a]	−0.06
Mg, mmol/l	0.17	0.06
Zn, μmol/l	0.05	−0.11
RBC concentrations		
Cu, μmol/g Hgb	−0.36	−0.26
Mg, mmol/g Hgb	0.12	−0.13
Zn, μmol/g Hgb	−0.12	0.31
Iron status		
Hematocrit, %	0.39	0.10
Hemoglobin, g/l	0.30	0.18
In (Ferritin), μg/l	0.53[a]	0.20
Transferrin, %	0.61[a]	−0.33
Copper status		
Cp-ENZ, mg/l	0.35	−0.47
SOD, U/g Hgb	0.33	0.36

[a] $p < 0.01$

thus, performance improves. Conversely, as nutritional status deteriorates, event times increase and performance declines. Therefore, the beneficial effect of nutritional status on event time is indicated with a negative correlation coefficient, and an adverse effect of compromised or impaired nutritional status is evidenced as a positive correlation coefficient.

The second hypothesis is that physical activity per se influences nutritional status. This may be envisaged as a decline in an index of nutritional status as the event or test time decreases and performance increases (Figure 3). This relationship also

**TABLE 4   Multiple Regression Equations to Predict
100-Yard Free-Style Swim Time in Female
and Male Swimmers**

I.

	Female Swimmers: Early and End of Season ($n = 20$)		
	Variable	**R^2**	**SEE**
X1	Transferrin, %	0.370	4.4
X2	Mg intake/1000 kcal	0.601	3.6
X3	Zn intake	0.685	3.3
X4	ln (Ferritin)	0.784	2.8
X5	Fe intake/1000 kcal	0.851	2.4
X6	RBC Mg	0.901	1.7
X7	SOD	0.951	1.2

$Y = 0.49X1 - 0.20X2 + 1.52X3 + 3.61X4 - 2.01X5 + 2.01X6 + 0.001X7 + 19.58$

II.

	Male Swimmers: Early and End of Season ($n = 12$)		
	Variable	**R^2**	**SEE**
X1	Plasma Fe	0.361	2.1
X2	Zn intake/1000 kcal	0.701	1.5
X3	Transferrin, %	0.816	1.2
X4	Cu intake/1000 kcal	0.930	0.8

$Y = 1.02X1 - 1.40X2 - 0.68X3 + 10.6X4 + 56.56$

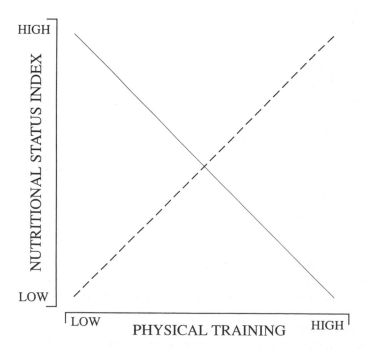

FIGURE 2.   Relationships between indicators of nutritional status and physical training.

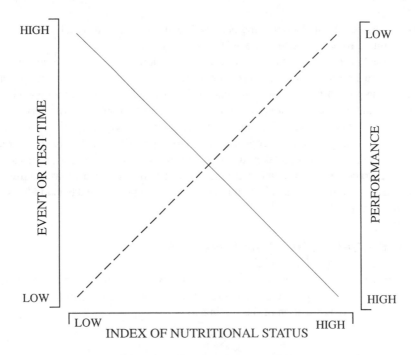

FIGURE 3. Relationships among nutritional status, performance, and event time.

may be described as a decline in a measure of nutritional status in relation to increased training or activity; it is shown as a negative correlation coefficient. Conversely, an increase in a status indicator associated with increased physical training would be indicated with a positive correlation coefficient.

Assessment of the capacity of individual indicators of mineral nutritional status to predict swim times indicated that only a few variables were important. Zinc intake was a significant predictor only in the men; mineral intakes were not significant predictors of swim time in the women. Blood biochemical measurements of iron status were significant predictors of swim time in the women, but not in the men.

The sign of the correlation coefficients relating measurements of nutritional status to swim time provides some indication of the interaction between nutritional status and physical activity. The negative correlation coefficient between swim time and zinc intake in the men indicates an inverse relationship between these variables. In contrast, the positive correlation coefficient between swim time and blood indices of iron status in the women signifies a direct relationship between iron nutriture and swim time. Because swim times decreased during the competitive season, one may interpret these findings to indicate that as swim time decreases, zinc intake increases among the men, and indices of iron nutriture decrease among the women. Because no significant differences were found in either mineral element intakes or blood biochemical indicators of mineral status, and all determinations of mineral intake and blood biochemical indices of nutritional status were within ranges of acceptable values, one could conclude that the observed relationships were functional adaptations without impaired mineral element nutritional status.

These findings indicate that if overt nutritional deficiency is not present, as was the case in the present study, then an integrated model of nutritional assessment might be useful to predict function or performance. Results of multiple regression analysis indicated that distinct nutritional variables could be used to predict swim times. For the women, intakes of iron, zinc, and magnesium, and blood biochemical measurements of iron, magnesium, and copper status were important predictors of swim time. Similarly, zinc and copper intakes, together with blood measurements of iron status, were used to estimate swim time in the men. These findings indicate that, regardless of gender, swim time is dependent on mineral element nutrient intake and indices of mineral nutritional status.

A. PHYSICAL ACTIVITY AND MINERAL ELEMENT NUTRITURE

Experimental evidence describing interrelationships among nutritional status and physical activity is available. However, differences in experimental designs complicate the interpretation of the findings.

1. Iron

It is well recognized that iron status can significantly influence human physiologic function and physical performance. Cross-sectional studies indicate that hemoglobin concentration is linearly related to peak oxygen consumption.[17] In addition, mild iron depletion has been shown to increase glycolytic metabolism of women without changing peak oxygen uptake.[18-20] Whereas these findings clearly indicate an impaired metabolic response during exercise in iron-deficient humans, the etiology of the iron deficiency observed in physically active people remains undefined.

The incidence of iron depletion and anemia in trained athletes is similar to that found in the general population, and the percentage of female athletes with iron deficiency is twice as large as the percentage in American women.[21] Studies of female swimmers and runners have failed to document inadequate iron intakes in the presence of anemia or hypoferritinemia.[22-24] It remains to be demonstrated whether female athletes in physical training have inadequate iron intakes or increased iron losses.

2. Copper

Evidence of an effect of physical training on human copper nutriture is limited. Comparisons of blood biochemical indices of copper status between nontraining controls and athletes participating in various sporting activities indicated no difference in measured copper status indicators.[25-27] However, longitudinal studies of swimmers provide conflicting data. In an early report, plasma copper and ceruloplasmin concentrations decreased significantly in male and female swimmers during 4 months of physical training.[28] Other reports found no significant changes in the plasma copper and ceruloplasmin concentrations of male and female swimmers during 5 months of training for competition;[22,23] comparisons with age- and gender-matched, nontraining controls indicated neither difference in blood biochemical measurements of copper status nor copper dietary intake. Among highly trained women runners, copper intake and plasma copper concentrations were within the ranges of acceptable values.[24]

3. Zinc

The role of physical activity on human zinc nutritional status also is ill-defined. A cross-sectional study found significantly decreased plasma zinc concentrations in male distance runners in comparison to untrained men. In a longitudinal study of young men training for nine months, serum zinc concentration decreased significantly.[29,30] In each of these studies, zinc intake was not estimated. Hypozincemia also has been reported in female distance runners whose mean zinc intake was about 65% of the recommended intake for American adults.[24] In contrast, other studies have not found differences in plasma zinc concentrations in either cross-sectional or longitudinal studies of collegiate athletes who consumed zinc intakes of about 70% of recommended values.[22,23] Interestingly, the observations of hypozincemia were made principally in runners, even those consuming what is considered an adequate amount of dietary zinc, in contrast to swimmers consuming a similar amount of zinc in the diet. It is unclear if type of physical activity affects zinc nutriture when dietary zinc is adequate by population standards.

4. Magnesium

The effects of intense physical activity or training on human magnesium status are not well characterized. Studies of athletes participating in endurance events[31,32] and of untrained men performing acute exercise[29] reveal significant decreases in plasma or serum magnesium concentrations during, or briefly after, exercise. These values are normalized on the days following the exercise bout. A cross-sectional study of athletes and non-athletes found no differences in plasma or erythrocyte magnesium concentrations by group.[27] However, a significant relationship was found between plasma magnesium concentration and peak oxygen consumption in athletes.

The interaction of magnesium intake, blood biochemical indices of magnesium status, and physical training has been studied.[33] Magnesium status, indicated by plasma and red blood cell concentrations of magnesium, was similar between athletes and non-athletes. Magnesium intake, expressed either in mg/d or mg/1000 kcal·d, was greater among the athletes.

V. SUMMARY AND CONCLUSIONS

In contrast to the majority of studies designed to evaluate the interactions among intakes of essential nutrients, nutritional status, and physical activity, the present investigation determined relationships among indicators of nutritional status and actual performance. Some individual measurements of mineral element intake and blood biochemical indices of mineral nutriture were found to be significant predictors of swim performance. In male swimmers, zinc intake was inversely related to swim time, suggesting that as zinc intake increased, swim time decreased. For the female swimmers, a positive relationship was observed between blood measurements of iron status and swim time; this indicates that iron status decreased in parallel with swim times. Because all of the measurements of mineral nutriture (intakes and biochemical values) were within established reference ranges, one can conclude that multiple nutritional variables might be interacting to influence swim performance. Multiple regression models using measurements of mineral element nutriture were developed to predict swim times for the female and male swimmers.

These findings emphasize that physical activity per se does not adversely affect mineral nutritional status when adequate amounts of mineral elements are consumed. Also, they indicate that recommended intakes of iron, copper, zinc, and magnesium, to meet the needs of physically active people, can be achieved without the use of dietary supplements.

REFERENCES

1. Costill, D. L., and Miller, J. M., Nutrition for endurance sport: carbohydrate and fluid balance, *Int. J. Sports Med.*, 1, 2, 1980.
2. Brotherhood, J. R., Nutrition and sports performance, *Sports Med.*, 1, 350, 1984.
3. Keen, C. L., and Hackman, R. M., Trace elements in athletic performance, in *Sport, Health and Nutrition*, Katch, F. I., Ed., Human Kinetics, Champaign, IL, 1986, 51.
4. Wolinsky, I., and Hickson, J. F., *Nutrition in Exercise and Sport*, Second Edition, CRC Press, Boca Raton, FL, 1994, 280.
5. Dallman, P. R., Biochemical basis for the manifestations of iron deficiency, *Annu. Rev. Nutr.*, 6, 13, 1986.
6. Mason, K. E., A conspectus of research on copper metabolism and requirements of man, *J. Nutr.*, 109, 1979, 1979.
7. Curzon, G., and O'Reilly, S., A coupled iron-caeruloplasmin oxidation system, *Biochem. Biophys. Res. Commun.*, 2, 284, 1960.
8. Beinert, H., Cytochrome c oxidase: present knowledge of the state and function of its copper components, in *Biochemistry of Copper*, Peisach, J., Aisen, P. and Blumberg, W. E., Eds., Academic Press, New York, 1966, 213.
9. McCord, J. M., and Fridovich, I., Superoxide dismutase. An enzymatic function for erythrocuprein (hemocuprein), *J. Biol. Chem.*, 244, 6049, 1970.
10. National Research Council, Subcommittee on Zinc, *Zinc*, University Park Press, Baltimore, MD, 1979, 123.
11. Chesters, J., Biochemical functions of zinc in animals, *World Rev. Nutr. Diet.*, 32, 135, 1978.
12. Lindskog, S., Henderson, L. E., Kannan, K. K., Liljas, A., Nyman, P. O., and Strandbert, B. Carbonic anhydrase, in *Enzymes*, Volume 5, *Hydrolysis, Sulfate Esters, Carboxyl Esters, Glycosides, Hydration*, 3rd ed., Boyer, P. D., Ed., Academic Press, New York, 1971, 587.
13. Vallee, B. L., and Wacher, W. E. C., Zinc, a component of rabbit muscle lactic dehydrogenase, *J. Am. Chem. Soc.*, 78, 1771, 1956.
14. Widdowson, E. M., McCance, R. A., and Spray, C. M., Chemical composition of the human body, *Clin. Sci.* 10, 113, 1951.
15. Wacker, W. E. C., and Parisi, A. F., Magnesium metabolism, *N. Engl. J. Med.*, 278, 658, 1968.
16. National Research Council, Food and Nutrition Board, Subcommittee on the Tenth Edition of the RDA's, *Recommended Dietary Allowances*, Washington, D.C., National Academy Press, 1989, 187.

17. Viteri, F. E., and Torun, B., Anemia and physical work capacity, *Clin. Haematol.*, 3, 609, 1974.
18. Schoene, R. B., Escourrou, P., Robertson, H. T., Nilson, K. L., Parsons, J. R., and Smith, N. J., Iron repletion decreases maximal exercise lactate concentrations in female athletes with minimal iron-deficiency anemia, *J. Lab. Clin. Med.* 102, 306, 1983.
19. Rowland, T. W., Deisworth, M. B., Green, G. M., and Kelleher, J. F., The effect of iron therapy on the exercise capacity of nonanemic iron-deficient adolescent runners, *Am. J. Dis. Child*, 142, 165, 1988.
20. Lukaski, H. C., Hall, C. B., and Siders, W. A., Altered metabolic response of iron-deficient women during graded maximal exercise, *Eur. J. Appl. Physiol.*, 63, 140, 1991.
21. Haymes, E., Proteins, vitamins and iron, in *Ergogenic Aids in Sport*, Williams, M. H., Ed., Champaign, IL, Human Kinetics, 1983, 27.
22. Lukaski, H. C., Hoverson, B. S., Milne, D. B., and Bolonchuk, W. W., Copper, zinc and iron status of female swimmers, *Nutr. Res.*, 9, 493, 1989.
23. Lukaski, H. C., Hoverson, B. S., Gallagher, S. K., and Bolonchuk, W. W., Physical training and copper, iron and zinc status, *Am. J. Clin. Nutr.*, 51, 1093, 1990.
24. Deuster, P. A., Kyle, S. B., Moser, P. B., Vigersky, R. A., Singh, A., and Schoomaker, E. B., Nutritional survey of highly trained women, *Am. J. Clin. Nutr.*, 44, 954, 1986.
25. Haralambie, G., and Keul, J., The response of serum ceruloplasmin and copper during prolonged athletic training, *Arzneim. Forsch.*, 24, 112, 1970.
26. Dressendorfer, R. H., and Sockolov, R., Hypozincemia in runners, *Phys. Sports Med.*, 8, 97, 1980.
27. Lukaski, H. C., Bolonchuk, W. W., Klevay, L. M., Milne, D. B., and Sandstead, H. H., Maximal oxygen consumption as related to magnesium, copper and zinc nutriture, *Am. J. Clin. Nutr.*, 37, 407, 1983.
28. Dowdy, R. P., and Burt, J. R., Effect of intensive long-term training on copper and zinc nutriture of man, *Fed. Proc.*, 39, 786, 1980.
29. Haralambie, G., Changes in electrolytes and trace minerals during long-lasting exercise, in *Metabolic Adaptation to Prolonged Physical Exercise*, Howard, H. and Poortmans J. R., Eds., Birkhauser Verlag, Basel, Switzerland, 1975, 340.
30. Couzy, F., Lafargue, P., and Guezennec, C. Y., Zinc metabolism in the athlete: influence of training, nutrition and other factors, *Int. J. Sports Med.*, 11, 263, 1990.
31. Rose, L. I., Carrol, D. R., Lowe, S. L., Peterson, E. W., and Cooper, K. H., Serum electrolyte changes after marathon running, *J. Appl. Physiol.*, 29, 449, 1970.
32. Refsum, H. E., Tveit, B., Meen, H. D., and Strom, S. B., Serum electrolyte, fluid and acid-base balance after prolonged heavy exercise at low environmental temperatures, *Scand. J. Clin. Lab. Invest.*, 32, 117, 1973.
33. Fogelholm, M., Laakso, J., Lehto, J., and Ruokonen, I., Dietary intake and indicators of magnesium and zinc status in male athletes, *Nutr. Res.*, 11, 1111, 1991.

Chapter 21

COMPARISON OF MINERAL INTAKE, EXCRETION, AND HEMATOLOGICAL PARAMETERS OF ANABOLIC STEROID USERS AND NONUSERS

————————————————————— Nweze Nnakwe

CONTENTS

I. ABSTRACT

Two groups of weight lifters were studied; twelve self-administered anabolic steroid users and thirteen nonusers. A 5-d dietary record was collected from each subject to determine dietary calcium, phosphorus, magnesium, fiber, and trace mineral intakes. Twenty-four-hour urine samples were collected on the same 5 d the dietary records were kept. Fasting blood samples were collected to determine plasma testosterone, iron, calcium, phosphorus, alkaline phosphatase, and hematological concentrations. There was no significant difference between the groups in either serum calcium, phosphorus, iron, alkaline phosphatase, or dietary calcium, phosphorus, iron, or magnesium intakes. In addition, there were no differences in urinary calcium, phosphorus, and magnesium excretion. Subjects on anabolic steroids had significantly higher serum testosterone, protein, and copper intakes. Results from this study could provide needed information on the effect of self-administered anabolic steroids on mineral utilization.

II. INTRODUCTION

Anabolic steroid use has become increasingly popular among athletes principally to develop strength and power. The use of anabolic steroids by athletes is quite controversial. The first major area of controversy is whether the steroids do indeed improve athletic performance. Many athletes having personal experience with these steroids insist that their performance is improved.[1,2] The second major area of controversy is whether anabolic steroids are harmful to the athlete. Many athletes seem to be able to recognize some side effects of the steroid, which include personality changes, irritability, and increased aggressiveness.[3] An increase in systolic blood pressure, heart rate, a decrease in protective levels of high-density lipoprotein cholesterol (HDL), and an increase in nonprotective levels of low-density lipoprotein cholesterol (LDL) have been reported.[4] When anabolic steroids are used by women, masculinizing changes, perhaps with irreversible results, are seen. Hair growth on the upper lip, chin, and cheeks, baldness, deepening of the voice, shrinkage of breast size, enlargement of the clitoris, and disruption of menstrual cycle have all been observed. Among the side effects suggested by several authors is failure to reach full stature (if taken during adolescence) because of premature closure of bone growth plates.[3,5-8]

Several authors have reported that a high protein diet plus anabolic steroid use appears to be associated with a significant increase in strength and muscle mass in body builders and football players,[9,10,11] However, the association of a high protein diet with anabolic steroids has not been effectively studied because of the lack of dietary history in most of the studies. The use of anabolic steroids and protein supplementation by body builders is widespread.[5,8] In a summary of data from nutritional surveys in the U.S., Pao[12] showed that dietary protein intake was well above the 1980 Recommended Dietary Allowances (RDA)[13] for both men and women, regardless of age. It has been well established that the ingestion of high dietary protein levels results in hypercalciuria in men, and that hypercalciuria is frequently accompanied by a negative calcium balance.[14,15] Meredith et al.[16] studied the effect of regular submaximal exercise on dietary protein requirements, whole body protein turnover, and urinary 3-methyl-histidine excretion of endurance trained men. The subjects consumed 0.6 g, 0.9 g, or 1.2 g of protein per kg body weight/d over three separate 10-d periods. Results showed negative nitrogen balance when 0.6g/kg/body weight/d was fed. Whole body protein turnover, using [^{15}N] glycine as a tracer, and 3-methyl-histidine excretion were not different in the groups. The author suggested that the protein requirement for athletes should be 0.94 g/kg body weight/d.

The trace minerals zinc, copper, and iron participate as cofactors for a variety of enzymes which are important during exercise. For example, zinc is an essential component of carbonic anhydrase and lactate dehydrogenase;[17] iron is a constituent of erythrocyte hemoglobin, muscle myoglobin, and the mitochondrial cytochrome complex.[17] Last, the copper metalloenzyme cytochrome-C-oxidase is required for electron transport and mitochondrial oxidation.[18] There is little information on how acute and/or chronic exercise influences the body's distribution of trace minerals. The relationship of zinc status and zinc intake has been studied. Bazzarre et al.[19] found that athletes have lower than adequate intakes of zinc, but blood levels were normal. But Couzy et al.[20] found that serum zinc was significantly decreased after 5 months of intensive training. Zinc is lost mainly from the body through sweat and urine. Anderson and Guttman[21] found an increase in urinary zinc excretion after a 6-mi run.

Lukaski[22] examined copper status of collegiate swimmers before and after the competitive season and found no difference in plasma copper levels or ceruloplasmin activity. However, Dowdy and Burt[23] found that serum copper levels were significantly lower after 6 months of swim training. Marrella et al.[24] also reported that resting copper concentrations were lower in triathletes compared to controls, but no differences were found for ceruloplasmin and total blood cell copper.

More studies have been done to assess iron status of athletes than for all other minerals combined. Assessment of iron status is generally done from blood samples, however, two studies are available that assessed iron status in bone marrow aspirations from runners.[25] Eleven male runners and one female runner in one study,[26] and eight male runners in the other study,[25] showed that the athletes had insufficient iron stores. Wishnitzer et al.[26] showed that serum iron levels, percentage iron saturation, and hemoglobin concentrations were normal despite the insufficient level for stored iron. Several studies have reported low serum iron levels in athletes. For example, low serum ferritin levels have been found in male middle- and long-distance runners,[27] female distance runners,[28] female endurance athletes,[19] and male and female endurance runners.[29] Information on the dietary intakes of zinc, copper, and iron in weight lifters is limited.

The primary importance of changes in sex steroid concentrations in the development of osteoporosis in postmenopausal women has been demonstrated by numerous studies showing that cessation of ovarian function results in acceleration of age-related bone loss.[30,31] However, the effect of changes in sex steroids on the development of bone disease in men has not been well studied, in spite of evidence suggesting a relationship between sex steroids and bone mass in men.[32,33] The prevalence of spinal osteoporosis in men 45 to 79 years of age is approximately 18%. By the ninth decade the cumulative incidence of fracture of the proximal femur in men is 17%.[33] The use of anabolic steroids and high protein intakes could promote the loss of important minerals. The objectives of this study were: (1) to investigate the dietary protein, mineral intakes, and excretion of male weight lifters; (2) to determine the hematological parameters, serum minerals, and testosterone levels.

III. MATERIALS AND METHODS

It was difficult to find an athlete who would admit to steroid use. This influenced the protocol in the sense that the drugs, dosage, and nutrient supplements that each participant used had to be accepted. Steroid users cycle the drug intake with the hope of alleviating some of the harmful side effects, while still experiencing the positive anabolic effects. The steroid cycle is implemented according to a pyramid scheme, from a low dose, or baseline, when steroid use may be abstained, then slowly increasing to a high dose when multiple preparations may be used, and then tapering off again, with the entire cycle lasting approximately 10 to 16 weeks. These dosages vary with the individual. Twenty-five male weight lifters volunteered for this study. Subjects were recruited from different weight lifting centers and were selected on the basis of steroid use and nonuse. All gave their consent in accordance with the procedures established by University Human Subjects Review Committee. All were in good health and received medical clearance through the University student health services.

Group A consisted of twelve weight lifters on self-administered anabolic steroids and nutritional supplements. Group B consisted of thirteen weight lifters taking only nutritional supplements. Data on the duration of training program periods were collected by means of a questionnaire. The subjects' height (in centimeters) and weight (in kilograms) were measured using a balance beam scale, and their age was recorded in years.

All subjects were trained to record their food and beverage intake accurately. Each participant completed a dietary record (diary method) for five consecutive weekdays using estimated household measures. In addition, subjects completed a 5-d 24-h urine sample at the same time dietary records were kept. Daily urinary creatinine levels were determined to assess the completeness of urine collection. Urine samples from one of the steroid users were not included in the data due to incomplete collections. Composites of 5-d urinary samples for each subject were used for analysis.

At the end of the dietary record period, subjects reported to the laboratory at 7:15 A.M. after an overnight fast. After a 20 min seated rest, a 15 ml sample of venous blood was drawn by a trained phlebotomist. One subject in the nonuser group refused to provide blood samples for analysis. Serum levels of calcium, phosphorus, iron, creatinine, the hematological concentrations, and alkaline phosphatase, which is a metalloenzyme that is sensitive to zinc deficiency, were determined photometrically by the method of Henry,[34] Winsten,[35] and Tietz.[36] Testosterone was determined using radioimmunoassay (Diagnostic Products Corporation).[37] The 5-d dietary intake was analyzed using N-squared Nutritionist III,[38] a computerized diet analysis program based on nutrient data standards from all the USDA Agricultural Handbooks.

IV. STATISTICAL ANALYSIS

A two-tailed *t*-test was used to compare differences between the steroid and nonsteroid groups using the SPSS-X computer package. An equal variance of the two groups was tested. When the *f*-test was significant at the $p < 0.05$ level, the separate variance estimate for *t*-test was used to determine the level of significance. Otherwise, the pooled variance estimate for the *t*-test was used.

V. RESULTS AND DISCUSSION

There were no differences between the groups in the mean age, height, weight, and physical activities (Table 1). A wide variety of steroids were self-administered. Eleven subjects used varieties of anabolic steroids, while only one subject reported using HCG (Human Chorionic Gonadotropin). The description and the patterns of steroids used by the subjects are summarized in Table 2. The subjects reported that other drugs were not used during the study period.

All the subjects followed strict and consistent dietary intakes throughout the study period. All the subjects supplemented their diets with either a single nutrient or combinations of nutrients shown in Table 3. There were no significant differences in either dietary fiber, calcium, magnesium, phosphorus, mean calcium to phosphorus ratio, zinc, or iron as presented in Table 4. However, steroid users' dietary protein and copper intakes were significantly higher at $p < 0.02$ and $p < 0.04$, respectively.

Athletes' diets do not seem to be deficient in copper, and widespread deficiencies in body status have not been documented. Although it has been shown that copper is lost in sweat,[39] this loss seems to be easily corrected by a well-balanced diet. The mean dietary copper intake for steroid users in this study was above the recommended amount, but nonusers' mean copper intake was within the recommended amount.

Table 5 illustrates the number of steroid users and nonusers consuming nutrients at various percent ranges of the 1980 Recommended Dietary Allowances (RDA). Twelve steroid users consumed over 100% of the RDA for energy, iron, and phosphorus. Eleven subjects and nine subjects consumed over 100% of the RDA for calcium and magnesium, respectively. Six subjects consumed over 100% for copper and four for zinc. However, eight nonusers consumed over 100% of the RDA for energy, twelve for calcium and iron; thirteen for phosphorus, nine for magnesium, and one for copper. One steroid user consumed 75% or less for copper, and three for zinc. Also one and five users consumed less than 50% of the RDA for magnesium and copper, respectively. Six, two, one, and three nonusers consumed 75% or less of the RDA for copper, iron, and zinc, respectively. Two consumed less than 75% for energy and magnesium. Two, three, and four nonusers consumed 50% or less for magnesium, zinc, and copper, respectively. Higher intakes of nutrients above the Recommended Dietary Allowances observed in this study is similar to that reported by Kleiner et al.[4] Kleiner et al.[4] reported that caloric consumption was 44% carbohydrate, 22% protein, and 34% fat for all the subjects studied. The percent of caloric consumption of 52% carbohydrate, 22% protein, and 24% fat for steroid users, and 48% carbohydrate, 17% protein, and 33% fat for nonusers, was observed in this study.

Serum testosterone, calcium, phosphorus, iron, creatinine, alkaline phosphatase, and hematological parameters are presented in Table 6. There were no significant

TABLE I   Mean Age, Physical Acitivity, Height,
           and Weight of Anabolic Steroid Users
           and Nonusers

	Anabolic Steroid Users (n = 12)	Nonusers (n = 13)
Age (y)	22.10 ± 0.87	23.51 ± 1.19
Height (cm)	176.42 ± 2.38	182.48 ± 1.93
Weight (kg)	90.18 ± 3.17	84.40 ± 2.88
Exercise (h/week)	11.25 ± 1.40	9.38 ± 1.30

Note: The data were expressed as mean ± SEM for each group.

TABLE 2   Dose Patterns of the Substances Used by Twelve Weightlifters

Drug/Chemical Name	Trade Name	Daily Dosage	Duration (months)	Number of Subjects/ Substance
Danazol	Novadex	50.0 mg.	3.0	2
Human chorionic gonadotropin	HCG	1000 unit	3.0	1
Methandrostenolone	Dianabol	1.0–45.0 mg	3.0	6
Nandrolone decanoate	Deca-Durabolin	14.0–100.0 mg	3.0	7
Testosterone cyclopentyl propionate	Depot-Testosterone Cypionate	57.0–58.0 mg	3.0	4
Norethandrolone	Nilevar	5.0–10.0 mg	3.0	1
Oxymetholone	Anadrol	42.0–43.0 mg	3.0	1
Andecyclenate	Equipose	100.0 mg	2.5	1
Oxandrolone	Anavar	2.0–17.5 mg	1.5–3.0	4
Stanozolol	Winstrol	20.0–120.0 mg	1.5	5

TABLE 3   Supplements Used by Both Groups

Supplement	Number of Subjects Using Supplements
Free-form amino acids	9
Carbo fuel[a]	1
Muscle fuel[a]	1
Multivitamin	9
B-complex vitamins	2
Liver tablet	1
Challenge liquid protein[b]	1
Milk/egg protein drink[b]	1

[a]   A carbohydrate powder
[b]   A protein drink

TABLE 4   Mean Mineral, Protein, Fat, Energy, and Fiber Intakes of Anabolic Steroid Users and Nonusers

	Anabolic Steroid Users (*n* = 12)	Nonuser (*n* = 13)
Energy intake (kcal/d)	3457.25 ± 164.92	3065.23 ± 358.69
Carbohydrate (g/d)	479.20 ± 38.46	397.04 ± 52.80
Fat (g/d)	45.49 ± 7.49	59.56 ± 8.11
Protein (g/d)	195.32 ± 17.18	143.08 ± 13.30
Calcium (mg/d)	1571.75 ± 216.62	1508.92 ± 325.76
Phosphorus (mg/d)	2214.25 ± 213.19	2012.69 ± 332.38
Magnesium (mg/d)	523.02 ± 70.00	380.91 ± 64.59
Fiber (g/d)	23.97 ± 4.87	16.75 ± 2.80
Phosphorus/calcium	1.67 ± 0.21	1.48 ± 0.13
Magnesium (mg/d)	523.02 ± 70.00	380.91 ± 64.59
Fiber (g/d)	23.97 ± 4.87	16.75 ± 2.80
Phosphorus/calcium	1.67 ± 0.21	1.48 ± 0.13
Iron (mg/d)	29.01 ± 4.06	22.15 ± 2.49
Zinc (mg/d)	14.02 ± 1.07	13.71 ± 2.13
Copper (mg/d)	3.14 ± 0.76	1.47 ± 0.23

Note: Data are expressed as mean ± SEM for each group. The difference in protein and copper intake were significant at $p < 0.02$ and $p < 0.04$, respectively.

TABLE 5   The Number of Anabolic Steroid Users and Nonusers Consuming Selected Nutrients at Selected Percent Ranges of the Recommend Dietary Allowances

Nutrients	Anabolic Steroid Users (*n* = 12)				
	Under 25%	26–50%	51%–75%	76–100%	Over 100%
Energy					12
Calcium				1	11
Phosphorus					12
Magnesium		1		2	9
Iron					12
Zinc			3	5	4
Copper		5	1	6	

Nutrients	Nonusers (*n* = 13)				
	Under 25%	26–50%	51–75%	76–100%	Over 100%
Energy			2	3	8
Calcium				1	12
Phosphorus					13
Magnesium		2	2		9
Iron			1		12
Zinc		3	3	2	5
Copper		4	6	2	1

TABLE 6   Serum Testosterone, Creatinine, Alkaline Phosphatase, Mineral Levels, and Hematological Parameters of Anabolic Steroid Users and Nonusers

	Anabolic Steroid Users ($n = 12$)	Nonusers ($n = 12$)
Testosterone (ng/dl)	2128.67 ± 532.97	738.35 ± 50.12
Calcium (mg/dl)	9.41 ± 0.16	9.80 ± 0.21
Phosphorus (mg/dl)	4.57 ± 0.22	4.45 ± 0.24
Alkaline Phosphatase (u/l)	92.00 ± 10.60	81.41 ± 5.76
Creatinine (mg/dl)	1.35 ± 0.04	1.27 ± 0.04
Hemoglobin (gm/dl)	16.29 ± 0.23	15.92 ± 0.38
Hematocrit (v%)	48.40 ± 0.80	46.43 ± 1.32
Total Protein (mg/dl)	6.77 ± 0.18	7.20 ± 0.22
Albumin (g/dl)	4.45 ± 0.09	4.72 ± 0.11
Iron (µg/dl)	93.83 ± 7.54	107.66 ± 11.07
RBC (× 106/mm3)	7.01 ± 1.62	5.10 ± 0.15
WBC (× 103/mm3)	9.10 ± 0.99	7.36 ± 0.53

Note: The data were expressed as mean ± SEM for each group. The difference in the serum testosterone was significant at $p < 0.02$.

differences between the groups in either serum calcium, phosphorus, or alkaline phosphatase. However, serum testosterone level was significantly higher for Group A at $p < 0.01$. There has been very little research on the effect of anabolic steroids on serum testosterone levels. However, some side effects generally recognized by steroid users, such as irritability, increased aggressiveness, and personality changes, could be attributed to the increase in serum testosterone levels.

The use of high dosage of anabolic steroids/testosterone has been said to lead to long-lasting impairment of normal testosterone endocrine function.[40] A study by Alen et al.[41] with five male power athletes showed that after 26 weeks of anabolic steroid and testosterone administration, serum testosterone concentrations increased 2.3-fold. However, the cessation of anabolic steroid administration brought about a reduction in serum testosterone levels below normal. This effect lasted throughout the 12 to 16 week follow-up period, indicating long-lasting impairment of testicular endocrine function. The impairment of the endocrine function may lead to testosterone deficiency, and subsequently to osteoporosis later in life.

Urinary calcium, phosphorus, magnesium, creatinine, and phosphorus to calcium ratio are summarized in Table 7. There were no differences between groups in the urinary calcium, phosphorus, magnesium, creatinine, and phosphorus to calcium ratio. However, anabolic steroid users excreted slightly higher urinary calcium than nonusers.

In conclusion, anabolic steroids are widely used by athletes seeking gains in muscle size and strength.[42,43,44] These drugs produce well-documented adverse medical effects but the effect of anabolic steroids on nutrient utilization have rarely been examined. This study showed slightly higher urinary calcium excretion in the steroid

TABLE 7   Urinary Mineral and Creatinine Excretions
of Anabolic Steroid Users and Nonusers

	Anabolic steroid users (n = 11)	Non-Users (n = 13)
Calcium (mg/d)	226.20 ± 44.20	189.30 ± 24.73
Phosphorus (mg/d)	1060.10 ± 127.41	1193.84 ± 69.50
Magnesium (mg/d)	7.80 ± 0.82	7.11 ± 0.64
Creatinine (mg/kg)	23.50 ± 1.60	23.63 ± 1.41
Phosphorus/calcium	6.22 ± 0.60	7.61 ± 1.10

Note: The data are expressed as mean ± SEM for each group.

users. High dosage of anabolic steroid resulted in high serum testosterone levels. It has been reported that serum testosterone levels decrease below normal after the cessation of anabolic steroids administration. If this decrease continues over a long period of time, a reduction in bone density may occur and osteoporosis might set in at an early age. Many athletes are taking supplements without regard for specific deficiencies, even after supplementation they remain deficient in certain nutrients. Parr et al.[45] found that those athletes who were familiar with dietary guidelines used them regularly. This suggests that if athletes become acquainted with proper nutrition education, they will make use of it. It would seems then, that an important task for exercise and health professionals is to provide athletes with proper nutrition information on sports nutrition so that they are not left to rely on some of the enticing, and sometimes misleading, information presented in the media.

REFERENCES

1. Freed, D. L. J., Bank, A. J., Longson, D., Anabolic steroids in athletics: crossover double-blind trial on weightlifters, *Br. Med. J.*, 2, 471, 1976.
2. Hervey, G. R., Are Athletes wrong about anabolic steroids?, *Br. J. Sports Med.*, 9, 74, 1975.
3. Grunby, P., A medical team goes to olympic, *J. Am. Med. Assoc.*, 252(4), 454, 1984.
4. Kleiner, S. M., Leonard, H., Calabrese, D. O., Karen, M., Fielder, H. K., Naito, C., and Skibinski, I., Dietary influences on cardiovascular disease risk in anabolic steroid-using and nonusing bodybuilders, *J. Am. Coll. Nutr.*, 8(2), 109, 1989.
5. Lamb, D. R., Anabolic steroids in athletics, How well do they work and how dangerous are they?, *Am. J. Sport Med.*, 12(1), 31, 1984.
6. Rosenballm, D. and Sutton, J. R., Drugs and exercise, *Med. Clin. N. Am.*, 69(1), 177, 1985.
7. Alen, M., Rahkila, P., Marniewm, J., Serum lipids in power athletes self-administering testosterone and anabolic steroids, *Int. J. Sport Med.*, 6(1), 24, 1985.
8. Lenders, J. W. M., Demacker, P. N. M., Jansen, J. S., Hoitsma V. L., Thien, T., Deleterious effects of anabolic steroids on serum lipoproteins, blood pressure, and liver function in amateur body builders, *Int. J. Sports Med.*, 9, 19, 1988.
9. Fahey, T. D. and Brown, C. H., The effects of an anabolic steroid on the strength, body composition, and endurance of college males when accompanied by a weight training program, *Med. Sci. Sports*, 5, 272, 1973.
10. Johnson, L. C., Fisher, G., Silvester, L. J., Anabolic steroid: effects on strength, body weight, oxygen uptake and spermatogenesis upon nature males, *Med. Sci. Sports*, 4, 43, 1972.

11. Williams, M. H., *Nutritional Aspects of Human Physical and Athletic Performance*, 2nd ed., Charles C. Thomas, Springfield, IL, 1985.
12. Pao, E. M. and Mickle, S. J., Changes in American food consumption patterns and their nutritional significance, *Food Technology*, 35, 43, 1981.
13. Food and Nutrition Board, National Academy of Sciences — National Research Council, Recommended Daily Allowances, 9th ed., Washington, D.C., Academy Press, 1980.
14. Johnson, N. E., Alcantara, E. N., Linkswiler, H., Effect of level of protein intake on urinary and fecal calcium and calcium retention of young adult males, *J. Nutr.*, 100, 1425, 1970.
15. Walker, R. and Linkswiler, H., Calcium retention in the adult human male as affected by protein intake, *J. Nutr.*, 102, 1297, 1972.
16. Meredith, C. N., Zackin, M. J., Frontera, W. R., Evans, W. J., Dietary protein requirements and body protein metabolism in endurance-trained men, *J. Appl. Physiol.*, 66(6), 2850, 1989.
17. Cousins, R. J., Absorption, transport, and hepatic metabolism of copper and zinc: special reference to metallothionein and celuloplasmin, *Physiol. Rev.*, 65, 238, 1985.
18. Kruse-Jarres, J. D., Clinical indication for trace element analyses, *J. Trace Elem. Electrolytes Health Dis.*, 1, 5, 1987.
19. Bazzarre T. L., Marquart, L. F., Izurieta, M., Jones, A., Incidence of poor nutritional status among triathletes, endurance athletes and control subjects, *Med. Sci. Sports Exercise*, 18(2), s446, 1986.
20. Couzy, F., Lafargue, P., Guezennec, C. Y., Zinc metabolism in the athlete: influence of training nutrition and other factors, *Int. J. Sports Med.*, 11, 263, 1990.
21. Anderson, R. A., and Guttman, H. N., Trace minerals and exercise, in *Exercise, Nutrition, and Energy Metabolism*, Horton E. and Terjung R.L., Eds., Macmillian, New York, 180, 1988.
22. Lukaski, H. C., Influence of physical training on human copper nutritional status, Abstract of the *Am. Chem. Soc.*, 197, 91, 1989.
23. Dowdy, R. P. and Burt, J., Effect of intensive, long-term training on copper and iron nutriture in man, *Fed. Proc.*, 39, 786, 1980.
24. Marrella, M., Guerrini, F., Tregnaghi, P. L., Nocini, S., Velo, G. P., Milanino, R., Effect of copper, zinc and ceruloplasmin levels in blood of athletes, metal ions in biology and medicine, *Proc. 1st Int. Symp.*, 16, 111, 1990.
25. Ehn, L. Carlmark, B., Hoglund, S., Iron status in athletes involved in intense physical activity, *Med. Sci. Sports Exercise*, 12, 61, 1980.
26. Wishnitzer, R., Vorst, E., Berrebi, A., Bone marrow iron depression in competitive distance runners, *Int. J. Sports Med.*, 4, 27, 1983.
27. Dufaux, B., Hoederath, A., Streitberger, I., Hollmann, W., Assmann, G., Serum ferritin, transferrin, haptoglobin, and iron in middle and long-distance runners, elite rowers, and professional racing cyclists, *Int. J. Sports Med.*, 2,43,1981.
28. Clement, D. B. and Asmundson R. C., Nutritional intake and hematological parameters in endurance runners, *Phys. Sports Med.*, 10, 37,1982.
29. Casoni, B. C., Cavicchi, A., Martinelli, S., Conconi, F., Reduced hemoglobin concentration and red cell hemoglobinization in Italian marathon and ultramarathon runners, *Int. J. Sports Med.*, 6, 176, 1985.
30. Chestnut, C. H., An appraisal of the role of estrogens in the treatment of postmenopausal osteoporosis, *J. Am. Geriat. Soc.*, 32, 604, 1984.
31. Avioli, L. V., Senile and postmenopausal osteoporosis, *Adv. Intern. Tiss. Int.*, 26, 103, 1978.
32. Odell, W. D. and Swerdlow, R. S., Male hypogonadism, *W. J. Med.*, 124, 446, 1976.
33. Baran, D. T., Bergfeld, M. A., Teitelbaum, S. L., Effect of testosterone therapy on bone formation in an osteoporotic hypogonadal male, *Calc. Tiss. Int.*, 26, 103, 1978.
34. Henry, D. S., *Clinical Chemistry Principles and Technics*, 2nd ed., Harper and Row, Hagerstown, MD., 1974.
35. Winsten S., Standard method, *Clin. Chem.*, 5, 1965, 1
36. Tietz, N., *Clinical Guide to Laboratory Tests*, W. B. Saunders, Philadelphia, 1983, 384, 386.
37. Radioimmunoassays, Diagnostic Product Cooperation, 5700 West 96th Street, Los Angeles, CA 90045.

38. N-Squared Computing Analytic Software, 5318 Forest Ridge Road, Silverton, Oregon 97381.
39. Gutteridge, J. M. C., Rowley, D. A., Halliwell, B., Cooper, D. F., Heeley, D. M., Copper and iron complexes catalytic for oxygen radical reactions in sweat from human athletes, *Clin. Chim. Acta,* 145, 267, 1985.
40. McArdle, W. D., Katch, F. I., Katch. V. L., *Exercise Physiology: Energy, Nutrition, and Human Performance,* 2 ed., Lea and Febiger, Philadelphia, 1986, 402.
41. Alen, M., Reinila, M., Vihko, R., Response of serum hormones to androgen administration in power athletes, *Med. Sci. Sports Exercise,* 17, 354, 1985.
42. Markku, A., Matti, R., Reijo, V., Androgen administration in power athletes, *Med. Sci. Sports Exercise,* 17, 354, 1985.
43. Harrison, G., Pope, H. G., Katz, D. L., Affective and psychotic symptoms associated with anabolic steroid use, *Am. J. Psych.,* 145, 487, 1988.
44. Haupt, H. A. and Rovere, G. D., Anabolic steroids: a review of the literature, *Am. J. Sports Med.,* 12, 469, 1984.
45. Parr, R. B., Porter, M. A., Hodgson, S. C., Nutrition knowledge and practices of coaches, trainers, and athletes, *Phys. Sports Med.,* 12, 126, 1984.

Chapter 22

MINERAL AND ENERGY STATUS OF GROUPS OF MALE AND FEMALE ATHLETES PARTICIPATING IN EVENTS BELIEVED TO RESULT IN ADVERSE NUTRITIONAL STATUS

Jean T. Snook
David Cummin
Philip R. Good
Jennifer Grayzar

CONTENTS

I. INTRODUCTION

Although good nutritional status is important for athletes striving for optimal athletic performance, there are athletes who are so concerned about body weight, especially as it affects performance, that dietary adequacy is of secondary interest. This chapter focuses on samples of two groups of athlete competing in varsity sports in a large midwestern university. The first sample is comprised of women competing in track events. Many female runners seem discontented with their weight and have the perception that thinner is faster.[1] Because female long-distance runners in particular appear to be at risk of developing amenorrhea and iron deficiency,[2,3] we compared diets and some biochemical parameters of nutritional status in three groups of women: long-distance runners, short-distance sprinters, and sedentary college women not participating in sports or exercise programs.

The wrestling community has an established tradition of weight loss prior to competition, and an entrenched belief that rapid weight loss will not decrease athletic performance. Prior to competition wrestlers lose 2 to 5 kg by a combination of techniques including dehydration, caloric reduction, and exercise.[4] With this cycle of weight loss occurring many times during a wrestling, the effect on health and nutritional status could be serious. We will report the results of a study of our second sample involving comparison of nutritional status of two groups of wrestlers. One group underwent weight cycling during the wrestling season to compete in a certain weight class. The second group practiced with the varsity wrestlers, but did not lose weight or compete. A novel aspect of this study is that the wrestlers were assessed at two points during the competitive season to determine if nutritional status declined with recurring weight loss.

II. SUBJECTS AND METHODS

A. SUBJECTS

This research was descriptive in nature. In the study of the women competing in varsity track, a sample of 7 long-distance runners and 12 sprinters from The Ohio State University women's track team were recruited. All active, uninjured members of the team participated with the encouragement of their coaches. Twenty sedentary women were also selected to serve as a control group. All subjects were fully informed about the protocol and signed a consent form approved by The Ohio State University Biomedical Human Subjects Review Committee. The sedentary control subjects did not exceed 35% body fat based upon bioelectric impedance assessment (RJL Systems, Detroit, MI). The sedentary subjects did not participate in vigorous exercise for greater than 30 min per week. Data were collected during the first half of the track and field season, from January to March.

The wrestlers were studied during the second half of the wrestling season which began in November and ended in March. A sample of 7 wrestlers who practiced weight cycling to compete in a specific weight class was compared to a sample of 8 wrestlers who practiced with the team but did not compete or lose weight. Data collections were conducted in the second week of January and the last week of February to assess the effects of additional cycles of weight loss on biochemical measures of nutritional status. All subjects signed an approved consent form before participating. After-practice weights of all participants were taken for 3 and 7 d, respectively, prior to the first and second blood drawings. A Toledo scale located in the wrestling team locker room was used to weigh the wrestlers.

B. METHODS

All subjects consumed self-selected diets and completed a 3-d diet record (one weekend day and two weekdays) prior to having their blood drawn. Detailed written and verbal instructions on how to complete the records were given. The women completed one 3-d record; the male wrestlers completed a 3-d record during each of the two collection periods coinciding with a time when competing wrestlers were restricting food energy to lose weight. Each diet was analyzed by a computerized nutrient data base, Food Processor II (ESHA Corporation, Salem, OR). All nutritional supplements consumed by the subjects were added to the nutrient data base and included in the diet analyses. Selenium intakes were calculated by hand using a data base compiled for foods grown and/or purchased in Ohio.[5]

Each subject completed a 7-d recall of activities at the time of blood drawing using a questionnaire developed by Blair et al.[6] To verify the accuracy of the recall an activity monitor (Caltrac, Hemokinetics, Inc., Madison, WI) was worn by each of the women subjects for a period of two weekdays. Caltrac is a motion sensor detector (accelerometer) worn on the belt; it can be programmed to calculate resting metabolic rate and to simultaneously give a value for total energy expenditure. The limitation of Caltrac seems to be its inability to measure isometric forms of activities and exercise in which the body is partially supported.[7]

For measurements of serum parameters, fasting venous blood samples were drawn without stasis from an antecubital vein into a evacuated tube containing either EDTA (for hemoglobin, hematocrit, and erythrocyte glutathione reductase activity) or no anticoagulant (for ferritin determination). Fresh whole blood samples were analyzed for hemoglobin by the cyanomethemoglobin method using a kit and control preparation obtained from Sigma Diagnostics (St. Louis, MO). Hematocrits were performed in a microhematocrit centrifuge. Ferritin concentrations were determined in serum previously frozen at $-80°C$ using a radioimmunoassay kit (Micromedic Systems, Inc., Horsham, PA). Plasma and whole blood selenium-dependent glutathione peroxidase were measured by a modification of the method described by Cantor and Tarino.[8] Riboflavin status was assessed by measuring erythrocyte glutathione reductase activity according to the method described by Tillotson and Baker.[9] Erythrocytes were isolated from fresh whole blood, washed three times with saline, and stored at $-80°C$ until the spectrophotometric *in vitro* analysis, which was performed with and without added riboflavin cofactor (FAD). The erythrocyte glutathione reductase activity coefficient (EGRAC) was determined by dividing the rate of change in absorbance of the assay mixture over a 10 min period with added FAD by the rate of change observed without added FAD. An EGRAC of 1.00 would indicate no stimulation, while a value of 1.20 is suggestive of inadequate riboflavin status.[9-11]

Standard two-tailed student's *t*-test and analysis of variance (Minitab, Inc. Data Analysis Software, State College, PA) were used to detect significant differences ($p < 0.05$) between the groups of wrestlers and groups of women, respectively.

III. RESULTS AND DISCUSSION

A. SUBJECT CHARACTERISTICS

The long-distance runners, sprinters, and sedentary control women did not differ in age, height, or weight (Table 1). Similarly, percent body fat, as determined by bioelectrical impedance assessment, did not differ significantly among the three groups although the sedentary women on average had a higher proportion of body fat. Average percentages of body fat were 22.4 ± 1.7 for the long-distance runner, 22.3 ± 1.1 for the sprinters, and 25.2 ± 0.9 for the sedentary women. Nutrient supplement use tended to be higher among the women competing in track events (Table 1). Reported incidence of irregular menses was highest in the long-distance runners (Table 1). Subjective reports on menstrual function will not identify all menstrual irregularities, e.g., luteal phase deficiency, since the respondents may not be aware of any abnormality.[12] Exercise-related menstrual dysfunction occurs in women participating in a variety of sports, but has been studied most often in runners.[12] One long-distance runner had a body fat percentage of 15.5. The other long-distance runners had body fat exceeding 20%. Thus, a low body fat content did not explain the incidence of irregular menses in the long-distance runners.

The competing and noncompeting groups of wrestlers did not differ significantly in age, height, or initial body weight as determined during the recruitment period, although the noncompeting wrestlers tended to be somewhat larger than the group that competed almost weekly in wrestling matches (Table 2). Percent body water was determined by bioelectric impedance in the two groups of wrestlers in both the dehydrated (after practice) and rehydrated state. Results suggested that the competing wrestlers maintained, on average, a higher proportion of body water than the nonweight loss wrestlers in both hydrated and dehydrated states, although differences were not statistically significant. Weight loss wrestlers averaged about $66 \pm 1\%$ water in both states whereas noncompeting wrestlers averaged 60.6 ± 3.0 and $63.3 \pm 2.0\%$ water in the dehydrated and rehydrated states, respectively. According to the instructions furnished by the manufacturer, the bioelectric impedance apparatus is not as accurate when water balance is abnormal; therefore, no effort was made to calculate body fat by this method. The accuracy of the body water measurements is not clear.

Four of the seven weight loss wrestlers consumed nutritional supplements during the study including a sport drink, multivitamins, and a protein supplement.

TABLE 1   Characteristics of Women Competing in Track and Sedentary Controls

Group	Age Years	Height cm	Weight kg	Irreg. Menses (%)	Supplement Use (%)
Long-distance	19 ± 0.4	169 ± 3	57 ± 3	57	43
runners (*n* = 7)	(18–20)[a]	(157–177)	(47–66)		
Sprinters	19 ± 0.3	167 ± 1	56 ± 1	10	40
(*n* = 12)	(18–21)	(157–173)	(49–65)		
Sedentary	21 ± 0.3	163 ± 1	57 ± 1	10	24
(*n* = 20)	(19–23)	(157–170)	(45–70)		

Note: Values are means ± SEM.

[a]   Range of values.

B. ENERGY INTAKE AND ESTIMATES OF PHYSICAL ACTIVITY

Energy expenditure, as estimated by activity recall and Caltrac activity monitor, was higher in the long distance runners than in the sprinters and sedentary women (Table 3). The Caltrac also predicted higher activity in sprinters than in sedentary women. The physical activity recall predicted higher mean energy expenditures than did Caltrac in all groups of subjects, although not in all individuals. Nevertheless, the correlation between the two methods was high in long-distance runners ($r = 0.95$) but was not significant in the other two groups. Since a more accurate criterion method of measuring energy expenditure, such as doubly labeled water, was not used in this study, it is difficult to assess whether 7-d activity recall or Caltrac most accurately estimated energy expenditure. One obvious conclusion is that these two methods cannot be used to quantitate energy expenditure in individuals but may accurately depict differences in energy expenditure between groups.

Energy intake, as determined by 3-d food records, tended to be lower in long-distance runners than in the other two groups of women, although differences among groups were not significant. Energy intake of all three groups was less than estimated energy expenditure. In previous studies of obese and nonobese adolescents and female athletes,[13,14] energy expenditure by the doubly labeled water technique considerably exceeded reported food energy intake. Other work involving measures of energy expenditure of elite female runners by doubly labeled water and indirect calorimetry imply that women competing in endurance events do not have energy needs that are lower than might be expected.[15] Although energy intake may not be optimal for the long-distance runners in this study, the discrepancy between intake and expenditure suggested by our data is probably not real considering that groups of subjects did not differ in body size.

Energy intake was significantly lower in the weight loss wrestlers than noncompeting wrestlers (Table 4). This result was not surprising considering the competing wrestlers were in the process of restricting food energy to make a particular weight category. The energy restriction, and probably also dehydration practices, applied during the days before competition, successfully resulted in weight loss in the competing group, although the changes in weight were not especially

TABLE 2 Characteristics of Subjects Participating in Study of Collegiate Male Wrestlers

Group	Age (years)	Height (cm)	Initial Weight (kg)
Weight loss (competing) (n = 7)	20 ± 1 (19–22)[a]	172 ± 3 (163–183)	70 ± 5 (54–88)
Not competing (n = 8)	21 ± 1 (19–27)	182 ± 4 (166–188)	82 ± 7 (59–123)

Note: Values are means ± SEM.

[a] Range of values.

TABLE 3 Energy Intake (3-d Records) and Daily Energy Expenditure Determined By 7-d Activity Recall and Caltrac Activity Monitor of Runners, Sprinters, and Sedentary Women (Means ± SEM)

Group	Energy Intake kcal × d⁻¹	Energy % from Carbohydrate	7-d Recall of Activity kcal × d⁻¹	Caltrac kcal × d⁻¹
Long-distance runners (n = 7)	1634 ± 250 (901–2712)[b]	61 ± 8 (35–79)	3290 ± 184[a] (2646–3943)	2594 ± 155[a] (2317–3100)
Sprinters (n = 11)	1890 ± 174 (1017–2341)	51 ± 3 (39–61)	2443 ± 184 (1974–3809)	2160 ± 42[c] (1964–2415)
Sedentary (n = 20)	1742 ± 96 (1133–2544)	51 ± 2 (35–64)	2120 ± 66 (1538–2704)	1793 ± 53 (1510–2314)

[a] Significantly higher ($p < 0.05$) than sprinters and sedentary group.
[b] Range of values.
[c] Significantly higher ($p < 0.05$) than sedentary group.

large. Again, physical activity recall predicted mean energy expenditures much greater than mean energy intakes even in the noncompeting group. In this case the mean energy expenditures predicted by physical activity recall appeared to be inaccurate in individuals, some of whom estimated they expended over 7000 kcal/d.

C. IRON INTAKE AND HEMATOLOGICAL PARAMETERS

Iron intake, including supplemental iron, was below 90% of the RDA of 15 mg/d in 50% of the long-distance runners and sedentary women (Table 5). Only 18% of the sprinters had iron intakes below 90% of the RDA. The incidence of marginal or unacceptable hemoglobin and hematocrit values was lower than the incidence of below standard iron intakes. Iron stores, as indicated by serum ferritin values, were unacceptable in 29% of the long distance runners and 18% of the sprinters. Unacceptable hematological measures were found in only one sedentary woman. These results agree with some similar work performed by other researchers. [16,17]

TABLE 4   Energy Intake (3-d Record), Weight Loss, and Physical Activity (7-d Activity Recall) of Collegiate Wrestlers at Two Times During the Competitive Season

Group	Energy Intake kcal × day⁻¹		Weight change[a] kg		Physical activity kcal × d⁻¹	
	Jan.	**Feb.**	**Jan.**	**Feb.**	**Jan.**	**Feb.**
Weight loss	2214 ± 405[b]	1942 ± 288[b]	–2.0 ± 0.4[b]	–2.5 ± 0.7[b]	4292 ± 601	4541 ± 597
(competing)	(1078,4183)[c]	(1049,3374)	(–3.2,0)	(–5,–1.1)	(3070,7525)	(2784,6871)
(n = 7)						
Not	3437 ± 355	3234 ± 520	0.6 ± 0.4	0.7 ± 0.4	4771 ± 525	4674 ± 529
competing	(2366,5131)	(1277,5613)	(–1.1,0.3)	(–0.9,2.3)	(2139,6505)	(2882,7012)
(n = 8)						

[a]   Jan. weight change was measured over 3 d prior to competition; Feb. weight change was measured for 6 d prior to competition.
[b]   Different from weight loss group (p <0.05).
[c]   Values in parentheses represent low and high values for the measurement.

TABLE 5   Hematological Status Data of Long-Distance Runners, Sprinters and Sedentary Women

Group	Hemoglobin g × dl⁻¹	Hematocrit %	Serum Ferritin ug × L⁻¹	Iron Intake[a] mg × d⁻¹
Long-distance	12.2 ± 0.2[b]	38.6 ± 0.6	28.7 ± 6.0[d]	20.2 ± 6.8
runners (n = 7)	(11.2–12.8)[c]	(36.5–40.0)	(10.0–55.0)	(5.0–42.3)
% unacceptable[e]	29	14	29	50
Sprinters	13.8 ± 0.5	39.7 ± 0.9	39.7 ± 8.3	16.0 ± 1.6
(n = 12)	(10.7–15.8)	(37.0–44.5)	(6.0–107.0)	(7.1–29.0)
% unacceptable[e]	8	0	18	18
Sedentary	13.8 ± 0.2	40.3 ± 0.4	56.6 ± 6.4	13.4 ± 1.1
(n = 20)	(11.9–15.3)	(36.0–43.0)	(11.0–106.0)	(6.3–26.3)
% unacceptable[e]	5	5	5	50

Note: Means ± SEM
[a]   From 3-d diet records (2 weekdays, 1 weekend day).
[b]   Significantly lower (p <0.05) than sprinters and sedentary group.
[c]   Range of values.
[d]   Significantly lower (p <0.05) than sedentary group.
[e]   Hemoglobin <12 mg/dl; hematocrit <37%; serum ferritin <18ug/l; iron intake <90% of the RDA.

Iron intake was less than 90% of the RDA in 2 to 3 of 7 of the competing wrestlers (Table 6). Nevertheless, hematocrit was unacceptable in only one competing wrestler during each of the data collection periods. Iron stores, as indicated by serum ferritin values, were acceptable in all of the competing wrestlers. Inexplicably, hematocrit values were below 44% in 4 of 7 noncompeting wrestlers during the February collection period; however, 3 of the 4 had values of 43%. Serum ferritin was unacceptable in one noncompeting wrestler during the January collection period. In

TABLE 6   Hematological and Iron Status Data of Collegiate Male Wrestlers at Two Times During the Competitive Season

Group	Iron Intake[a] mg × d⁻¹		Hematocrit %		Serum Ferritin ug × L⁻¹	
	Jan.	Feb.	Jan.	Feb.	Jan.	Feb.
Weight loss	18.0 ± 4.1	14.5 ± 1.9	46 ± 1	45 ± 2	93 ± 13	107 ± 23
(competing)	(5.6–26.1)[b]	(8.5–20.5)	(43–49)	(38–49)	(36–105)	(29–220)
(*n* = 7)						
< standard[c]	2/7	3/7	1/7	1/7	0/7	0/7
Not competing	27.0 ± 2.8	28.0 ± 7.4	46 ± 1	44 ± 1	111 ± 40	84 ± 9
(*n* = 8)	(17.9–39.8)	(7.4–67.5)	(43–49)	(41–49)	(13–380)	(38–120)
< standard	0/8	0/8	1/7	4/7	1/8	0/8

Note: Values are means ± SEM.

[a]   From 3-day diet records.
[b]   Range of values.
[c]   Iron intake < 90% of RDA, hematocrit below 44%, serum ferritin <18 ug × l⁻¹.

general, it appeared that recurring energy restriction and weight loss did not impair hematological status in the competing wrestlers.

D. STATUS IN SELECTED MINERALS OTHER THAN IRON

Data were also collected on dietary intakes of selected minerals previously shown to be a problem in athletes competing in aerobic events (Table 7). Zinc, copper, and calcium intakes were below 90% of the RDA, or suggested intake, in 50 to 85% of the long-distance runners, sprinters, and sedentary women. Mean intakes of these minerals were below standard in all groups even though supplements were taken by some of the women. The incidence of low zinc and copper intakes was greater than 80% from food alone and greater than 50% with food and supplements in a study of female triathletes, while calcium intake was adequate in at least 80% of the women.[18]

Selenium status was of interest to our research group at the time the wrestling study was performed. Selenium intakes were below 90% of the RDA in almost half of the competing wrestlers and in only 1 of 8 noncompeting wrestlers (data not shown). Biochemical measures of selenium status (plasma and red blood cell glutathione peroxidase activities) indicated all of the wrestlers were in good selenium status despite the repeated bouts of low dietary intakes by the competing wrestlers.

E. RIBOFLAVIN INTAKE AND ERYTHROCYTE GLUTATHIONE REDUCTASE ACTIVITY

Based on the 3-d dietary record, all groups of female subjects reported adequate mean riboflavin intakes (Table 8). Although the long-distance runners and sprinters reported a mean daily intake of over 1.90 mg, two of the long-distance runners and one sprinter did not meet even 70% of the RDA. Likewise the sedentary women's mean daily riboflavin intake was 1.66 mg; yet, three subjects also did not meet 70%

TABLE 7   Daily Intakes (3-d Records) of Selected Minerals
of Runners, Sprinters, and Sedentary Women
(Means ± SEM)

Group	Zinc mg × d⁻¹	Copper mg × d⁻¹	Calcium mg × d⁻¹
Long-distance	8.7 ± 1.5	1.3 ± 0.2	802 ± 245
runners (n = 7)	(2.4–12.1)[a]	(0.6–1.9)	(228–1927)
% low intake[b]	67	50	83
Sprinters	9.7 ± 0.9	1.2 ± 0.1	837 ± 149
(n = 11)	(5.0–12.7)	(0.4–1.9)	(176–1990)
% low intake	45	64	82
Sedentary	8.7 ± 0.7	1.3 ± 0.1	808 ± 58
(n = 20)	(5.2–17.4)	(0.8–2.4)	(466–1355)
% low intake	70	60	85

[a] Range of values.
[b] Below 90% of RDA or suggested intake.

TABLE 8   Daily Intake (3-d Records) of Riboflavin and Erythrocyte
Glutathione Reductase Activity Coefficients (EGRAC) of
Runners, Sprinters, and Sedentary Women (Mean ± SEM)

Group	Riboflavin mg × d⁻¹	EGRAC (*in vitro* activity with added ribo. × activity without added ribo.⁻¹)
Long-distance	1.95 ± 0.55	1.05 ± 0.04
runners (n = 7)	(0.53–3.59)[a]	(0.94–1.21)
% unacceptable[b]	50	14
Sprinters (n = 11)	1.96 ± 0.23	1.08 ± 0.02
	(0.58–3.39)	(0.95–1.19)
% unacceptable	9	0
Sedentary (n = 20)	1.66 ± 0.12	1.12 ± 0.02
	(0.66–2.57)	(1.00–1.27)
% unacceptable	15	15

[a] Range of values.
[b] Below 90% of RDA or an EGRAC of 1.20.

of the RDA. Erythrocyte glutathione reductase was used to check riboflavin status. Only one long-distance runner and three sedentary women displayed marginal status. Unlike our results suggesting poor iron status in some women athletes, our study did not indicate that either group of women athletes was deficient in riboflavin. This concern stemmed from two studies which inferred that active young women may require more riboflavin than the current RDA of 0.6 mg × 1000 kcal⁻¹.[10,11]

The wrestlers had higher mean riboflavin intakes with respect to the RDA than the groups of women we studied (Table 9). Nevertheless, individual riboflavin intakes were below 90% of the RDA in up to 30% of some collection groups. Biochemical evidence of marginal or unacceptable riboflavin status was also found

TABLE 9 Daily Intake (3-d Records) of Riboflavin and Erythrocyte Glutathione Reductase Activity Coefficients (EGRAC) of Male Collegiate Wrestlers (Means ± SEM)

| | Riboflavin Intake mg × d^{-1} | | EGRAC | |
Group	Jan.	Feb.	Jan.	Feb.
Weight loss	2.67 ± 0.73	1.83 ± 0.24	1.14 ± 0.08	1.09 ± 0.04
(competing)	(0.84–6.81)[a]	(0.96–2.74)	(0.95–1.62)	(0.96–1.26)
(n = 7)				
Below standard[b]	1/7	2/7	1/7	1/7
Not competing	3.76 ± 0.50	3.85 ± 1.10	1.13 ± 0.03	1.11 ± 0.04
(n = 8)	(1.45–5.42)	(1.13–9.17)	(1.02–1.28)	(0.98–1.35)
Below standard	1/8	2/8	1/8	2/8

[a] Range of values.
[b] Riboflavin intake below 90% of the RDA; EGRAC >1.20.

in the wrestlers and in some individuals was worse than that seen in individual women. For the most part, subjects with unacceptable EGRAC values consumed little or no milk and dairy products in their diets. However, the correlation between riboflavin intake and EGRAC values for both the weight loss and the nonweight loss groups of wrestlers was weak and nonsignificant ($r = -.242$). Thus, the dietary information could not be used to predict riboflavin status in these subjects.

III. SUMMARY AND CONCLUSIONS

In these studies of athletes believed to have special concerns about body weight and to be at risk of nutritional inadequacies we found that mean reported energy intake of long-distance runners, but not sprinters or sedentary women, was 40 to 50% lower than mean energy expenditures estimated by activity recall or monitor. Mean energy intake of wrestlers experiencing recurring weight loss was also 40 to 50% of mean energy expenditure estimated by activity recall.

Long-distance runners were in poorer hematologic status and had poorer iron stores than sprinters and sedentary women. Wrestlers who lost weight regularly to compete were not in poorer iron status than wrestlers who did not lose weight or compete. Mean intakes of zinc, copper, and calcium were low for all groups of exercising and sedentary college women. Biochemical evidence of poor riboflavin status was found in almost all female and male groups studied but it was not worse in the groups believed most at risk — long-distance runners and wrestlers experiencing recurring weight loss — than in control groups.

We concluded that women who compete in long-distance running events are at more risk nutritionally and physiologically than women who do not participate in endurance events and require special attention from nutritionists, coaches, and sports physicians. The sample of collegiate wrestlers at The Ohio State University was, for the most part, in adequate nutritional status despite recurring weight loss during the competitive season. More investigations are needed to determine the effects of weight loss on other samples of wrestlers, including high school wrestlers, who have adverse weight loss practices.

REFERENCES

1. Clark, N., Nelson, M., and Evans, W., Nutrition education for elite female runners, *Phys. Sportsmed.*, 16, 124, 1988.
2. Manore, M. M., Besenfelder, P. D., Wells, C. L., Carroll, S. S., and Hooker, S. P., Nutrient intakes and iron status in female long distance runners during training, *J. Am. Dietet. Assoc.*, 89, 257, 1989.
3. Barr, S. I., Women, nutrition and exercise: a review of athletes' intakes and a discussion of energy balance in active women, *Progress Food Nutr. Sci.*, 11, 307, 1987.
4. Tipton, C. M., Iowa wrestling study: weight loss in high school students, *J. A. M. A.*, 214, 1269, 1970.
5. Snook, J. T., Kinsey, D., Palmquist, D. L., Delany, J. P., Vivian, V. M., and Moxon, A. L., Selenium Content of foods purchased in Ohio, *J. Am. Dietet. Assoc.*, 87, 744, 1987.
6. Blair, S. N., Haskell, W. L., Ho, P., Paffenbarger, R. S. Jr., Vranizan, K. M., Farquhar, J. W., and Wood, P. D., Assessment of habitual physical activity by a seven-day recall in a community survey and controlled experiments, *Am. J. Epidemiol.*, 122, 794, 1985.
7. Montoye, H. J., Washburn, R., and Servais, S., Estimation of energy expenditure by a portable accelerometer, *Med. Sci. Sports Exercise*, 15, 403, 1983.
8. Cantor, A. H., and Tarino J. Z., Comparative effects of inorganic and organic dietary sources of selenium on selenium levels and selenium-dependent glutathione peroxidase activity in blood of young turkeys, *J. Nutr.*, 112, 2187, 1982.
9. Tillotson, M. S., and Baker, E. M., An enzymatic measurement of the riboflavin status in man, *Am. J. Clin. Nutr.*, 25, 425, 1972.
10. Belko, A. Z., Obarzanek, E., Kalkwarf, H. J., Rotter, M. A., Bogusz, S., Miller, D., Haas, J. D., and Roe, D. A., Effects of exercise on riboflavin requirements of young women, *Am. J. Clin. Nutr.*, 37, 509, 1983.
11. Roe, D. A., Bogusz, S., Sheu, J., and McCormick, D. B., Factors affecting riboflavin requirements of oral contraceptive users and nonusers, *Am. J. Clin. Nutr.,* 35, 495, 1982.
12. Otis, C. L., Exercise-associated amenorrhea, *Clin. Sports Med.*, 11, 351, 1992.
13. Bandini, S. G., Schoeller, D. A., Cyr, H. N., and Dietz, W. H., Validity of reported energy intake in obese and nonobese adolescents, *Am. J. Clin. Nutr.*, 52, 421, 1990.
14. Haggerty, P., McGaw, B., Maughan, R. J., and Fenn, C., Energy expenditure of elite female athletes measured by the doubly labelled water method, *Proc. Nutr. Soc.*, 47 (Abstr.), 35A, 1988.
15. Schulz, L. O., Alger, S., Harper, I., Wilmore, J. H., and Ravussin, E., Energy expenditure of elite female runners measured by respiratory chamber and doubly labeled water, *J. Appl. Physiol.*, 72, 23, 1992.
16. Haymes, E. M., and Spillman D. M., Iron status of women distance runners, sprinters, and control women, *Int. J. Sports Med.*, 10, 430, 1989.
17. Risser, W. L., Lee, E. J., Poindexter, H. B. W., West, M. S., Pivarnik, J. M., Risser, J. M. H., and Hickson, J. F., Iron deficiency in female athletes: its prevalence and impact on performance, *Med. Sci. Sports Exercise*, 20, 116, 1988.
18. Worme, J. D., Doubt, T. J., Singh, A., Ryan C. J., Moses, F. M., and Deuster, P. A., Dietary patterns, gastrointestinal complaints, and nutrition knowledge of recreational triathletes, *Am. J. Clin. Nutr.*, 51, 690, 1990.

Chapter 23

THE RELATION OF CALORIE AND FIBER INTAKE AND METABOLIC RATE TO ATHLETIC AMENORRHEA

Joan E. Benson
Patricia A. Eisenman
Katherine K. Heinrich

CONTENTS

I. INTRODUCTION

In the past few years, female athletes and their medical problems have received more than perfunctory interest. In particular, the medical consequences of inadequate nutrition, calorie restriction, vegetarianism, and rigorous training among these athletes have come into question. Athletic amenorrhea has been thought to be a consequence of the extraordinary training and dietary practices of female athletes. Female athletes experience a high incidence of menstrual abnormalities, such as secondary amenorrhea, irregular cycles, and anovulatory cycles.[1] Nearly 20 years ago, reports suggested that exercise-induced menstrual irregularity is common, and it was speculated that between 25 and 40% of highly trained endurance athletes report fewer than three menses per year.[2] More recently, the high incidence of amenorrhea and irregular menses among female athletes and dancers has been documented.[3] In the study by Cohen et al.,[1] 32 professional, full-time female ballet dancers were compared to nonathletic age-matched controls regarding menstrual history. Dancers had significantly fewer menses per year than controls ($p < 0.001$). A high frequency of amenorrhea and/or irregular cycles (11 of the 32, or 34%) has also been reported among dancers in a study by Calabrese et al.[4]

Nonmenstruating athletes may be at greater risk of developing osteopenia when compared to normally menstruating athletes or nonathletic, normally cycling females.[5,6] This decrease in bone mass is associated with an increased frequency of stress fractures of a lower extremity.[7,8] Attempts to explain athletic amenorrhea in the past have focused on loss of body fat or weight, reduced calorie intake, and excessive exercise as etiologic factors. However, the evidence linking these factors to menstrual dysfunction has been contradictory and confusing.

In this chapter we review those factors that have historically been linked to menstrual abnormalities in athletes, such as weight loss, reduced body fat, and excessive exercise. We then present the following as possible causative factors in athletic amenorrhea: reduction in metabolic rate as a consequence of restricted caloric intake in the face of increased caloric output, loss of body fat at metabolically specific sites, and vegetarianism and/or increased fiber intake.

II. CAUSES OF ATHLETIC AMENORRHEA

A. WEIGHT LOSS

In several early studies simple weight loss was suggested as a factor in producing amenorrhea among sedentary women.[9] Frisch and McArthur[10] proposed a "critical weight concept", stating that there is a set amount of body weight required to initiate and maintain menses. In their study, ballet dancers with amenorrhea and with irregular cycles had significantly lower body weights for height than dancers reporting regular cycles. The dancers experiencing menstrual dysfunction in the study by Cohen et al.[1] had significantly lower percent ideal body weights than dancers without menstrual dysfunction. In another survey by Frisch et al.,[11] 89 ballet dancers completed questionnaires on age, height, weight, duration of training, age of menarche, and menstrual periodicity. Fifteen percent of the group reported secondary amenorrhea, and 30% reported irregular cycles. Mean weights of the dancers with secondary amenorrhea and irregular cycles were 44.9 kg and 45.9 kg respectively, vs. 47.0 kg for the dancers with regular cycles ($p < .05$). Brooks-Gunn et al.[12] compared anthropometric measures of 56 professional dancers and also found that amenorrheic subjects were significantly lower in body weight ($p < 0.05$), weight/height ($p < 0.01$) and were below percent of ideal weight to a greater extent than normally cycling dancers. The nature of the relationship between weight loss and menstrual dysfunction is not well understood. Women with weight loss associated amenorrhea have been reported to have abnormalities in gonadotropin and estrogen secretion[13] and peripheral steroid metabolism.[14] Nonmenstruating athletes lack the typical pulsatile pattern of luteinizing hormone (LH) secretion from the pituitary that is typical in cyclic athletes and sedentary controls. It is possible that the menstrual disruption observed in athletes originates in the hypothalamus. The gonadotrope cells of the pituitary of amenorrheic athletes are actually more sensitive to stimulation by exogenous gonadotropin-releasing hormone (GnRH) when compared to eumenorrheic athletes[15] or nonathletic controls.[16] Therefore, it is likely that the GnRH generator in the hypothalamus is failing to stimulate gonadotropin release by the pituitary in amenorrheic athletes. Other possible mechanisms for amenorrhea suggested by Frisch[17] depend on the role of adipose in the aromatisation of estrogens and the potential effects of estrogens on hypothalamic regulatory centers. Fishman et al.[14] theorized that as body weight decreases, estrogen metabolism shifts from the normal 16-hydroxylation to 2-hydroxylation (catechol estrogens). Catechol estrogens are steroids that structurally resemble estrogens, but have only a weak estrogenic effect.[18]

B. LOW BODY FAT LEVELS

Body fat has also been proposed as a predictor of menstrual dysfunction. Frisch and McArthur[10] hypothesized that body fat must reach 17% of body weight before menstruation begins, and a minimum of 22% for menstruation to resume when secondary amenorrhea results from weight loss. However, when Carlberg et al.[19] followed 42 college-aged runners, swimmers, and basketball players to detect differences in body composition and/or exercise intensity in those who were regularly menstruating compared to those who experienced menstrual abnormalities, the results were at odds with this contention. Although the authors found that amenorrheic athletes indeed had significantly lower body fat levels than normal subjects (13.1% vs. 16%), the regularly menstruating subjects had percent body fat levels well below the critical level proposed by Frisch.[10] Exercise intensity and duration among the groups was found to be the same, but the amenorrheic athletes were significantly lower in total body weight and lean weight, prompting the authors to conclude that menstrual dysfunction is associated with lower total body weight as opposed to percent body fat.

Lack of differences in percent body fat between amenorrheic (AM) and eumenorrheic (EU) athletes has been consistently reported by other researchers as well. Sanborne et al.[20] examined runners with similar training programs for differences in body fat measures in AM vs. EU athletes and found none. Kaiserauer et al.[21] compared amenorrheic runners, regularly menstruating runners, and regularly menstruating sedentary controls for plasma hormone levels, physical characteristics, and nutrient intakes. While the AM subjects consumed less fat, red meat, and total calories than did the regularly menstruating subjects, there was no difference in body fat, body weight, or degree of exercise between the two groups. Deuster et al.[22] compared weight, percent body fat, training distance, and several dietary parameters in highly trained runners. Those who were amenorrheic had the same percent fat as normally cycling subjects (11.2% vs. 12.2%), as well as the same weight, and training distance. However, dietary fat intake of AM runners was significantly lower than that of EU runners (66 g vs. 97 g/d), and, the authors note, the fiber intake particularly high.

While it appears that menstrual disturbance is not a function of total body fat as a percentage of body weight, these data do suggest that a combination of low body weight, variable nutrient or calorie intake, and exercise exert synergistic effects in the development of menstrual problems. There is also the possibility that total body fat does not affect menstrual function so much as degree of fat at specific body sites, which in turn may directly influence gonadal function.

C. LOSS OF SPECIFIC FAT STORES

In their review of the weight regulation practices of athletes, Brownell et al.[23] suggested that specific fat deposits, rather than total body fat, may be key determinants of menstrual function. Research has shown that metabolic activity of the adipose tissue of women differs by region during pregnancy and lactation.[24] Lipolytic activity of adipose tissue is higher in the femoral region than in the abdominal region in pregnant and lactating women. In addition, the femoral region exhibits higher lipoprotein lipase (LPL) activity in both nonpregnant and pregnant women, but is particularly pronounced during pregnancy.

These findings suggest that femoral adipose deposits (fat found in the hips, buttocks, and thighs) play a key role in female reproductory process, such that when these fat stores fall below a certain level, pregnancy and lactation may not be viable. Depletion of these specific fat deposits in female athletes could possibly account for menstrual abnormalities, by providing a signal that the body cannot sustain fertility. It is not known whether patterns of fat distribution differ between athletes with and without menstrual irregularities, but if differences exist, this could explain the conflicting results of studies exploring the relationship between body fat and amenorrhea.

D. EXCESSIVE EXERCISE

Exercise, alone or in conjunction with decreased body weight, may contribute to the development of menstrual abnormalities. In the study by Cohen et al.,[1] 6 out of the 8 women (75%) who currently had oligomenorrhea had fewer menstrual cycles or more menstrual irregularities associated with increased dancing loads during the ballet season. Seven out of nine (78%) had more menstrual cycles or increased regularity during the off-season (a period of 3 to 4 months). Warren[25] also noted a relationship between exercise and amenorrhea in her group of ballet students. Menses resumed in a group of amenorrheic dancers during rest intervals, even though body weight or percent body fat had not changed.

The same correlation between degree of exercise and amenorrhea was reported by Dale, et al.[26] in female distance runners. Frisch et al.[27] studied the age at menarche and menstrual periodicity of 21 college swimmers and 17 runners. They found that 61% of the athletes who had begun training before menarche had menstrual irregularities (cycles differing in length by 9 d or more), and 22.4% were amenorrheic. Only 16.7% had regular cycles.

Bullen et al.[28] investigated exercise-induced menstrual disorders in a group of university students with well-established menstrual function. For 6 months, these subjects engaged in a training program that included 3.5 h/d of sports activity, such as bicycling, volley ball, tennis, and a running program. In addition, the subjects were expected to run 4 mi/d during the first week and increase the distance by 1.5 mi per week in successive weeks, attaining a distance of 10 mi/d by the fifth week, a level held constant thereafter. The normalcy of menses was assessed by the comparison of its characteristics with those of the subjects control cycle. The term "delay of menses" was employed to describe a suspension of flow extending over at least one full cycle length for any given subject. Those exercising subjects who also experienced weight loss (−4 kg) had significantly more delayed menses than those subjects who maintained their weight during the test period. It is likely that increased exercise affects menses only when it is accompanied by weight loss. A hypothesized mechanism by which exercise may affect menstrual cycle involves the hypothalamic-pituitary-adrenal axis.[29] Research on athletes has shown that cortisol levels in amenorrheic athletes are elevated about 25% while sedentary and cyclic athletes experience little change in a 24 h period.[29] In addition, pituitary secretion of ACTH in response to exogenous CRH has been shown to be reduced in athletes, and the amount of cortisol secretion by the adrenal cortex for a given amount of stimulation by ACTH appears to be increased in amenorrheic athletes. Loucks has described past research on animals showing that the GnRH pulse generator in the hypothalamus can be inhibited by corticotropin releasing hormone, the hormone which initiates the activation of the adrenal cortex during stress, such as exercise stress. Other animal research has found the inhibition of gonadotropin secretion by ACTH to occur only in the presence of intact adrenals, suggesting a direct effect of cortisol on the reproductive system.

E. NUTRITIONAL INADEQUACY

Insufficient caloric intake,[30,31] even in the absence of physical training, has been proposed as a factor contributing to menstrual dysfunction.[32,33] The relationship between nutritional intake and exercise training remains elusive. Brooks et al.[30] monitored cyclic ovarian function with daily hormonal measurements and serial ultrasound determinations of follicular development in a group of 17 recreational athletes and 13 sedentary controls. While 11 of the 13 controls demonstrated estradiol (E2) and progesterone (P4) concentrations as well as luteal phase lengths which met the normal criteria, only 10 of 17 athletes satisfied these criteria. The athletes with disturbed menstrual function ($n = 7$) and the athletes meeting the normal criteria ($n = 10$) had significantly lower E2 concentrations in all phases of the menstrual cycle. The P4 concentrations were significantly lower for the athletes with disturbed menstrual function. Both groups of athletes had similar aerobic capacities, indicating similar training levels. These researchers also noted that there was no difference in caloric consumption between the groups. Since the athletes were expending more energy due to training, the reported caloric intake values indicated that, as a group, they had failed to increase energy intake appropriately. Thus the researchers speculated that inadequate nutritional adaptation may have been a factor contributing to menstrual dysfunction.

This lack of difference in caloric intake has also been noted by others comparing female athletes and sedentary controls, as well as for comparisons of eumenorrheic and amenorrheic athletes.[31,34-36] An apparently negative energy balance, without a change in body weight, could be explained by a significant reduction in metabolic rate during nontraining hours, or an increased metabolic efficiency during exercise.

The reduction in resting metabolic rate (RMR) that accompanies caloric restriction is a well-documented occurrence.[37-40] In most cases, the decline in RMR can be attributed solely to losses of lean body mass. Although exercise is commonly believed to offset the reduction in RMR that results from calorie restriction, this is not always the case. Van Dale et al.[40] found that exercise, when added to an energy restricted diet, did not prevent a reduction in RMR, although it did lessen the reduction when compared to the diet-only group. In support of this discovery, Hill et al.[39] showed that after 8 weeks of a 500 kcal/d diet, the total decline in RMR for exercising subjects was 19.1% and for nonexercising subjects was 17.3%. A similar effect was observed by Phinney et al.[41]

Evidence that some amenorrheic athletes consume less energy than regularly menstruating athletes, coupled with the discovery that exercise does not necessarily lead to elevation of RMR, suggests that an athlete with menstrual irregularities may be characterized by negative energy balance and reduced RMR. This hypothesis was supported by a recent study which documented that the RMR of amenorrheic runners was significantly lower than that of eumenorrheic runners and sedentary controls.[42] There were no significant differences between the two groups of runners in age, anthropometric characteristics, weekly running mileage, and $\dot{V}O_2$ max. Additionally, the dietary intakes of all three groups were similar in terms of macro- and micronutrients. The authors concluded that amenorrheic runners are able to maintain energy balance and stable weight through a reduction in RMR. This discovery raises interesting questions about metabolic changes occurring in amenorrheic women.

Apparently not all women athletes experience the same metabolic changes. There are studies which report no differences in the training load or energy intake for amenorrheic and eumenorrheic athletes. These findings detract from the premise that caloric deficit is the only factor which causes menstrual dysfunction. Caloric deficits could work in a synergistic fashion with training intensity and impact ovarian function, or it might be that alterations in the composition of macronutrient consumption instead of caloric deficit is the determining variable. In a study with 6 normal weight women,[43] a reduction in dietary fat from 40% of 1800 total calories to 25% of calories resulted in a significant shift away from the 16α-hydoxylated estrogen metabolites toward the catechol estrogens. Anderson et al.,[44] has also noted that alterations in the composition of the macronutrients results in shifts in 16α-hydroxylase activity and 2-hydroxylase activity. These differences in metabolic pathways are of potential significance because of the differences in peripheral activity of the metabolites which result from 16α- and 2-hydroxylation. C-2 products have virtually no uterotropic activity while C16α-products are potent uterotropic agents.[45]

Although there are data to support that athletes do consume a diet that is lower in fat content than many sedentary control groups, and so a resultant increase in E2 2-hydroxylase oxidation might explain menstrual function differences between the athletes and sedentary subjects, the reports of groups of athletes whose dietary fat intakes do not differ, and yet their menstrual function responses to increased training loads differ, negate the premise that percent of dietary fat is the only regulating factor. Snow et al.[46] monitored estrogen metabolism and menstrual function in two groups of oarswomen. Each group progressed through a 3 month period of low-intensity training. Group A ($n = 5$) experienced no disruptions in menstrual function, in spite of alterations in training intensity. Group B ($n = 5$) exhibited menstrual dysfunction during the high-intensity training period. A control group of subjects also experienced no menstrual disruptions during the course of the study. Estrogen metabolism oxidative pathways were evaluated by monitoring the appearance of $^3H^2O$ in the plasma water after administration of $[2\text{-}^3H]E_2$ or $[16\alpha\text{-}^3H]E^2$, respectively. During all three phases of the study, Group B oarswomen metabolized a significantly greater fraction of E^2 by 2-hydroxylase oxidation than did Group A oarswomen or the control subjects. There were no differences in 16α-hydroxylase oxidation between any of the groups at any point in the study. The oarswomen consumed diets with similar levels of dietary fat, and this fat percentage was lower than for the control subjects.

Snow et al.[46] had no explanation for why the Group B oarswomen had increased 2-hydroxylase oxidation as compared with the equally well-trained women in Group A. They did speculate that the increased 2-hydroxylase oxidation among the Group B athletes became limiting, at least in terms of menstrual function, during the high-intensity training when body fat percentage dropped to lower values. These results, along with many of the other seemingly contradictory data, suggest that individual variability with respect to metabolism interacts with external variables such as diet and training to induce menstrual dysfunction.

F. VEGETARIANISM

Another of the possible external variables influencing menstrual function is vegetarianism. Brooks, et al.[47] noted that, in previous studies, most female runners with amenorrhea were vegetarians. They analyzed in detail the diets of 11 amenorrheic, and 15 regularly menstruating, runners. The results suggested the runners who had regular menstrual cycles ate five times more meat than the amenorrheic runners. If a runner ate less than 200 g per week of meat (any combination of poultry or red meat) she was classified as a vegetarian. Of the amenorrheic group, 9 (82%) were vegetarians, whereas only two (13%) of the regularly menstruating runners were vegetarians. The only other dietary difference was in fat consumption (regularly menstruating runners ate 98 g/d, amenorrheic runners ate 68 g/d, $p < 0.05$). Kaiserauer et al.[48] reported that a greater percentage (25%) of AM runners were considered to be vegetarians using the same criteria as above than were EU runners (11%). The two groups differed in average energy intake as well, with the AM runners consuming significantly less energy than the EU runners (1582 kcal/d vs. 2490 kcal/d). Slavin, et al.[49] reported similar findings in exercising women and in competitive cyclists. Thirty-one percent of the 45 vegetarian athletes had secondary amenorrhea (defined as less than three menstrual cycles during the previous year), whereas only 4% of the 84 women who consumed a "balanced four food group" diet had less than three menstrual cycles yearly, and 1 of them had lost more than 9 kg during the previous year, which could explain the menstrual difficulties. The authors speculate that aspects of the diets, such as trace elements or plant hormones, may affect menstruation.

Lloyd et al.[49] examined the effects of several nutritional factors on menstrual function and bone density in collegiate athletes. Dietary fiber intake was significantly elevated in the oligomenorrheic athletes (5.74 g/d) compared to the normally cycling athletes (3.62 g/d), and the bone density of oligomenorrheic athletes tended to be lower (158 mg/ml) than that of the eumenorrheic athletes (184 mg/ml). Kcalorie intake and percent body fat (EU = 18.2%; Oligo = 15.6%) did not differ between the two groups. The authors concluded that increased dietary fiber intake is associated with menstrual dysfunction and a lower bone density in these college athletes. In a study of nonathletes, Snow et al.[50] found that oligomenorrheic women consumed significantly more dietary fiber and significantly less saturated fat than their EU classmates. The groups did not differ in aspects of body composition or weight.

How fiber affects menstrual function is unclear. Past studies have shown that vegetarian women who consumed twice as much fiber as nonvegetarian women had reduced circulating estrone and estradiol levels, and significantly greater fecal excretion of estrogens.[52] Dietary fiber increases fecal bulk, which in turn decreases the concentration of intestinal β-glucuronidase,[53] an enzyme that hydrozlyzes the bile acid-steroid complex, an event necessary for the reabsorption of estrogens. Some fibers may also bind nonpolar estrogens in the intestinal lumen,[54] reducing their reabsorption. Preliminary results in the large "Finland study" have revealed positive correlations between intake of total fiber and plasma concentration of sex hormone binding globulin (SHBG), and negative correlations between fiber and plasma percent free estradiol (%FE)[55] The result could be a reduction in the bioavailability of the hormone for reproductive and other functions.

Plant lignins and isoflavonic phytoestrogens have been observed to be excreted in large amounts in the urine of Finnish subjects consuming large amounts of whole grains, vegetables, and berries, and by Japanese persons consuming the typical Japanese diet, which consists of large quantities of soy products.[54] Particularly low excretion of isoflavonic phytoestrogens has been observed in subjects consuming a diet low in whole grains and beans.[51] Several of these lignins and isoflavones have weak estrogenic activity and may compete with estradiol for binding sites. It also has been suggested that lignins and isoflavones stimulate the synthesis of SHBG in the liver, thereby reducing %FE, and subsequently the biological activity of estradiol.[54]

In summary, the inability of research to consistently show that calorie deficits, body fat losses, or excessive exercise are causes of menstrual dysfunction may be explained by the failure to consider the adjustments to metabolic rate, specific body fat stores, or both that may accompany exercise training in certain individuals. Similar training routines, coupled with lower energy intakes, when compared to those with normal menstrual cycles, raises the possibility of an energy deficit in amenorrheic athletes. In addition, while the evidence linking dietary fat and calorie intake levels to menstrual dysfunction is inconsistent, the failure to consider fiber and or vegetable intake in these analyses may explain the inconsistency in findings.

REFERENCES

1. Cohen, J. L., Chung, S. K., May, P. B., Exercise, body weight, and amenorrhea in professional ballet dancers, *Phys. Sportsmed.*, 10, 92, 1982.
2. Feicht, C. B., Johnson, T. S., Martin, B. J., Sparkes, K. E., Wagner, W. W., Secondary amenorrhea in athletes, *Lancet*, 2, 1145, 1978.
3. Cook, S. D., Harding, A. F., Thomas, K. A., Morgan, E. L., Schnurpfeil, K. M., Haddad, R. J., Trabecular bone density and menstrual function in women runners, *Am. J. Sports Med.*, 15, 503, 1987.
4. Calabrese, L. H., Kirkendall, D. T., Floyd, M., Menstrual abnormalities, nutritional patterns and body composition in female classical ballet dancers, *Phys. Sportsmed.*, 11, 86, 1983.
5. Cann, C. E., Martin, M. C., Genant, H. K., *Detection of premenopausal women at risk for the development of osteoporosis,* (abstract), 64th Annual Meeting of the Endocrine Society, San Fransisco, CA, 1982.
6. Drinkwater, B. L., Milson, K., Chesnut, C. H. III., Bone mineral content of amenorrheic and eumenorrheic athletes, *N. Engl. J. Med.*, 311, 277, 1984.
7. Lindberg, J. S., Fears, W. B., Hunt, M. M., Exercise induced amenorrhea and bone density, *Ann. Intern. Med.*, 101, 647, 1984.
8. Markus, R., Cann, C., Madvig, P., Minkoff, J., Goddard, M., Bayer, M., Martin, M., Gaudianin, L., Haskell, W., Genant, H., Menstrual function and bone mass in elite women distance runners: Endocrine and metabolic features, *Ann. Intern. Med.*, 102, 158, 1985.
9. Fries, H., Nillius, S. J., Pettersson, F., Epidemiology of secondary amenorrhea. II. A retrospective evaluation of etiology with special regard to psychogenic factors and weight loss, *Am. J. Obstet. Gynecol.*, 118, 473, 1974.
10. Frisch, R. E., McArthur, J. W., Menstrual cycles: fatness as a determinant of minimum weight for height necessary for their maintenance or onset, *Science*, 185, 949, 1974.
11. Frisch, R. E., Wyshak, G., Vincent, L., Delayed menarch and amenorrhea in ballet dancers, *N. Engl. J. Med.*, 303, 17, 1980.

12. Brooks-Gunn, J., Warren, M. P., Hamilton, L. H., The relation of eating problems and amenorrhea in ballet dancers, *Med. Sci. Sports Exercise,* 19(1), 41, 1987.

13. Knuth, U. A., Hall, M. G. R., Jacobs, H. S., Amenorrhea and loss of weight, *Br. J. Obstet. Gynaecol.,* 84, 801, 1977.

14. Fishman, J., Boyar, R. M., Hellman, L., Influence of body weight on estradiol metabolism in young women, *J. Clin. Endocrinol. Metab.,* 41, 989, 1975.

15. Yahiro, J., Glass, A. R., Fears, W. B., Ferguson, E. W., Vigersky, R. A., Exaggerated gonado-tropin response to luteinizing hormone-releasing hormone in amenorrheic runners, *Am. J. Obstet. Gynecol.,* 156, 586, 1987.

16. Vedhuis, J. D., Evans, W. S., Demers, L. M., Thorner, M. O., Wakat, D., Rogol, A. D., Altered neuroendocrine regulation of gonadotropin secretion in women distance runners, *J. Clin. Endocrinol. Metab.,* 61, 557, 1985.

17. Frisch, R. E., Body fat, menarche, and reproductive ability, *Semin. Reprod. Endocrinol.,* 3, 45, 1985.

18. Mishell, D. R., Reproductive endocrinology, in *Comprehensive Gynecology,* Droegemueller, W., Herbst, A. L., Mishell, D. R., Stenchever, M. A., Eds., C. V. Mosby, Co., St. Louis, 1987, 76.

19. Carlberg, K. A., Buckman, M. T., Peake, G. T., Riedesel, M. L., Body composition of oligo/amenorrheic athletes, *Med. Sci. Sports Exercise,* 15, 215, 1983.

20. Sanborn, C. F., Albrecht, B. H., Wagner, W. W., Athletic amenorrhea: lack of association with body fat, *Med. Sci. Sports Exercise,* 19, 207, 1987.

21. Kaiserauer, S., Snyder, A. C., Sleeper, M., Zierath, J., Nutritional, physiological, and menstrual status of distance runners, *Med. Sci. Sports Exercise,* 23, 15, 1991.

22. Deuster, P. A., Kyle, S. B., Moser, P. B., Vigersky, R. A., Singh, A., Schoomaker, E. B., Nutritional intakes and status of highly trained amenorrheic and eumenorrheic women runners, *Fertil. Steril.,* 46, 639, 1986.

23. Brownell, K. D., Steen, S. N., Wilmore, J. H., Weight regulation practices in athletes: analysis of metabolic and health effects, *Med. Sci. Sports Exercise,* 19, 546, 1987.

24. Rebuffe-Scrive, M., Enk, L., Crona, N., et al., Fat cell metabolism in different regions in women, *J. Clin. Invest.,* 75, 1973, 1985.

25. Warren, M. P., The effects of exercise on pubertal progression and reproductive function in girls, *J. Clin. Endocrinol. Metab.,* 51, 1150, 1980.

26. Dale, E., Gerlach, D. H., Martin, D. E., Wilhite, W. L., Menstrual dysfunction in distance runners, *Obstet. Gynecol.,* 54, 47, 1979.

27. Frisch, R. E., Gotz-Welbergen, A. V., McArthur, J. W., Albright, T., Witschi, J., Bullen, B., Birnholz, J., Reed, R. B., Hermann, H., Delayed menarche and amenorrhea of college athletes in relation to age on onset of training, *J. Am. Med. Assoc.,* 246, 1559, 1981.

28. Bullen, B. A., Skrinar, G. S., Beitins, I. Z., Mering, G., Turnbull, B. A., McArthur, A. W., Induction of menstrual disorders by strenuous exercise in untrained women, *N. Engl. J. Med.,* 312, 1349, 1985.

29. Loucks, A. B., Effects of exercise training on the menstrual cycle: existence and mechanisms, *Med. Sci. Sports Exercise,* 22, 275, 1987.

30. Brooks, A., Pirke, M., Schweiger, U., Tuschi, R. J., Laessle, R. G., Strowitzki, T., Hori, E., Haas, W., Jeschke, K., Cyclic ovarian function in recreational athletes, *J. Appl. Physiol.,* 68, 2083, 1990.

31. Drinkwater, B. L., Nilson, K., Chestnut, C. H., Bremner, W. J., Shainholtz, S., Southworth, M. B., Bone mineral content of amenorrheic and eumenorrheic athletes, *N. Engl. J. Med.,* 311, 277, 1984.

32. Durser, M. S., Calloway, D. H., Effects of energy deprivation on sex hormone patterns of healthy menstruating women, *Am. J. Physiol.,* 251 (Endocrinology Metabolism, 14), E483, 1986.

33. Schweiger, U., Laessle, H., Pfister, H., Hoehl, C., Schwingerschloegel, M., Schweiger, M., Pirke, K. M., Diet-induced menstrual irregularities: effects of age and weight loss, *Fert. Steril.,* 48, 746, 1987.

34. Marcus, R. C., Cann, C., Madvig, P., Minkoff, J., Goddardy, M., Bayer, M., Martin, M., Gaudianan, L., Haskell, W., Genant, H., Menstrual function and bone mass in elite women distance runners, *Ann. Intern. Med.,* 102, 158, 1985.

35. Nelson, M. E., Fischer, E. C., Catsos, P. D., Meredith, C. N., Turksoy, R. N., Evans, W. J., Diet and bone status in amenorrheic runners, *Am. J. Clin. Nutr.*, 43, 910, 1986.
36. Dahlstrom, M., Jansson, E., Nordevang, E., Kaijer, L., Discrepancy between estimated energy intake and requirement in female dancers, *Clin. Physiol.*, 10, 11, 1990.
37. Davies, H. J. A., Baird, I. M., Fowler, J., et al., Metabolic response of low- and very-low-calorie diets, *Am. J. Clin. Nutr.*, 49, 745, 1989.
38. Mole, P. A., Stern, J. S., Schultz, C. L., Berneauer, E. M., Hocomb, J. J., Exercise reversed depressed metabolic rate produced by severe caloric restriction, *Med. Sci. Sports Exercise*, 21, 29, 1989.
39. Hill, J. O., Sparling, P. B., Shields, T. W., Heller, P. A., Effects of exercise and food restriction on body composition and metabolic rate in obese women, *Am. J. Clin. Nutr.*, 46, 622, 1987.
40. Van Dale, D., Saris, W. H. M., Schoffelen, P. F. M., Hoor, F. T., Does exercise give an additional effect in weight reduction regimens, *Int. J. Obesity*, 9, 39, 1985.
41. Phinney, S. D., LaGrange, B. M., O'Connell, M., Danforth, E., Effects of aerobic exercise on energy expenditure and nitrogen balance during very low calorie dieting, *Metabolism*, 37, 758, 1988.
42. Myerson, M., Gutin, B., Warren, M. P., May, M. T., Contento, I., Lee, M., Pi-Sunyer, F. X., Piersn, R. N., Brooks-Gunn, J., Resting metabolic rate and energy balance in amenorrheic and eumenorrheic runners, *Med. Sci. Sports Exercise*, 23, 15, 1991.
43. Longscope, G., Gorbach, S., Goldin, B., Woods, M., Dwyer, J., Morrill, A., Warram, J., The effect of a low fat diet on estrogen metabolism, *J. Clin. Endocrinol. Metab.*, 64, 1246, 1987.
44. Anderson, K. E., Kappas, A., Conney, A. H., Bradlow, H. L., Fishman, J., The influence of dietary protein and carbohydrate on the principal oxidative biotransformations of estradiol in normal subjects, *J. Clin. Endocrinol. Metab.*, 59, 103, 1984.
45. Fishman, J., Martucci, C., Biological properties of 16 - Hydroxyestrone: implications in estrogen physiology and pathophysiology, *J. Clin. Endocrinol. Metab.*, 51, 611, 1980.
46. Snow, R. C., Barbieri, R. L., Frisch, R., Estrogen 2-hydroxylase oxidation and menstrual function among elite oarswomen, *J. Clin. Endocrinol. Metab.*, 69, 369, 1898.
47. Brooks, S. M., Sanborn, C. F., Albrecht, B. H., Wagner, W. W., Diet in athletic amenorrhoea, *Lancet*, March 10, 559, 1984.
48. Slavin, J., Lutter, J., Cushman, S., Amenorrhea in vegetarian athletes, *Lancet*, June 30, 351, 1984.
49. Lloyd, T., Triantafyllou, S. J., Baker, E. R., et al., Women athletes with menstrual irregularity have increased musculoskeletal injuries, *Med. Sci. Sports Exercise*, 18, 374, 1986.
50. Snow, R. C., Schneider, J. L., Barbieri, R. L., High dietary fiber and low saturated fat intake among oligomenorrheic undergraduates, *Fertil. Steril.*, 54, 632, 1990.
51. Goldin, R. R., Aldercruetz, H., Gorbach, S. L., et al., Estrogen secretion patterns and plasma levels in vegetarian and omnivorous women, *N. Engl. J. Med.*, 307, 1542, 1982.
52. Aldercreutz, H., Does fiber rich food containing animal lignin precursors protect against both colon and breast cancer? An extension of the fiber hypothesis, *Gastroenterology*, 86, 761, 1984.
53. Schultz, T. D., Howie, B. J., *In vitro* binding of steroid hormones by natural and purified fibers, *Nutr. Cancer*, 8, 141, 1986.
54. Aldercreutz, H., Western diet and Western disease: some hormonal and biochemical mechanisms and associations, *Scand. J. Lab. Invest.*, 50 (Suppl. 201), 3, 1990.

Chapter **24**

FREE RADICALS IN SPORTS

Okezie I. Aruoma
Barry Halliwell

CONTENTS

I. ABSTRACT

Reactive oxygen species (ROS) are implicated in the molecular and tissue damage arising from increased oxidative metabolism associated with strenuous exercise. This chapter discusses the current status of the role of free radicals in sports.

II. INTRODUCTION

The subject area of "free radical" biochemistry has captured the imagination of scientists. A free radical may be defined as any species capable of independent existence, possessing one or more unpaired electrons, an unpaired electron being one that is alone in an orbital. The conventional radical dot (·) designates the presence of one or more of the unpaired electrons. Examples of free radicals are hydroxyl (OH·), superoxide (O_2^-, an oxygen centered radical), peroxyl (RO_2·, radical intermediates arising as a result of lipid oxidation), trichloromethyl (·CCl_3, a carbon centered radical), and nitric oxide (NO·). Examples of nonradical oxygen-derived species are hypochlorous acid (HOCl), hydrogen peroxide (H_2O_2), singlet oxygen ($^1O_2$) and ozone (O_3, a pale blue gas which serves as an important protective shield against solar radiation in the atmosphere). Free radicals and other reactive oxygen species are constantly formed in the human body (for reviews see References 1 to 4). Reactive oxygen species (ROS) are also increasingly implicated in the oxidative metabolism associated with strenuous exercise.[5,6,7] Exercise causes an increased oxygen (O_2) consumption *in vivo*. O_2 is a toxic gas. Indeed, humans and other aerobes can only tolerate it because antioxidant defenses to protect against the toxic effects of O_2 evolved in line with the evolution of the electron transport chains. A small part of the oxygen consumed by the human body leads to the formation of reactive oxygen species. However, excessive production of ROS beyond the antioxidant defense capacity of the human body can cause oxidative stress.[1-3] Table 1 shows a representative list of human clinical conditions in which a role for free radical mechanism has been implicated.

III. IRON AND COPPER IN FREE RADICAL REACTIONS: RELEVANCE TO SPORTS

It is generally accepted that much of the toxicity of O_2^- and H_2O_2 in living organisms is due to their conversion into OH· and into reactive-radical-metal ion complexes. These processes are often referred to as either the iron-catalyzed Haber-Weiss reaction (I), or the superoxide-driven Fenton reaction (II).[8-11]

$$\text{Haber-Weiss} \qquad H_2O_2 + O_2^- \quad \xrightarrow[\text{catalyst}]{\text{Fe/Cu}} \quad O_2 + OH· + OH^- \qquad (I)$$

$$\text{Fenton} \qquad Fe^{2+} + H_2O_2 \rightarrow \text{intermediates} \rightarrow Fe^{3+} + OH· + OH^- \qquad (II)$$

TABLE 1   Some Clinical Conditions in Which Oxygen Free Radicals Are Thought to be Involved

Brain
   Parkinson's disease
   Neurotoxins
   Vitamin E deficiency
   Hyperbaric oxygen
   Hypertensive cerebrovascular injury
   Aluminium overload
   Allergic encephalomyelitis (demyelinating diseases)
   Potentiation of traumatic injury
Eye
   Photic retinopathy
   Occular hemorrhage
   Cataractogenesis
   Degenerative retinal damage
   Retinopathy of prematurity
Heart and cardiovascular system
   Atherosclerosis
   Adriamycin cardiotoxicity
   Keshan disease (selenium deficiency)
   Alcohol cardiomyopathy
Kidney
   Metal ion-mediated nephrotoxicity
   Aminoglycoside nephrotoxicity
   Autoimmune nephrotic syndromes
Gastrointestinal tract
   NSAID-induced GI tract lesions*
   Oral iron poisoning
   Endotoxin liver injury
   Diabetogenic actions of alloxan
   Halogenated hydrocarbon liver injury
   FFA-induced pancreatitis*
Cancer
Inflammatory-immune injury
   Rheumatoid arthritis
   Glomerulonephritis
   Autoimmune diseases
   Vasculitis (hepatitis B virus)
Alcoholism
Aging
Radiation injury
Iron overload
   Nutritional deficiencies (Kwashiorkor)
   Thalassemia and other chronic anemias treated with multiple blood transfusions
   Dietary iron overload (red wine, beer brewed in iron pots)
   Idiopathic hemochromatosis
Red blood cells
   Fanconi's anemia
   Sickle cell anemia
   Favism
   Malaria
   Protoporphyrin photo-oxidation

TABLE 1 (continued)   Some Clinical Conditions in Which Oxygen Free Radicals Are Thought to be Involved

Lung
  Bronchopulmonary dysplasia
  Mineral dust pneumoconiosis
  Bleomycin toxicity
  Hypoxia
  Cigarette-smoke effect
  Emphysema
  ARDS* (some forms)
  Oxidant pollutants (ozone, SO_2, NO_2^-)
Ischemia-reperfusion
  Stroke/myocardial infarction
  Organ transplantation

Note: Skin injury due to solar radiation, porphyria, contact dermatitis, and photosensitizers may also involve free radical mechanisms.

* ARDS: adult respiratory distress syndrome, NSAID: non-steroidal anti-inflammatory drug, FFA: free fatty acid

Pure O_2^- and H_2O_2 are poorly reactive in aqueous solutions. They do not oxidize membrane lipids or degrade DNA.[12] H_2O_2 *in vivo* can be generated by the dismutation of O_2^- and by several enzymes. For reviews on the biochemistry of O_2^- see References 13 and 14. On production *in vivo*, OH reacts at its site of formation. Thus in the case of OH generation by Fenton-type chemistry, the extent of OH formation is largely determined by the availability and location of the metal ion catalyst. Iron salts have been widely studied as catalysts of free radical reactions *in vivo*, but copper ions may also be important. When the roles of copper ions and iron ions in causing damage to DNA in systems containing H_2O_2 are compared, added copper ions were significantly more reactive in causing DNA damage. This catalytic ability suggests that the availability of "free" iron and copper ions in the human body should be carefully controlled. This is indeed the case.

The average human body contains much less copper (0.08 g) than iron (4.5 g). Iron ions are absorbed from the gut and transported to iron-requiring cells by the protein transferrin. In contrast, most or all of the plasma copper in humans is attached to the protein ceruloplasmin. Iron specifically bound to transferrin will not participate in free radical reactions.[15] The protein ceruloplasmin similarly does not stimulate OH formation from H_2O_2.[16] The consequences of uncontrolled iron availability can be seen in 'iron-overload' diseases, such as idiopathic hemochromatosis, where there is a progressive increase in total body iron stores of iron in the parenchymal cells of the liver.[1,17]

There is much current interest in metal metabolism during human exercise,[18-24] particularly in relation to "sports anemia". It would seem that physiological processes that could cause an imbalance in the distribution of iron and/or copper might be of some significance in oxidative damage.[25] By comparing the plasma levels of zinc, iron, and copper before and after a period of controlled exercise, with losses of the metals in sweat together with changes in plasma volume and hematocrit, it may be possible to gain an insight into the significance of metal metabolism in exercise.

In one such investigation where the effect of a 30 or 40 min exercise on a cycle ergometer upon concentrations of zinc, iron, and copper in plasma from healthy male athletes were studied.[19] Appreciable amounts of iron are lost during exercise and this varies between different parts of the human anatomy.[19] Appreciable amounts of copper are lost via the sweat route. Given the relatively low pool of copper *in vivo*, these losses could be biologically significant. There is a tendency for losses of copper in sweat from the abdomen, arm, chest, and back to be greater than losses of iron, although there is considerable variation between subjects.[19] The variability, even between male subjects of similar age and body mass in such parameters as sweat rate, plasma volume changes, and changes in the metal contents of plasma, suggests that real "sports anemia" may be a feature only of certain individuals.[19] If the loss of iron in sweat was a significant contributor to sports anemia, then depletion of copper would also be expected since the body pool of copper is less than that of iron. A number of reports exist in the literature implicating oxidative stress in exercise.[5-7,24-26]

Generation of highly reactive oxygen species requires catalytic metal complexes, especially those of iron. However, proving that oxidative damage in biological systems is due to OH˙ radical is extremely difficult. This highly reactive radical, once generated, will combine very quickly with adjacent molecules and so is almost impossible to scavenge.

When cells are damaged (e.g., muscle injury as a result of exercise) iron ions are released. Heme proteins may also be liberated, and these can be powerful pro-oxidants. Hence, biological systems must sequester iron to prevent it from circulating around in free form. *In vivo*, iron is normally bound to transport and storage proteins, transferrin, lactoferrin, ferritin, and hemosiderin. Indeed, at pH 7.4, apotransferrin and apolactoferrin are able to bind to iron ions and protect against OH˙ radical generation promoted by iron added as $FeCl_3$, by iron released from ferritin in the presence of ascorbate, or a superoxide radical generating system, hence supporting the proposal that under normal conditions, iron binding proteins function as antioxidants *in vivo*.[15]

A. COMMENTS ON METHODOLOGY

The development of effective and accurate methods for measuring free radical generation, or free radical damage, in humans would contribute towards a greater understanding of the role of reactive oxygen species in disease pathology.

A number of methods for detection of hydroxyl radicals have been discussed in the literature.[27-32] One of the methods which could be applied to sports research for the measurement of free radical reaction *in vivo*, aromatic hydroxylation, involves the use of a nontoxic aromatic compound (aspirin for example) with a high rate constant for reaction with OH˙ The end products of OH˙ attack must be stable *in vivo* and not identical with those produced *in vivo* via normal enzyme mechanisms. Another method in use involves the measurement of the levels of uric acid and its oxidation products allantoin, cyanuric, parabanic acid, and oxonic acids. Uric acid is a product from the degradation of purines. This would serve as a potential index of free radical attack *in vivo*.[15,28,29]

For salicylate hydroxylation, three major products are usually identified: catechol (~11%), 2,3-dihydroxybenzoate (~49%), and 2,5-dihydroxybenzoate (~40%). 2,3-dihydroxybenzoate is the main product of interest in attempts to use salicylate as a detector of OH generation. Analysis of uric acid and its product has been applied to exercising adult humans.[25] There is a rise in uric acid levels, which may be accounted for by observed changes in plasma volume and increased purine breakdown.

IV. OXIDATIVE DAMAGE AND ANTIOXIDANT STRATEGIES

Our premise in this chapter that the antioxidant status of exercising subjects and/or training athletes is important, and that biological systems must tend towards avoidance of environments harboring excessive ROS formation, is well established. There is a need to delineate the contribution of nutrients to modulation of the pathological consequences of free radicals in the human body. It would seem that use of a range of antioxidants, combined with new methods for measuring free radical damage *in vivo*, and the effect of dietary antioxidants upon it, is the way forward.

For the training athlete or exercising individuals, antioxidant status is important. Antioxidant supplementation to prevent exercise induced oxidative stress[26] and to minimize the consequences of ROS-to-human clinical conditions[4,33-37,41] has been suggested. Eating a balanced diet is indeed prudent, since good food will provide most, if not all, of the nutrients required for normal body function. Antioxidant defenses in humans are afforded by the enzymes superoxide dismutase, catalase, glutathione peroxidase and its substrate glutathione (GSH), and a number of low molecular mass compounds such as ascorbate, α-tocopherol, and possibly carotenoids.

By definition, antioxidants, when present at low concentrations, compared with that of an oxidizable substrate, significantly delay or prevent the oxidation of that substrate. A number of important questions must be addressed when formulating an antioxidant cocktail. These include:

1. What biomolecules are the antioxidants supposed to protect? An inhibitor of lipid peroxidation is unlikely to be useful if damage is mediated by oxidative attack upon proteins (e.g., in muscle) or DNA. In other words, can antioxidants cause damage in biological systems different from those in which they exert protection?
2. For naturally occurring antioxidants, is antioxidant protection the primary biological role of the molecule or a secondary one?
3. If the antioxidants act by scavenging a ROS, can the antioxidant derived radicals themselves do biological damage?

Thus the potential antioxidant, and possible pro-oxidant, actions of the antioxidant should be fully characterized using established assays.[38-40] It is also important to consider the physiological state of the athlete during antioxidant supplementation.[25,41] Bioavailability of drugs, for example, is determined by their pharmacokinetics, determined by absorption, metabolism, distribution, and elimination. Although antioxidant supplements are not drugs within the broad definition of drugs, they must become available to the consumer following ingestion. Thus, how much of the consumed antioxidant supplement becomes available to the athlete depends on the chemical nature of the antioxidant, the effect of other nutrient components in the antioxidant cocktail, diet, and the physiological state of the subject.

ACKNOWLEDGMENTS

We are grateful to the U.K. Sports Council, the U.K. Ministry of Agriculture, Fisheries, and Foods, and Nestec SA, Switzerland, for research support.

REFERENCES

1. Halliwell, B. and Gutteridge, J.M.C., *Free Radicals in Biology and Medicine,* 2nd ed. Clarendon Press, Oxford, 1989.
2. Slater, T.F., Free radicals in medicine, *Free Rad. Res. Commun.,* 7, 119, 1989.
3. Sies, H., *Oxidative Stress,* Academic Press, London, 1985.
4. Aruoma, OI., *Free Radicals in Tropical Diseases,* Harwood Academic Publishers, London, 1993.
5. Jenkins, R.R., Free radical chemistry: relationship to exercise, *Sports Med.* 5, 156, 1988.
6. Jenkins, R.R., Symposium: oxidant stress, aging and exercise. *Med. Sci. Sports Exercise,* 25, 210, 1993.
7. Packer, L., Oxygen radicals and antioxidants in endurance exercise, in *Biochemical Aspects of Physical Exercise,* G. Benzi, Packer, L. and Siliprandi, N., Eds., Elsevier, Amsterdam, 1986, 73-92.
8. Fenton, H.J.H., Oxidation of tartaric acid in the presence of iron, *J. Chem. Soc.,* 65, 899, 1894.
9. Haber, F. and Weiss, J.J., The catalytic decomposition of hydrogen peroxide by iron salts, *Proc. Roy. Soc. London Ser. A.,* 147, 332, 1943.
10. Walling, C., Fenton's reagent revisited, *Acc. Chem. Res.,* 8, 125, 1975.
11. Halliwell, B. and Gutteridge, J.M.C., Biologically relevant metal ion-dependent hydroxyl radical generation, *FEBS Lett.,* 307, 108, 1992.
12. Halliwell, B. and Aruoma, O.I., DNA damage by oxygen derived species. Its mechanism and measurement in mammalian systems, *FEBS Lett.,* 281, 9, 1991.
13. Fridovich, I., Superoxide radical: an endogenous toxicant. *Annu. Rev. Pharmacol. Toxicol.,* 23, 239, 1983.
14. McCord, J., Human disease, free radicals and the oxidant-antioxidant balance, *Clin. Biochem.,* 26, 351, 1993.
15. Aruoma, O.I. and Halliwell, B., Superoxide-dependent and ascorbate-dependent formation of hydroxyl radicals from hydrogen peroxide in the presence of iron. Are lactoferrin and transferrin promoters of hydroxyl radical generation? *Biochem. J.,* 241, 273, 1987.
16. Halliwell, B. and Gutteridge, J.M.C., Role of free radicals and catalytic metal ions in human diseases: an overview, *Methods Enzymol.,* 186, 1, 1990.
17. Lauffer, R.B., Ed., *Iron and Human Disease,* CRC Press, Boca Raton, 1992.

18. Mouton, G., Sluse, F.E., Bertrand, A., Welter, A., Cabay, J.L. and Camus, G., Iron status in runners of various running specialities, *Arch. Int. Physiol. Biochem.,* 98, 103, 1990.
19. Aruoma, O.I., Reilly, T., MacLaren, D. and Halliwell, B., Iron, copper and zinc concentrations in human sweat and plasma: the effect of exercise, *Clin. Chim. Acta,* 177, 81, 1988.
20. Lukaski, H.C., Hoverson, B.S., Gallagher, S.K. and Bolonchuk, W.W., Physical training and copper, iron and zinc status in swimmers, *Am. J. Clin. Nutr.,* 51, 1093, 1990
21. Balaban, E.P., Cox, J.V., Snell, P., Vaughan, R.H. and Frenkel, E.P., The frequency of anaemia and iron deficiency in the runner, *Med. Sci. Sports Exercise,* 21, 643, 1989.
22. Magnusson, B., Hallberg, L., Rossander, L. and Swolin, B., Iron metabolism and 'sports anaemia', *Acta Med. Scand.,* 216, 149, 1984.
23. Lamanca, J.J., Haymes, E.M., Daly, J.A. and Waller, M.F., Sweat iron loss of male and female runners during exercise, *Int. J. Sports Med.,* 9, 52, 1988.
24. Meydani, M., Evans, W.J., Handelman, G., Biddle, L., Fielding, R.A., Meydani, S.N., Burrill, J., Fiatarone, M.A., Blumberg, J.B. and Cannen, J.G., Protective effect of vitamin E on exercise-induced oxidative damage in young and older adults, *Am. J. Physiol.,* 264, R992, 1993.
25. Aruoma, O.I., Free radicals and antioxidant strategies in sports, *J. Nutr. Biochem.,* 5, 370, 1994.
26. Goldfarb, A.H., Antioxidants: role of supplementation to prevent exercise-induced oxidative stress, *Med. Sci. Sports Exercise,* 25, 232, 1993.
27. Halliwell, B., Grootveld, M. and Gutteridge, J.M.C., Methods for the measurements of hydroxyl radicals in biochemical systems: deoxyribose degradation and aromatic hydroxylation, *Meth. Biochem. Anal.,* 33, 59, 1989.
28. Grootveld, M. and Halliwell, B., Measurement of allantoin and uric acid in human body fluids. A potential index of free radical reactions *in vivo, Biochem. J.,* 243, 803, 1987.
29. Kaur, H. and Halliwell, B., Action of biologically-relevant oxidizing species upon uric acid. Identification of uric acid oxidation products, *Chem.-Biol. Interac.,* 73, 235, 1990.
30. Rice-Evans, C., Diplock, A.T. and Symons, M.C.R., Eds., *Techniques in Free Radical Research,* Elsevier Applied Science, London, 1991.
31. Aruoma, O.I., Experimental tools in free radical biochemistry, in *Free Radicals in Tropical Diseases,* O.I. Aruoma, Ed., Harwood Academic Publishers, London, 1993, 233.
32. Greenwald, R.A., *Handbook of Methods for Oxygen Radical Research,* CRC Press, Boca Raton, Florida, 1985.
33. Rice-Evans, C.A. and Diplock, A.T., Current status of antioxidant therapy, *Free Rad. Biol. Med.,* 15, 77, 1993.
34. Halliwell, B., Evans, P. J., Kaut, H., and Aruoma, O. I., Free radicals, tissue injury, and human disease: a potential for therapeutic use of antioxidants?, in *Organ Metabolism and Nutrition,* J. M. Kinney and H. N. Tucker, Eds., Raven Press, New York, 1994, 425.
35. Halliwell, B., Gutteridge, J.M.C., and Cross, C.E., Free radicals, antioxidants and human disease: where are we now?, *J. Lab. Clin. Med.,* 119, 598, 1992.
36. Riemersma, R.A., Wood, D.A., Macintyre, C.C., Elton, R.A., Gey, K.F. and Oliver, M.F., Risk of angina pectoris and plasma concentrations of vitamins A, C and E and carotene, *Lancet,* 337, 1, 1991.
37. Waldron, K.W., Johnson, I.T. and Fenwick, G.R., Eds., *Food and Cancer Prevention: Chemical and Biological Aspects,* Special Publication 123, Royal Society of Chemistry, London, 1993.
38. Halliwell, B., How to characterize a biological antioxidant, *Free Rad. Res. Commun.,* 9, 1, 1990.
39. Aruoma, O. I., Nutrition and health aspects of free radicals and antioxidants, *Fd. Chem. Toxic.,* 32, 671, 1994.
40. Aruoma, O. I., Murcia, A., Butler, J., and Halliwell, B., Evaluation of the antioxidant actions of gallic acid and its derivatives, *J. Agric. Food Chem.,* 41, 1880, 1993.
41. Maxwell, S. R. J., Jakeman, P., Thomsen, H., Leguen, C., and Thorpe, G. H. G., Changes in plasma antioxidant status during eccentric exercise and the effect of vitamin supplementation, *Free Rad. Res. Commun.,* 19, 191, 1993.

INDEX

A

Acid-base regulation, see pH
Aerobic exercise
  magnesium status and, 159–166,
    179–186
  magnesium supplementation and,
    179–186
  plasma chromium concentration and,
    199–202
  plasma/erythrocyte magnesium
    concentration and, 179–186
Amenorrhea, 305–313, see also Athletic
    amenorrhea
American Chemical Society, 1–2
American College of Sports Medicine, see
    ASCM
Anabolic steroids
  mineral nutriture in users vs. nonusers,
    282–289
  properties, 281–282
Anaerobic exercise
  iron deficiency and, 66–77
  magnesium status and, 166, 179–186
  magnesium supplementation and,
    179–186
Anemia, see also Hematologic status; Iron
  and athletic performance, 89–90
  in distance runners vs. sprinters, 5–11
  and endurance/anaerobic sports
    activities, 66–67
  sports, 18–19
Antioxidants, 322–323, see also Free
    radicals
Aruoma, Okezie I., vii, 317–323
ASCM dehydration/fluid replacement
    guidelines, 226–229
Athletic amenorrhea
  excessive exercise and, 308–309
  loss of specific fat stores and, 308
  low body fat level and, 307–308
  nutritional inadequacy and, 309–311
  vegetarianism and, 311–313
  weight loss and, 306–307

B

Balke Index, 219–220
Basal metabolic rate

and athletic amenorrhea, 310–311
  iron deficiency and, 21, 25–26
Beard, John L., vii, 13–28, 33–44
Benson, Joan E., vii, 305–313
Body fat and athletic amenorrhea,
    307–308
Brilla, Lorraine R., vii, 139–169

C

Calcium
  anabolic steroid use and, 285–289
  dietary content of selected foods, 126
  ferrous fumate/calcium carbonate
    interactions, 121–128
  intake and metabolism in cerebral palsy
    and visual impairment, 98–102
  and iron bioavailability, 108–117
  and iron supplementation in women,
    51–55
  supplementation, 109–117, 123
  weight loss/weight cycling and, 300
Caloric intake
  anabolic steroid use and, 285–289
  athletic amenorrhea and insufficient,
    309–311
  iron deficiency and, 20–21
Carbohydrates
  early studies, 236–238
  prolonged exercise and
    digestion and absorption, 248–252
    hepatic glucose appearance,
      252–253
    muscle oxidation of glucose, 253
    replacement beverage
      recommendations, 254–256
  recognition of importance, 239–240
  sports drinks in dehydration, 215–230
  water vs. carbohydrate replacement,
    238–239
Cardiovascular system, magnesium and,
    157–158
Carroll, Steven S., vii, 179–186
Castellani, Walter, vii, 179–186, 199–202
Cerebral palsy, dietary calcium and iron
    intake in, 98–102
Chen, Chaunn-Show, vii, viii, 5–11
Chloride, comparative status of athletes
    and nonathletes, 205–213